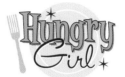

CLEAN & HUNGRY

OBSESSED!

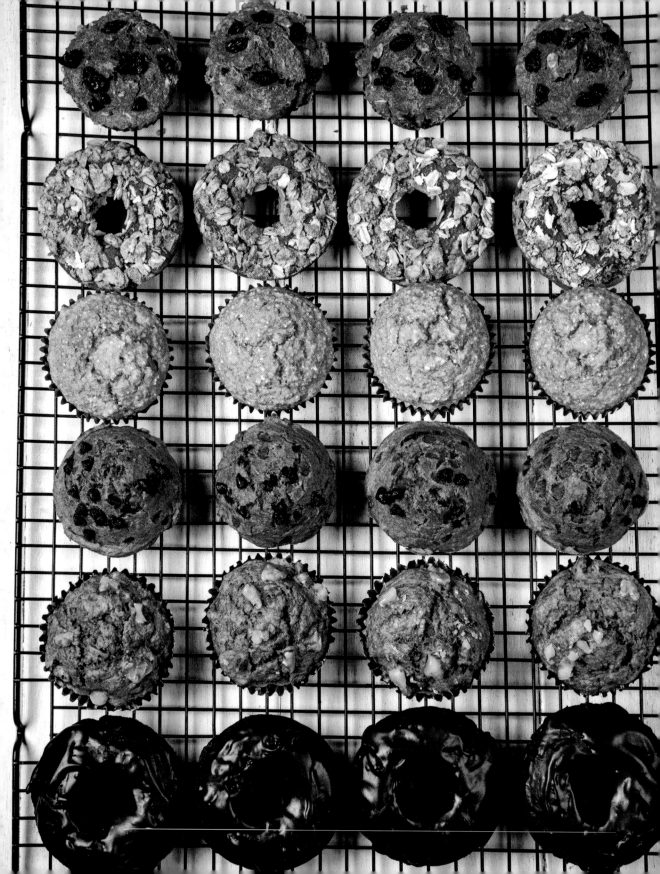

Also by Lisa Lillien

HUNGRY GIRL:
Recipes and Survival Strategies for Guilt-Free Eating in the Real World

HUNGRY GIRL 200 UNDER 200:
200 Recipes Under 200 Calories

HUNGRY GIRL 1-2-3:
The Easiest, Most Delicious, Guilt-Free Recipes on the Planet

HUNGRY GIRL HAPPY HOUR:
75 Recipes for Amazingly Fantastic Guilt-Free Cocktails & Party Foods

HUNGRY GIRL 300 UNDER 300:
300 Breakfast, Lunch & Dinner Dishes Under 300 Calories

HUNGRY GIRL SUPERMARKET SURVIVAL:
Aisle by Aisle, HG-Style!

HUNGRY GIRL TO THE MAX!
The Ultimate Guilt-Free Cookbook

HUNGRY GIRL 200 UNDER 200 JUST DESSERTS:
200 Recipes Under 200 Calories

THE HUNGRY GIRL DIET

THE HUNGRY GIRL DIET COOKBOOK:
Healthy Recipes for Mix-n-Match Meals & Snacks

HUNGRY GIRL CLEAN & HUNGRY:
Easy All-Natural Recipes for Healthy Eating in the Real World

HUNGRY GIRL: THE OFFICIAL SURVIVAL GUIDES:
Tips & Tricks for Guilt-Free Eating
(audio book)

HUNGRY GIRL CHEW THE RIGHT THING:
Supreme Makeovers for 50 Foods You Crave
(recipe cards)

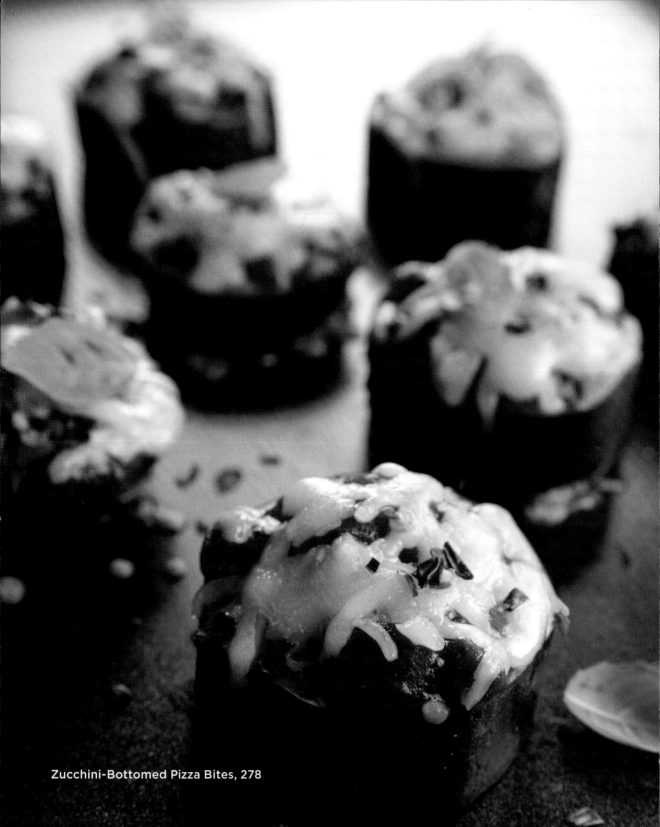

Zucchini-Bottomed Pizza Bites, 278

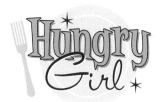

CLEAN &
HUNGRY

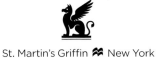

OBSESSED!

ALL-NATURAL RECIPES FOR
THE FOODS YOU CAN'T
LIVE WITHOUT

Lisa Lillien

St. Martin's Griffin ⚞ New York

HUNGRY GIRL CLEAN & HUNGRY OBSESSED! ALL-NATURAL RECIPES FOR THE FOODS YOU CAN'T LIVE WITHOUT. COPYRIGHT © 2017 by Hungry Girl, Inc. All rights reserved. Printed in the United States of America. For information, address St. Martin's Press, 175 Fifth Avenue, New York, N.Y. 10010.

www.stmartins.com

Cover design by Julie Leonard
Book design by Ralph Fowler
Illustrations by Jack Pullan
Food styling by Cindy Epstein
Food photography by Carl Kravats
Author photography by Jay Lawrence Goldman

Library of Congress Cataloging-in-Publication Data is available upon request.

ISBN 978-1-250-08725-6 (trade paperback)
ISBN 978-1-250-08726-3 (e-book)

Our books may be purchased in bulk for promotional, educational, or business use. Please contact your local bookseller or the Macmillan Corporate and Premium Sales Department at (800) 221-7945, extension 5442, or by e-mail at MacmillanSpecialMarkets@macmillan.com.

First Edition: September 2017

10 9 8 7 6 5 4 3 2 1

This book is dedicated to
the memory of my mother-in-law,
CAROL SCHNEIDER.

I miss your silly, sharp wit, your endless knowledge,
and your unparalleled creme brûlée.

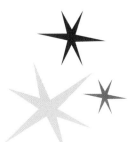

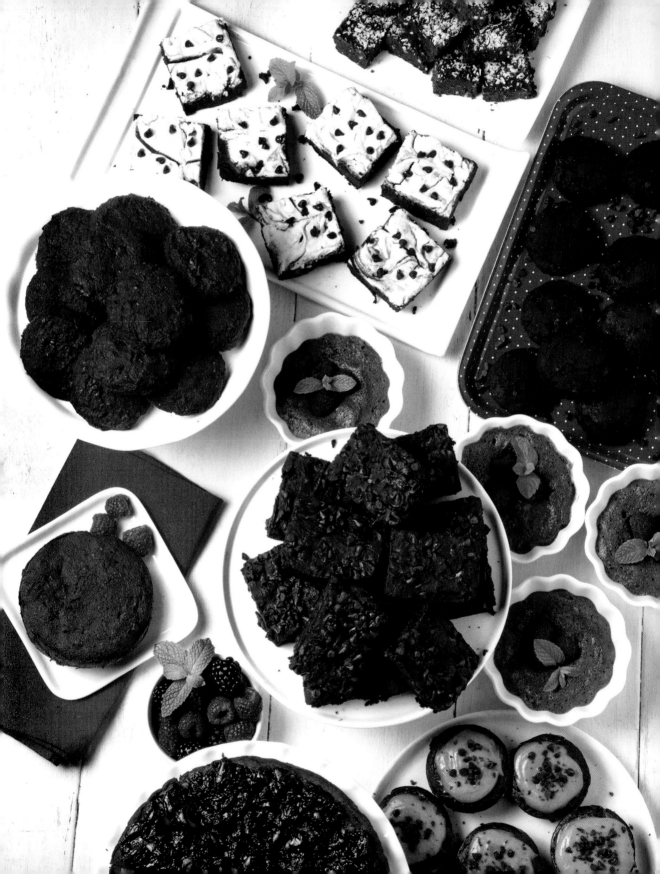

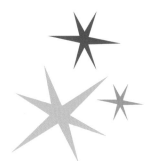

Get More Hungry Girl

For guilt-free recipes, food news, tips 'n tricks, and more . . .

Sign up for free daily emails at hungry-girl.com!

Plus . . .

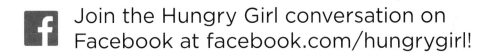

Join the Hungry Girl conversation on Facebook at facebook.com/hungrygirl!

And follow Hungry Girl on Instagram under the name hungrygirl!

Check out Hungry Girl on Pinterest at pinterest.com/hungrygirl!

Follow @hungrygirl on Twitter for behind-the-scenes fun!

Contents

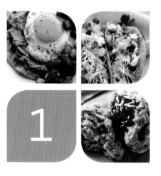

Wake-Up Call!

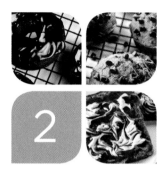

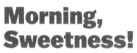

Morning, Sweetness!

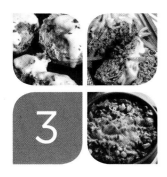

3

Mom's the Word!

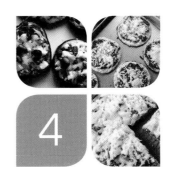

4

You Wanna Pizza Me?

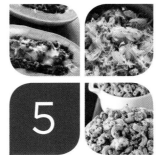

5

Noodle This!

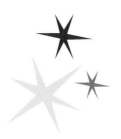

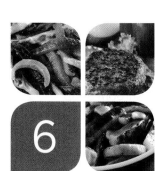

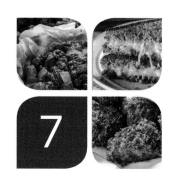

7

I Kid You Not!

6

Welcome to Goodburger

8

Mmmmm, Mexican!

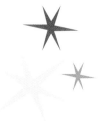

9

Chinese, Please!

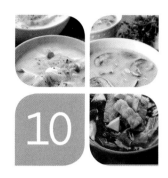

10

Souped Up!

11

Raising the Bar!

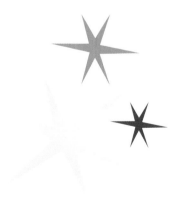

12

Party Hearty!

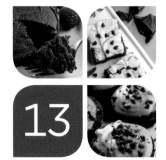

13

Choc' It to Me!

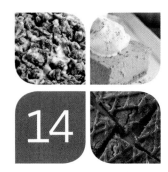

14

Totally Desserted!

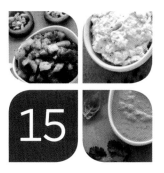

15

Clean & Hungry Staples

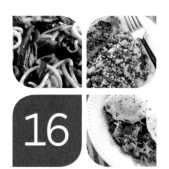

16

How-Tos for Clean & Hungry Obsessions

17

Shop It Up! Grocery Guide & Ingredient FAQs

18

HG Obsessions! Recipes at a Glance

Acknowledgments

Jamie Goldberg—You put everything you've got into everything you do! I'm lucky (and thrilled!) that you're OBSESSED with perfection and fully committed to helping me put out the best content ever. A million thank-yous for all you do.

Huge thank-yous go out to the incredible HG team members who always strive for publishing perfection. This book simply would not exist without you . . .

Lynn Bettencourt
Dana DeRuyck
Erin Norcross
Katie Killeavy
Julie Leonard
Dyana Goldman
Dana Olsen

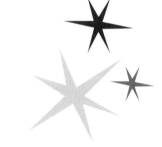

Special thanks to the following HGers for their constant support and hard work!

Alison Kreuch
Gina Muscato
Erika Wells
Cindy Sloop
Olga Gatica

Immense appreciation goes out to the extended Hungry Girl family . . .

John Vaccaro
Neeti Madan
Jennifer Enderlin
John Karle

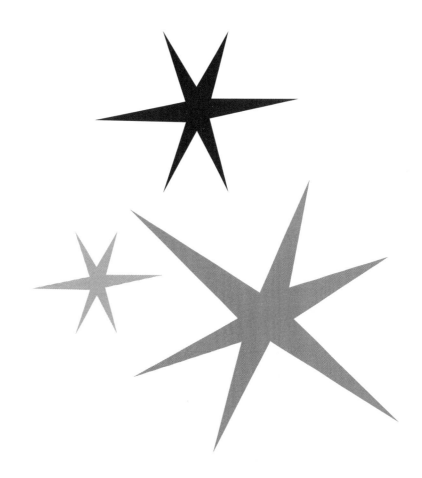

Anne Marie Tallberg
Brant Janeway
Elizabeth Catalano
Caitlin Dareff
James Sinclair
Cheryl Mamaril
Tracey Guest
Bill Stankey
Tom Fineman
Steve Younger
Jeff Becker
Susan Garcia
Jackie Mgido
Jennifer Fleming
Emily Warren

I also want to send a big-time shout-out to these creative superstars!

Ralph Fowler
Carl Kravats
Cindy Epstein
Jack Pullan

And last but not least, endless gratitude to my loving and super-supportive husband and family . . .

Daniel Schneider
Florence and Maurice Lillien
Meri Lillien
Jay Lillien
Lolly and Jordan

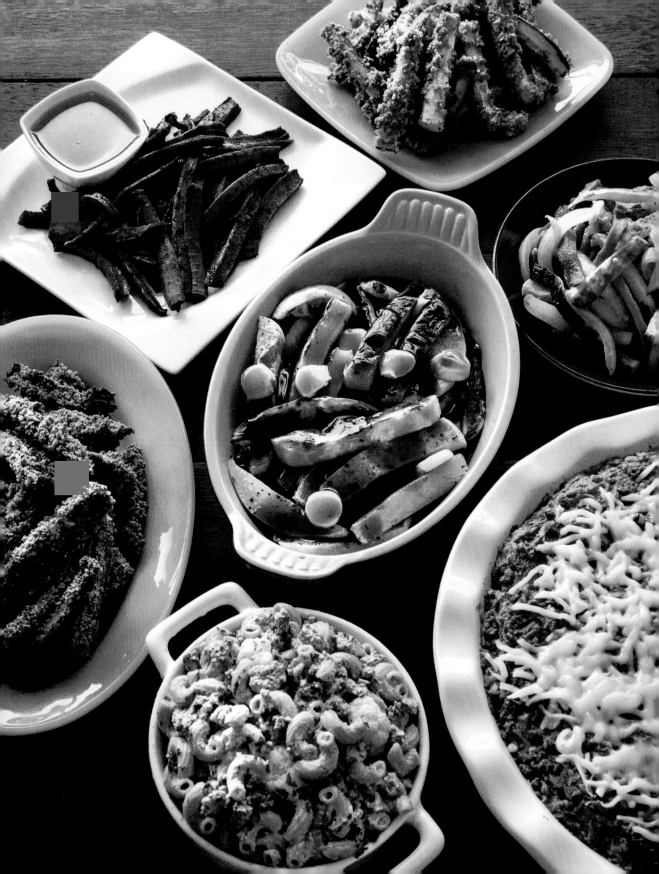

Hi!

I'm obsessed with food. I'll be the first to admit it. I've felt this way ever since I was a toddler. I remember my mom pushing me in a stroller and feeding me special ice cream sundaes from a local department store in Brooklyn. I can recall the *exact* taste and texture of the chocolate chip cookies served in my elementary school cafeteria. And I especially remember loving those Swanson frozen dinner mashed potatoes once some of the apple goo from the cobbler bubbled over into it in the toaster oven. I was the 8-year-old who ordered surf & turf at family celebration dinners (thanks, Dad!) and the kid who was completely fixated on reading the packages of every item in every vending machine I passed since the day I could read.

Pretty much all of my first memories involve food. In fact, the very first thing about my entire life that I can recall vividly is being in a playpen, barely able to stand, and hobbling over to the edge to greet my big sister who had walked over eating a slice of pizza. I wanted that pizza. Badly. And when I was told I couldn't have it (I was toothless!), I started to cry.

These days, I've perfected the whole standing and walking thing. And the reason I don't eat certain foods is less about not having teeth and more about not wanting to consume all the artery-clogging fat and the insane number of calories those foods contain. But instead of crying about it, I simply create healthier versions of these foods. My complete and total obsession with all things chewable has turned me into Hungry Girl. And this, my 12th Hungry Girl book, is packed solid with recipes for things that we all crave. Nachos. Brownies. Quesadillas. Pizza. Mashed potatoes. Cheesecake. Lasagna. Pie. They're all here. And they're all made with healthy ingredients and clock in with less than 375 calories.

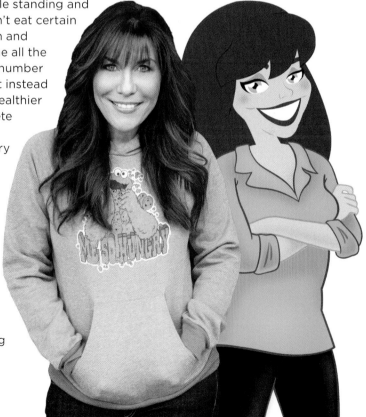

I hope you love these recipes as much as I do . . . and I have a feeling you will!

Lisa :)

FAQs

Who and what is Hungry Girl?

That's me! I'm Lisa Lillien, a.k.a. Hungry Girl. I'm not a nutritionist . . . I'm just hungry. I like to call myself a "foodologist," because I've devoted my life to finding ways to enjoy the world's most craveable foods without popping a pants button. And since nothing makes me happier than sharing my knowledge of guilt-free food with other people, I created the Hungry Girl brand.

It all started back in 2004, when I launched Hungry Girl as a free daily email. Today, millions of Hungry Girl fans access HG content—as subscribers to the emails (sign up at hungry-girl.com), on social media, in magazines, on television, and more. Hungry Girl serves up calorie-slashed recipes, food finds, and tips & tricks. The goal is to help people eat better, lose weight, and maintain their weight in a fun, real-world way. And it's working!

What's Clean & Hungry?

A few years ago, people became very interested in clean eating, which focuses on pure and natural foods like fresh fruits and veggies, whole grains, and minimally processed protein. Unfortunately, most approaches to clean eating at the time were rigid and intimidating. Many also failed to address the importance that calorie consumption plays in maintaining a healthy body weight. So I decided to create my own version of clean eating; one that's relatable, realistic, and helpful with weight management.

In April of 2016, I released my eleventh book, *Hungry Girl Clean & Hungry: Easy All-Natural Recipes for Healthy Eating in the Real World* . . . and it instantly became a *New York Times* Best Seller! The Clean & Hungry concept combines the best of Hungry Girl with the best of clean eating. The recipes are low in calories and starchy carbs;

the portions are huge; and the ingredients are easy to find and 100 percent natural. Clean & Hungry recipes are also free of heavily processed foods, they contain little to no added sugar, and they're often high in protein and fiber. It's a delicious, satisfying, real-world approach to eating clean and staying lean!

Why Clean & Hungry Obsessed?

The first Clean & Hungry book introduced people to my style of clean eating with simple, fresh, and fantastic meals and snacks. But one thing immediately became clear: People were hungry for more! So I decided to dive in a little deeper. It was time to re-create the beloved comfort foods that Americans are OBSESSED with.

It's a known fact that Americans struggle with obesity and other diseases linked to poor food choices. And while many of us know how to fix the problem—consume fewer calories and eat less junk—it's easier said than done! Temptation is everywhere, and we want to indulge in the foods we crave.

There are certain foods that Americans can't live without, and I decided to identify them and give them Clean & Hungry makeovers! French toast, lasagna, fried chicken, quesadillas, fudge . . . No food is off-limits. And all of them contain less than 375 calories.

Where can I find the Weight Watchers SmartPoints® values for the recipes in this book?

Here at HG, we're fans of Weight Watchers, and we know many of you are too! So we're providing the Weight Watchers SmartPoints® value* for each recipe in this book online. Visit hungry-girl.com/books for all the values!

Don't miss the Ingredient FAQs in Chapter 17!

*The SmartPoints® values for these recipes were calculated by Hungry Girl and are not an endorsement or approval of the recipe or developer by Weight Watchers International, Inc., the owner of the SmartPoints registered trademark.

Go-To Recipe Guide

Looking for recipes with short ingredient lists, fast recipes, vegetarian recipes, and/or gluten-free recipes? Find these symbols throughout the book. To make things even easier, we've put together a complete guide on the following pages . . .

5i   Recipes with 5 Ingredients or Less

15m   Recipes in 15 Minutes or Less

30m   Recipes in 30 Minutes or Less

V   Vegetarian Recipes

GF   Gluten-Free Recipes

P.S. Also check out Chapter 18: HG Obsessions! Recipes at a Glance (page 361) for a guide to some categories for craveables: slow-cooker recipes, chicken dishes, peanut butter treats, and more!

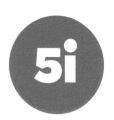

Recipes with 5 Ingredients or Less

You read that right! These recipes have no more than FIVE main ingredients. (Salt, pepper, no-calorie sweeteners, and basic dried seasonings aren't factored into the ingredient totals.) Easy peasy . . .

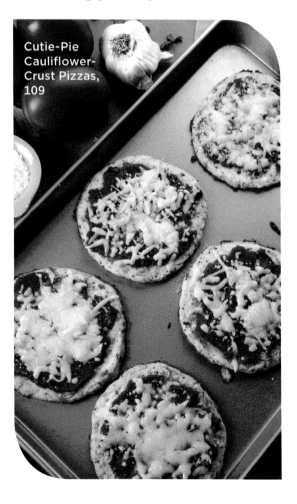

Cutie-Pie Cauliflower-Crust Pizzas, 109

15m Recipes in 15 Minutes or Less

Every recipe here takes 15 minutes or less to make. So speedy!

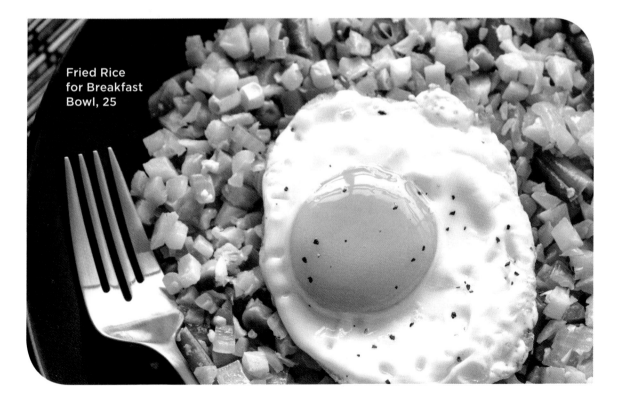

Fried Rice for Breakfast Bowl, 25

Recipes in 30 Minutes or Less

Each of these recipes will take you half an hour max from start to finish! How great is that?

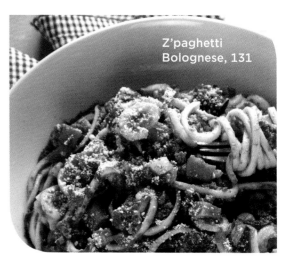

Z'paghetti Bolognese, 131

Vegetarian Recipes

These recipes are lacto-ovo vegetarian: no red meat, poultry, seafood, or any ingredients made with those foods (like chicken broth). They aren't necessarily vegan, however, and may include dairy and/or egg products.

Heads Up

When it comes to ingredients, although the food itself may be vegetarian friendly, some brands add ingredients derived from animals. For example, some yogurt contains gelatin. Always read labels carefully!

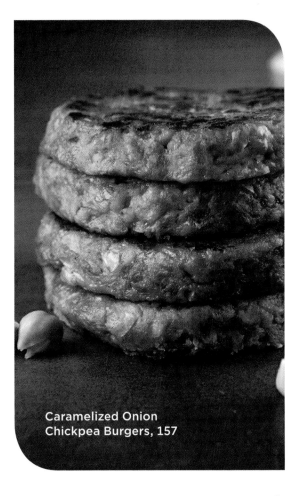

Caramelized Onion Chickpea Burgers, 157

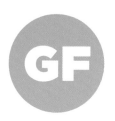

GF Gluten-Free Recipes

Each of these recipes calls for only ingredients that are naturally gluten-free. Pizza, cupcakes, pie, and more!

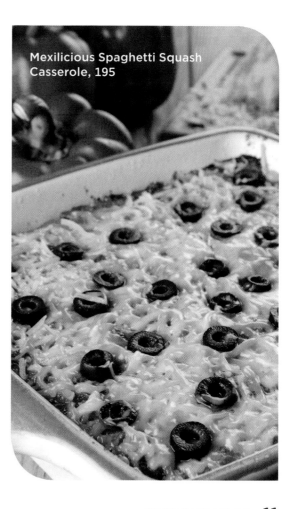

Mexilicious Spaghetti Squash
Casserole, 195

Heads Up

Even naturally gluten-free foods may contain a hint of gluten due to cross contamination. For example, oats are gluten-free, but some companies warn they may contain gluten due to sharing equipment with gluten-containing grains. And about half of the soy sauces found on supermarket shelves have gluten added to them. Check those labels!

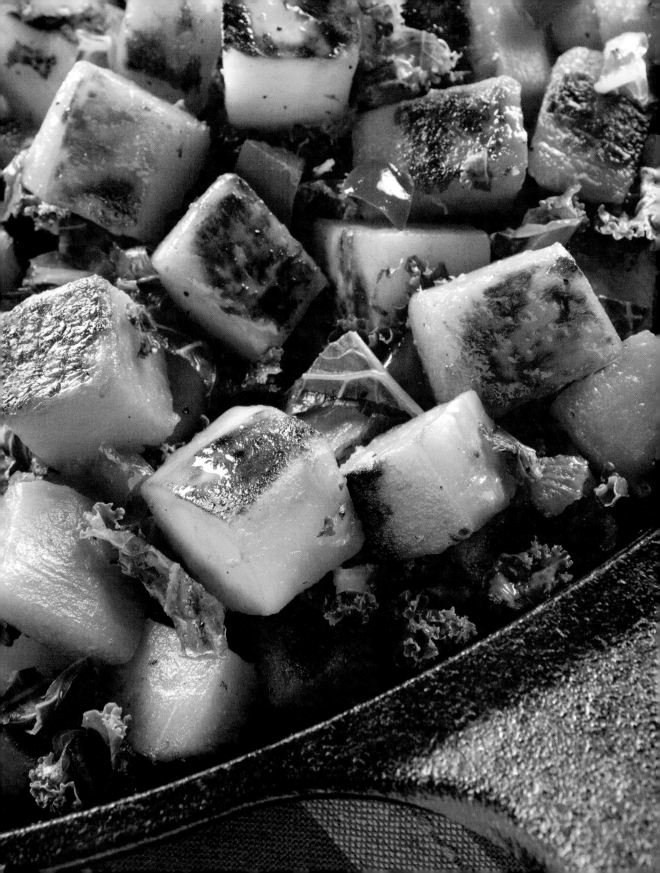

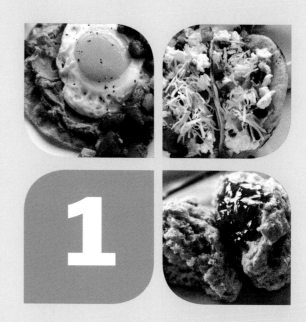

Wake-Up Call!

Research shows that people who eat a morning meal tend to weigh less than those who skip one. In this chapter, you'll find recipes for some of the most-craved savory breakfast foods EVER . . .

Best-Ever Breakfast Sandwich

260 cal

15m Now THIS is one delicious way to start the day! Hot, savory, and protein packed . . .

1 Breakfast Sausage Patty (recipe on page 17)

2 slices whole-grain bread with 60 to 80 calories per slice

¼ cup spinach leaves

1 large tomato slice

¼ cup egg whites (about 2 large eggs' worth)

⅛ teaspoon garlic powder

Optional topping: Clean & Hungry Ketchup (recipe and store-bought alternatives on page 343)

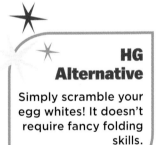

HG Alternative

Simply scramble your egg whites! It doesn't require fancy folding skills.

Entire recipe: 260 calories, 5.5g total fat (1.5g sat fat), 599mg sodium, 29.5g carbs, 5.5g fiber, 5g sugars, 25g protein

You'll Need: medium-small skillet, nonstick spray, microwave-safe plate (optional)

Prep: 5 minutes • **Cook:** 10 minutes

Plus prep and cook times for sausage patty if not made in advance.

1. If needed, reheat sausage patty, either over medium heat in a medium-small skillet sprayed with nonstick spray (for about 2 minutes per side) or on a microwave-safe plate in the microwave (for about 30 seconds).

2. Toast bread. Top one slice with spinach, tomato, and sausage patty.

3. Bring a medium-small skillet sprayed with nonstick spray to medium heat. (Clean skillet, if used to reheat sausage.) Add egg whites, and tilt skillet so they coat the bottom. Sprinkle with garlic powder. Cook until solid enough to flip, about 2 minutes.

4. Carefully flip. Cook for about 1 minute, until cooked through.

5. Fold omelette in half twice, and place over sausage patty.

6. Top with remaining bread slice.

MAKES 1 SERVING

Chew on This . . .

Nearly every fast-food chain, coffee shop & café offers egg & sausage breakfast sandwiches. But the average one has around 500 calories & 30g fat. Unacceptable!

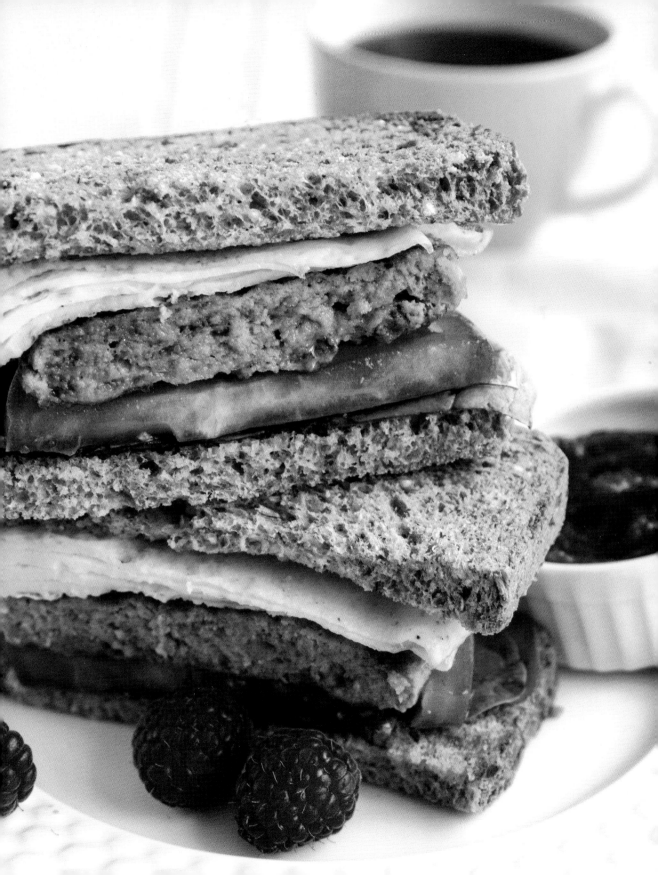

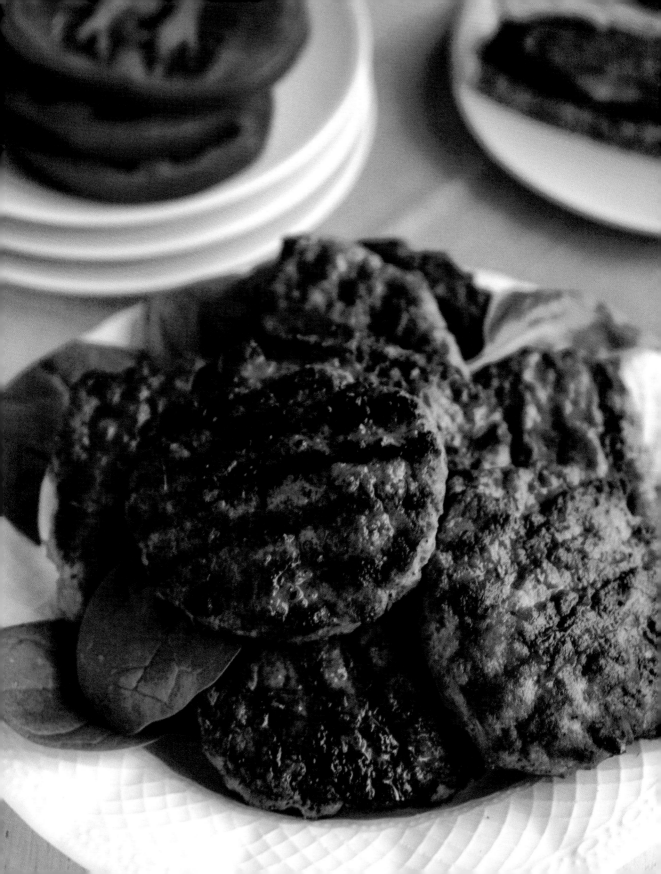

Breakfast Sausage Patties

85 cal

5i **30m** **GF** DIY sausage is a thing! These are totally natural and contain approximately 60 percent less fat than your average breakfast sausage.

1 pound raw lean ground turkey (7% fat or less)

¼ cup egg whites (about 2 large eggs' worth)

¾ teaspoon ground thyme

¾ teaspoon ground sage

¾ teaspoon salt

¼ teaspoon black pepper

⅛ teaspoon ground nutmeg

⅛th of recipe (1 patty): 85 calories, 4g total fat (1.5g sat fat), 277mg sodium, <0.5g carbs, 0g fiber, 0g sugars, 12g protein

You'll Need: large bowl, grill pan (or large skillet), nonstick spray

Prep: 10 minutes • **Cook:** 15 minutes

1. In a large bowl, combine all ingredients. Mix thoroughly.

2. Evenly form into 8 patties, each about ¼ inch thick.

3. Bring a grill pan (or large skillet) sprayed with nonstick spray to medium-high heat. Lay 4 patties in the pan. Cook for about 3 minutes per side, until golden brown and cooked through, using a spatula to flatten them as they cook.

4. Remove pan from heat; clean, if needed. Re-spray, and repeat with remaining 4 patties.

MAKES 8 SERVINGS

Perfect Portabella Benedict

 157 cal

  30m **V** **GF** Replacing bread with a mushroom cap results in miraculously impressive calorie and carb counts!

1 large portabella mushroom cap (stem removed)

1 tablespoon fat-free plain Greek yogurt

1 teaspoon Dijon mustard

1 teaspoon whipped butter

1 drop lemon juice

1 cup spinach leaves

¼ cup chopped tomatoes

⅛ teaspoon garlic powder

⅛ teaspoon each salt and black pepper

1 teaspoon white vinegar

1 large egg

HG FYI

The vinegar helps the egg stay together during the poaching process. You can't taste it!

Entire recipe: 157 calories, 7.5g total fat (2.5g sat fat), 520mg sodium, 11g carbs, 3g fiber, 5g sugars, 12g protein

You'll Need: baking sheet, nonstick spray, small microwave-safe bowl, medium microwave-safe bowl, medium pot, small shallow bowl, slotted spoon, paper towels

Prep: 10 minutes • **Cook:** 20 minutes

1. Preheat oven to 400 degrees. Spray a baking sheet with nonstick spray.

2. Place mushroom cap on the baking sheet, rounded side down. Bake until slightly tender, about 8 minutes.

3. Meanwhile, make the sauce: In a small microwave-safe bowl, combine yogurt, mustard, butter, and lemon juice. Mix until mostly uniform.

4. In a medium microwave-safe bowl, microwave spinach for 45 seconds, or until wilted. Blot away excess moisture. Add tomatoes, garlic powder, salt, and pepper. Microwave for 30 seconds, or until hot.

5. Blot away excess moisture from mushroom cap. Fill with spinach-tomato mixture.

6. Fill a medium pot with 2 inches of water. Add vinegar, and bring to a boil.

7. Reduce to a simmer. Crack egg into a small shallow bowl. Stir water, and gently add egg. Cook until egg white is mostly opaque, 3 to 5 minutes.

8. With a slotted spoon, carefully transfer egg to a layer of paper towels. Once excess water has been absorbed, transfer egg to the mushroom cap.

9. Microwave sauce until hot, about 20 seconds, and stir. (For a thinner sauce, add water.) Spoon over egg.

MAKES 1 SERVING

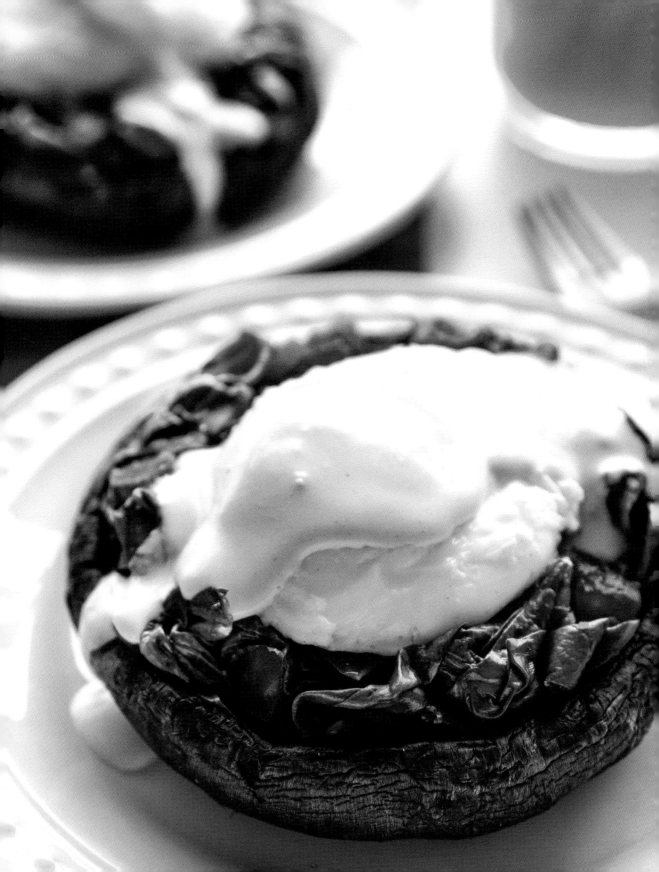

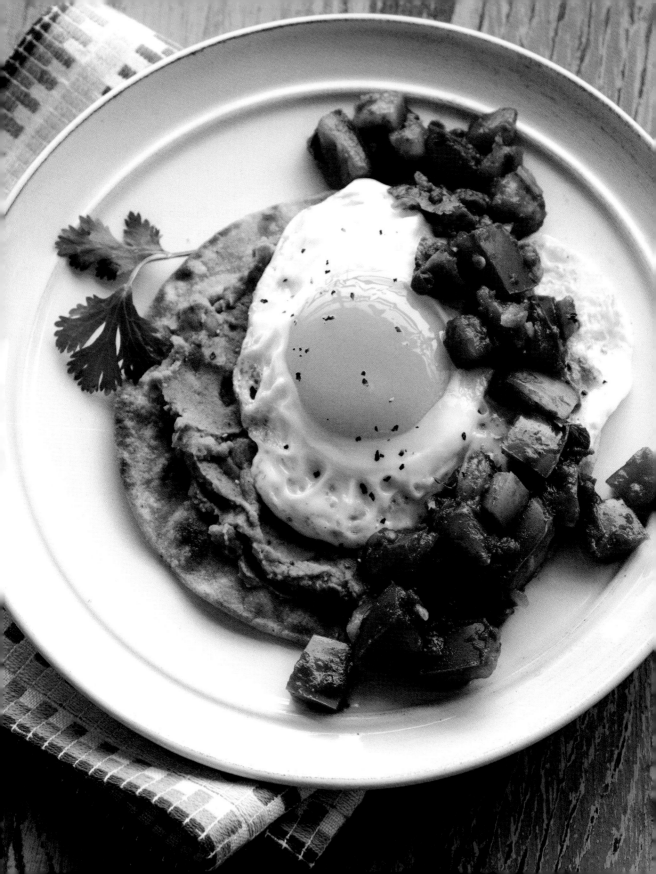

Uno Huevo Ranchero

 236 cal

   This is one saucy egg dish . . . It's CRAZY how good it is!

SAUCE

¼ **cup chopped bell pepper**

2 **tablespoons chopped onion**

½ **cup chopped tomatoes**

¼ **cup canned crushed tomatoes**

2 **tablespoons canned diced green chiles (not drained)**

½ **teaspoon chopped garlic**

⅛ **teaspoon chili powder**

⅛ **teaspoon ground cumin**

⅛ **teaspoon salt**

Dash black pepper

1 **tablespoon chopped fresh cilantro**

BASE

1 **teaspoon whipped butter**

One 6-inch corn tortilla

2 **tablespoons refried beans**

1 **large egg**

Optional topping: additional chili powder

Entire recipe: 236 calories, 8.5g total fat (3g sat fat), 748mg sodium, 30g carbs, 6.5g fiber, 7.5g sugars, 11.5g protein

You'll Need: skillet, nonstick spray, small bowl, plate

Prep: 10 minutes • **Cook:** 15 minutes

1. Bring a skillet sprayed with nonstick spray to medium-high heat. Add bell pepper and onion. Cook and stir until softened and lightly browned, about 3 minutes.

2. Reduce heat to medium low. Add all remaining sauce ingredients *except* cilantro. Cook and stir until hot and well mixed, about 1 minute.

3. Stir in cilantro. Transfer to a small bowl, and cover to keep warm.

4. Clean skillet. Add butter, and return to medium-high heat. Once butter has coated the bottom of the skillet, cook tortilla until lightly browned, about 2 minutes per side.

5. Plate tortilla, and spread with beans.

6. Remove skillet from heat, spray with nonstick spray, and bring to medium heat. Cook egg sunny-side up or over easy, 1 to 2 minutes.

7. Place egg over the tortilla, and top with sauce.

MAKES 1 SERVING

Vegetarian FYI

Not all refried beans are vegetarian friendly. If you avoid animal products, check the can's ingredient list!

Spaghetti Squash Your Hunger B-fast Bowl

5i **30m** **V** **GF** Spaghetti squash for breakfast?! Yup! I'm so obsessed with the stuff, you'll find four more spaghetti-squash recipes on page 363!

½ cup chopped bell pepper

¼ cup chopped onion

2 cups cooked spaghetti squash, drained of excess moisture

⅛ teaspoon garlic powder

⅛ teaspoon each salt and black pepper

2 large eggs

¼ cup chopped tomato

Optional toppings: additional salt and black pepper

Entire recipe: 271 calories, 10.5g total fat (3.5g sat fat), 495mg sodium, 30.5g carbs, 7g fiber, 13.5g sugars, 16g protein

You'll Need: skillet, nonstick spray, medium bowl

Prep: 10 minutes • **Cook:** 10 minutes

Plus prep and cook times for spaghetti squash (page 350) if not made in advance.

1. Bring a skillet sprayed with nonstick spray to medium-high heat. Add bell pepper and onion. Cook and stir until softened, about 4 minutes.

2. Add spaghetti squash, and sprinkle with seasonings. Cook and stir until hot and well mixed, about 2 minutes. Transfer to a medium bowl, and cover to keep warm.

3. Remove skillet from heat; clean, if needed. Re-spray, and bring to medium-low heat. Cook eggs sunny-side up or over easy, 1 to 2 minutes.

4. Add tomato to the bowl, and top with eggs.

MAKES 1 SERVING

Chew on This...

I've read that Americans consume around 76.5 billion eggs per year. This delicious morning meal uses only two!

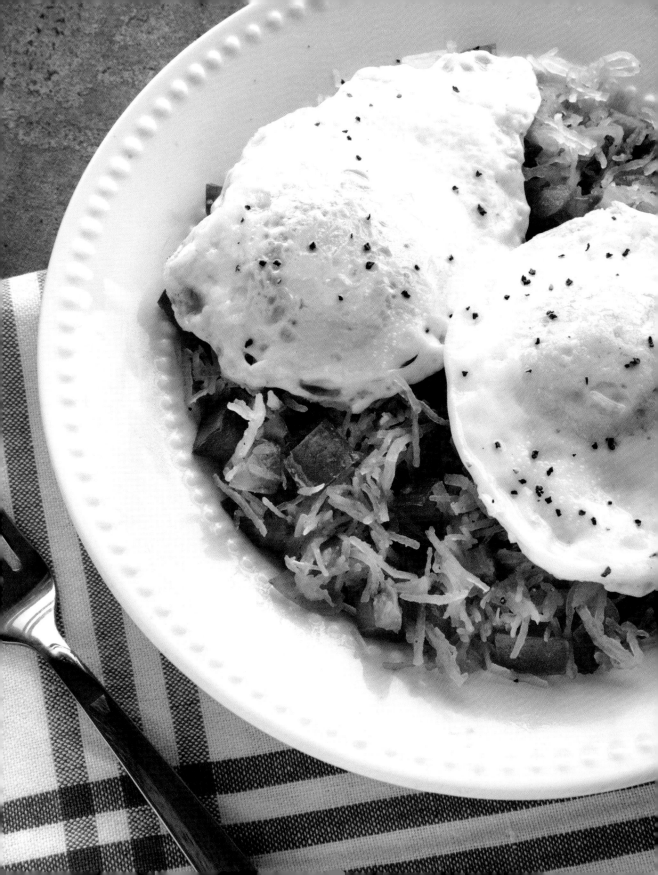

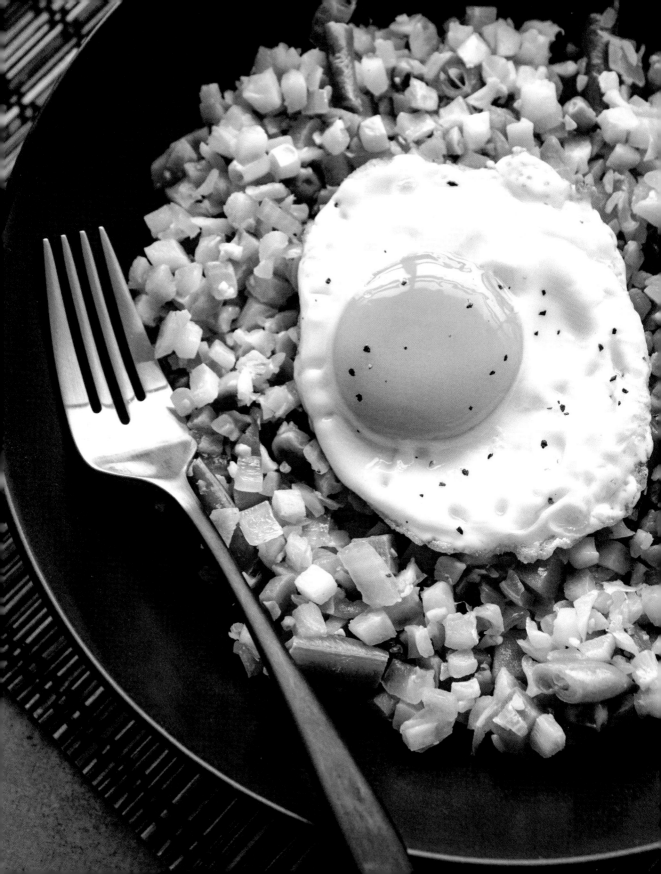

Fried Rice for Breakfast Bowl

239 cal

🕐15m Ⓥ GF Obsession confession: I was inspired to make this recipe after eating another HG "fried rice" recipe for breakfast! This is the first of many cauliflower-rice creations in this book; flip to page 362 for more.

½ cup frozen petite mixed vegetables

1½ cups cauliflower rice/crumbles

½ cup chopped onion

1 teaspoon sesame oil

½ teaspoon chopped garlic

1 tablespoon Clean & Hungry Teriyaki Sauce (recipe and store-bought alternatives on page 342)

1 large egg

Optional: salt, black pepper, reduced-sodium/lite soy sauce

Entire recipe: 239 calories, 10g total fat (2.5g sat fat), 257mg sodium, 26g carbs, 7g fiber, 10g sugars, 13g protein

You'll Need: large skillet with a lid, nonstick spray, large bowl

Prep: 5 minutes • **Cook:** 10 minutes

1. Bring a large skillet sprayed with nonstick spray to medium-high heat. Add frozen veggies and 2 tablespoons water. Cover and cook for 2 minutes, or until thawed.

2. Add cauliflower rice/crumbles, onion, oil, and garlic. Cook and stir until veggies have mostly softened, 4 to 5 minutes.

3. Add teriyaki sauce. Cook and stir until hot and well mixed, about 1 minute. Transfer to a medium bowl, and cover to keep warm.

4. Remove skillet from heat; clean, if needed. Re-spray, and bring to medium heat. Cook egg sunny-side up or over easy, 1 to 2 minutes.

5. Place egg over the contents of the bowl.

MAKES 1 SERVING

✴ Gluten FYI

Some soy sauce contains gluten. If you avoid gluten, check the ingredient lists. Or grab a product marked gluten-free.

Need-to-Know Info

Use store-bought cauliflower crumbles/rice, or DIY! See page 346 for the 411.

That's Good Stuffed Breakfast Peppers

V **GF** Having these scramble-stuffed peppers for breakfast will make your day 86 percent more enjoyable (unofficially, of course)!

2 large bell peppers

½ cup chopped mushrooms

½ cup chopped onion

1 cup egg whites (about 8 large eggs' worth)

¼ teaspoon garlic powder

¼ teaspoon onion powder

¼ teaspoon each salt and black pepper

½ cup shredded reduced-fat cheddar cheese

2 tablespoons chopped scallions

Optional topping: Clean & Hungry Salsa (recipe and store-bought alternatives on page 334)

½ of recipe (2 stuffed pepper halves): 212 calories, 6.5g total fat (3.5g sat fat), 712mg sodium, 15.5g carbs, 4g fiber, 8.5g sugars, 23g protein

You'll Need: 8-inch by 8-inch baking pan, nonstick spray, large skillet

Prep: 15 minutes • **Cook:** 40 minutes

1. Preheat oven to 350 degrees. Spray an 8-inch by 8-inch baking pan with nonstick spray.

2. Halve bell peppers. Remove and discard seeds and stems. Place pepper halves in the pan, cut sides up.

3. Bake until soft, 25 to 30 minutes. Blot away excess moisture.

4. Bring a large skillet sprayed with nonstick spray to medium-high heat. Add mushrooms and onion. Cook and stir until mostly softened, about 4 minutes.

5. Add egg whites to the skillet, and sprinkle with seasonings. Scramble until fully cooked, about 2 minutes.

6. Remove skillet from heat, and fold in cheese.

7. Fill pepper halves with egg scramble, and top with scallions.

MAKES 2 SERVINGS

Chew on This . . .

According to a recently reported survey, 77 percent of consumers have eaten eggs for breakfast in the past two weeks. Have YOU?

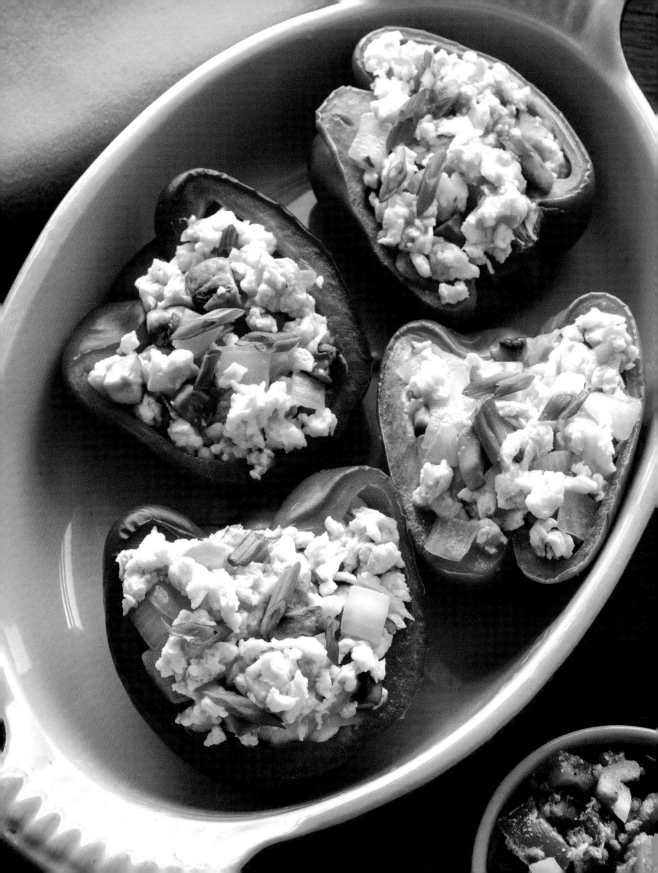

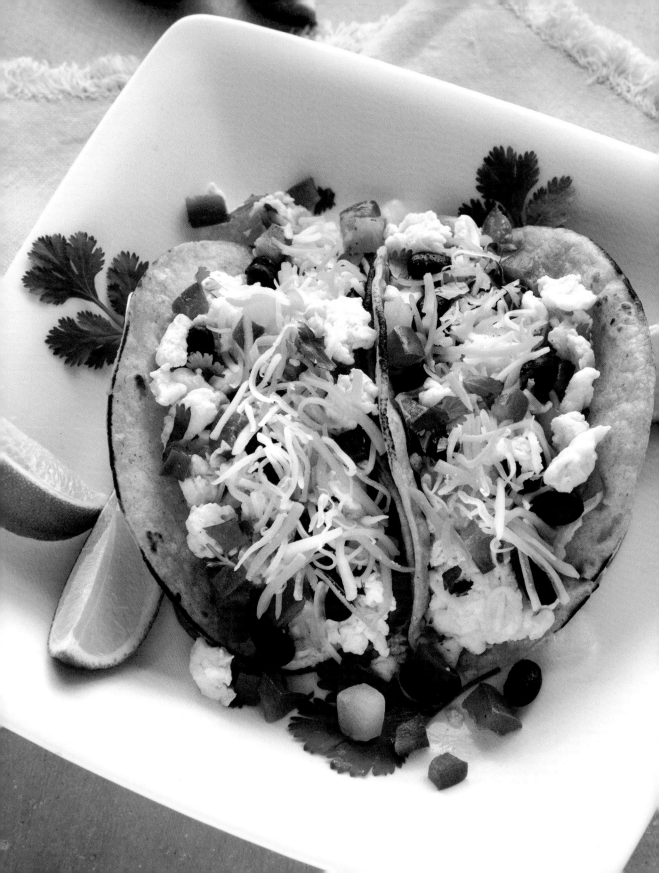

Rise & Shine Breakfast Tacos

288 cal

30m **V** **GF** Why limit tacos to the afternoon and evening hours? This a.m. version is a home run! For more Mexican food, check out Chapter 8: Mmmmm, Mexican!

¼ cup finely chopped onion

¼ cup finely chopped red bell pepper

½ cup egg whites (about 4 large eggs' worth)

⅛ teaspoon garlic powder

⅛ teaspoon salt

Dash ground cumin

Dash chili powder

¼ cup canned black beans, drained and rinsed

Two 6-inch corn tortillas

2 tablespoons shredded reduced-fat Mexican-blend cheese

1 tablespoon chopped fresh cilantro

Optional topping: Clean & Hungry Salsa (recipe and store-bought alternatives on page 334)

Entire recipe: 288 calories, 5g total fat (1.5g sat fat), 773mg sodium, 37.5g carbs, 6.5g fiber, 5.5g sugars, 23g protein

You'll Need: skillet, nonstick spray, microwave-safe plate
Prep: 10 minutes • **Cook:** 10 minutes

1. Bring a skillet sprayed with nonstick spray to medium-high heat. Add onion and pepper. Cook and stir until mostly softened, about 4 minutes.

2. Reduce heat to medium. Add egg whites, and sprinkle with seasonings. Scramble until fully cooked, about 2 minutes.

3. Add beans, and cook and stir until hot, about 1 minute.

4. On a microwave-safe plate, microwave tortillas for 20 seconds, or until warm.

5. Divide egg scramble between tortillas, and top with cheese and cilantro.

MAKES 1 SERVING

HG Alternative

If you like, brown your tortillas in the skillet before cooking your scramble!

Totally Turnip Home Fries

75 cal

5i **30m** **V** **GF** These slimmed-down home fries are made with turnips instead of potatoes. Major calorie saver!

4 cups peeled turnips cut into ¾-inch cubes (about 1½ turnips)

1 cup chopped bell pepper

½ cup chopped onion

2 teaspoons olive oil

¾ teaspoon salt

½ teaspoon garlic powder

½ teaspoon onion powder

¼ teaspoon black pepper

Optional toppings: Clean & Hungry Salsa, Clean & Hungry Ketchup (recipes and store-bought alternatives on pages 334 and 343)

¼th of recipe (about ¾ cup): 75 calories, 2.5g total fat (0.5g sat fat), 525mg sodium, 13g carbs, 3.5g fiber, 7g sugars, 1.5g protein

You'll Need: large skillet with a lid, nonstick spray

Prep: 15 minutes • **Cook:** 15 minutes

1. Bring a large skillet sprayed with nonstick spray to medium heat. Add turnips and ¼ cup water. Cover and cook for 7 minutes, or until turnips have mostly softened and water has evaporated.

2. Add bell pepper and onion. Drizzle with oil, and sprinkle with seasonings. Cook and stir until veggies have browned and softened, about 8 minutes.

MAKES 4 SERVINGS

Chew on This...

Rumor has it the average American consumes about 110 pounds of potatoes per year. That's nearly 40,000 calories' worth!

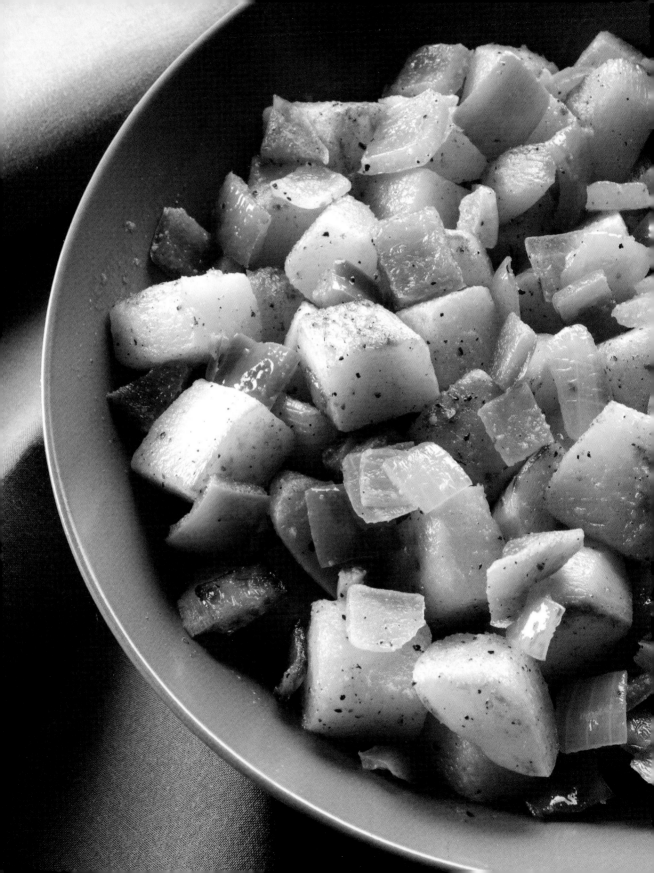

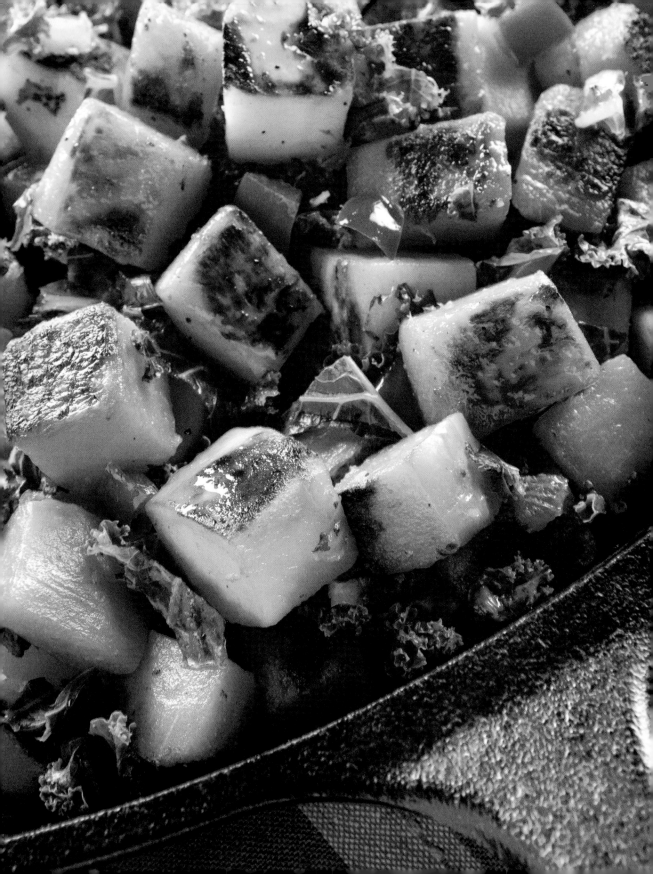

Squashed & Sweet Potatoed Home Fries

91 cal

🕐30m ⓥ ⒼⒻ This sweet & sassy side will knock your socks right off . . . Find six more unconventional fry recipes starting on page 158!

2 cups (about ½ medium) butternut squash cut into ¾-inch cubes

5 ounces (about ½ medium) sweet potato cut into ¾-inch cubes

1 cup finely chopped kale

¼ cup chopped red bell pepper

¼ cup chopped onion

2 teaspoons olive oil

¼ teaspoon salt

⅛ teaspoon black pepper

Dash paprika

Dash cayenne pepper

Optional seasonings: additional black pepper and cayenne pepper

¼th of recipe (about ¾ cups): 91 calories, 2.5g total fat (<0.5g sat fat), 170mg sodium, 17.5g carbs, 3g fiber, 4g sugars, 1.5g protein

You'll Need: large skillet with a lid, nonstick spray

Prep: 10 minutes • **Cook:** 20 minutes

1. Bring a large skillet sprayed with nonstick spray to medium heat. Add squash, sweet potato, and ¼ cup water. Cover and cook for 8 minutes, or until squash and sweet potato have mostly softened and water has evaporated.

2. Add kale, bell pepper, and onion. Drizzle with oil, and sprinkle with seasonings. Cook and stir until veggies have browned and softened, about 10 minutes.

MAKES 4 SERVINGS

Cauliflower Power Biscuit Bakes

106 cal

5i **V**   OMG: These are like the lovechild of a traditional biscuit and a sourdough roll! They're great dipped in soup or topped with butter or jam. You really can't taste the cauliflower at all . . .

1 cup roughly chopped cauliflower

1 cup whole-wheat flour

¾ cup fat-free plain Greek yogurt

1 tablespoon whipped butter, room temperature

2 teaspoons baking powder

¼ teaspoon salt

⅙th of recipe (1 biscuit): 106 calories, 1.5g total fat (0.5g sat fat), 286mg sodium, 17.5g carbs, 3g fiber, 2g sugars, 6g protein

You'll Need: baking sheet, nonstick spray, food processor, large microwave-safe bowl, fine-mesh strainer, clean dish towel (or paper towels)

Prep: 10 minutes • **Cook:** 15 minutes • **Cool:** 10 minutes

1. Preheat oven to 450 degrees. Spray a baking sheet with nonstick spray.
2. Pulse cauliflower in a food processor until reduced to the consistency of coarse breadcrumbs.
3. In a covered large microwave-safe bowl, microwave cauliflower crumbs for 2 minutes. Uncover and stir. Re-cover and microwave for another 2 minutes, or until hot and soft.
4. Transfer to a fine-mesh strainer to drain and cool, about 10 minutes.
5. Using a clean dish towel (or paper towels), firmly press out as much liquid as possible.
6. Return cauliflower crumbs to the large bowl. Add remaining ingredients, and thoroughly mix.
7. Evenly form into 6 mounds (about ⅓ cup each), and place on the baking sheet, evenly spaced.
8. Bake until tops are golden brown and insides are cooked through, about 10 minutes.

MAKES 6 SERVINGS

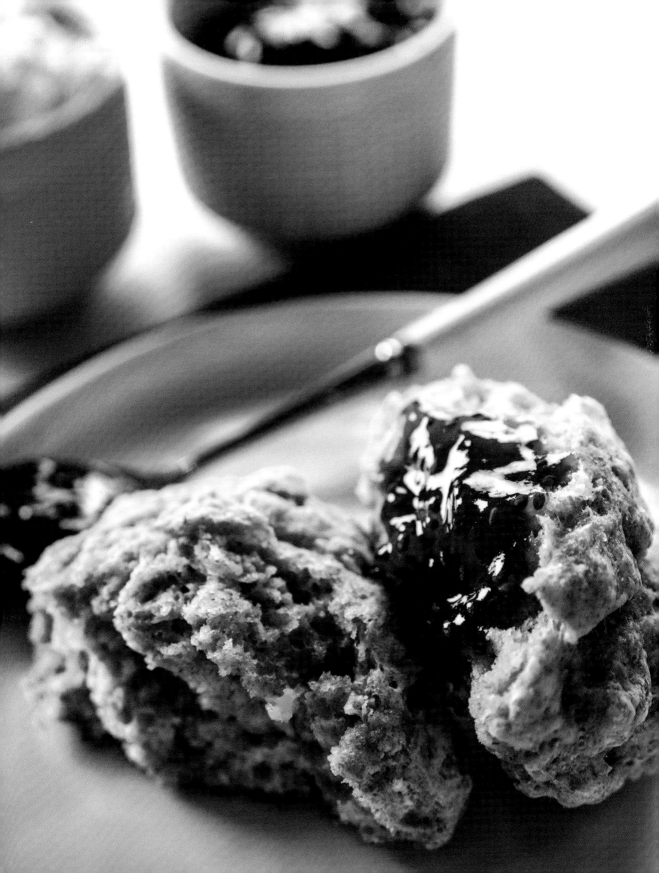

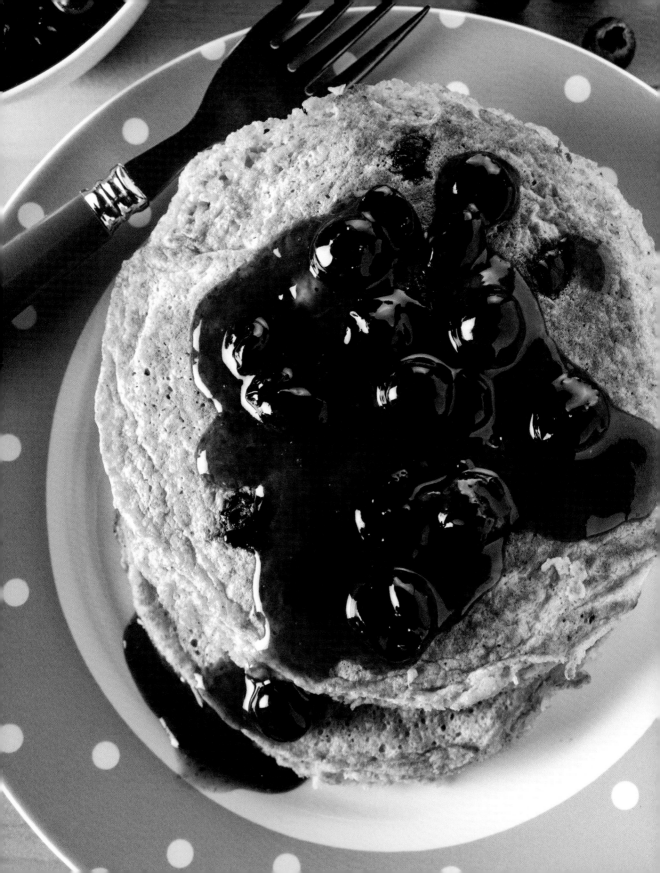

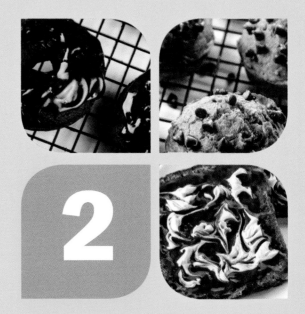

2

Morning,
Sweetness!

Research suggests eating something sweet for breakfast can help curb sweet-tooth cravings later on. But don't just reach for any ol' pastry! Those things can be loaded with sugar and fat. Instead, whip up these lean 'n clean muffins, donuts, and more . . .

Crammed with Chocolate Chip Muffins

152 cal

(V) Chocolate for breakfast . . . YES! And chocoholics: Don't miss the Chocolate Chocolate Donuts on page 46, plus an entire chapter of chocolate desserts, starting on page 286!

2 cups whole-wheat flour

2 teaspoons baking powder

½ teaspoon baking soda

¼ teaspoon salt

1½ cups canned pure pumpkin

½ cup egg whites (about 4 large eggs' worth)

¼ cup Truvia spoonable no-calorie sweetener (or another natural brand about twice as sweet as sugar)

¼ cup whipped butter, room temperature

¼ cup unsweetened vanilla almond milk

1 teaspoon vanilla extract

⅓ cup plus 2 tablespoons mini (or chopped) semi-sweet chocolate chips

¹⁄₁₂th of recipe (1 muffin): 152 calories, 5g total fat (3g sat fat), 221mg sodium, 27g carbs, 4g fiber, 6g sugars, 4.5g protein

You'll Need: 12-cup muffin pan, foil baking cups (or nonstick spray), large bowl, medium-large bowl, whisk

Prep: 20 minutes • **Cook:** 20 minutes

1. Preheat oven to 350 degrees. Line a 12-cup muffin pan with foil baking cups, or spray it with nonstick spray.

2. In a large bowl, combine flour, baking powder, baking soda, and salt. Mix well.

3. In a medium-large bowl, combine all remaining ingredients *except* chocolate chips. Whisk until uniform.

4. Add contents of the medium-large bowl to the large bowl, and mix until uniform. (Batter will be thick.)

5. Fold in ⅓ cup chocolate chips. Evenly fill muffin pan with batter, and smooth out the tops.

6. Sprinkle with remaining 2 tablespoons chocolate chips, and lightly press to adhere.

7. Bake until a toothpick inserted into the center of a muffin comes out clean, 18 to 20 minutes.

MAKES 12 SERVINGS

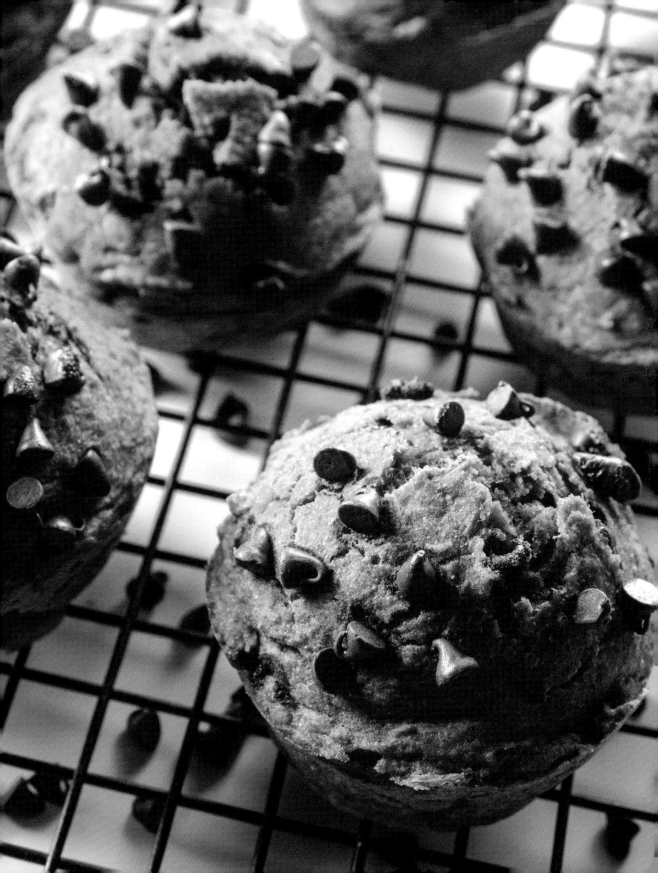

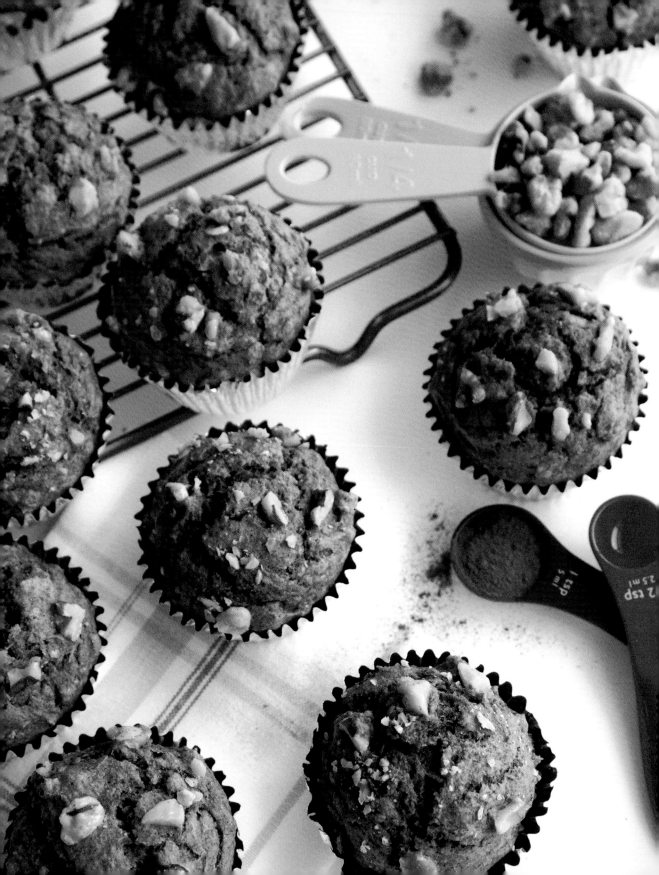

Banana Bread Bonanza Muffins

135 cal

 PSA: These muffins are PHENOMENAL, and you NEED them in your life!

2 cups whole-wheat flour

2 teaspoons baking powder

1 teaspoon cinnamon

½ teaspoon baking soda

¼ teaspoon salt

1 cup mashed very ripe bananas (about 3 medium bananas)

½ cup canned pure pumpkin

½ cup egg whites (about 4 large eggs' worth)

¼ cup Truvia spoonable no-calorie sweetener (or another natural brand about twice as sweet as sugar)

¼ cup whipped butter, room temperature

¼ cup unsweetened vanilla almond milk

1 teaspoon vanilla extract

1 ounce (about ¼ cup) chopped walnuts

¹⁄₁₂th of recipe (1 muffin): 135 calories, 4g total fat (1.5g sat fat), 220mg sodium, 25g carbs, 3.5g fiber, 3g sugars, 4.5g protein

You'll Need: 12-cup muffin pan, foil baking cups (or nonstick spray), large bowl, medium-large bowl, whisk

Prep: 20 minutes • **Cook:** 20 minutes

1. Preheat oven to 350 degrees. Line a 12-cup muffin pan with foil baking cups, or spray it with nonstick spray.

2. In a large bowl, combine flour, baking powder, cinnamon, baking soda, and salt. Mix well.

3. In a medium-large bowl, combine all remaining ingredients *except* walnuts. Whisk until uniform.

4. Add contents of the medium-large bowl to the large bowl, and mix until uniform. (Batter will be thick.)

5. Fold in ½ ounce (about 2 tablespoons) walnuts. Evenly fill muffin pan with batter, and smooth out the tops.

6. Sprinkle with remaining ½ ounce (about 2 tablespoons) walnuts, and lightly press to adhere.

7. Bake until a toothpick inserted into the center of a muffin comes out clean, 18 to 20 minutes.

MAKES 12 SERVINGS

Chew on This . . .

Bananas come in their own carrying case. No wonder they're so popular!

OMG Oatmeal
Raisin Muffins

128 cal

V Oatmeal and raisins are the Lucy and Ricky of the baking world. These muffins are so moist and delicious!

1½ cups whole-wheat flour

½ cup old-fashioned oats

2 teaspoons cinnamon

2 teaspoons baking powder

½ teaspoon baking soda

¼ teaspoon ground nutmeg

¼ teaspoon salt

1½ cups canned pure pumpkin

½ cup egg whites (about 4 large eggs' worth)

¼ cup Truvia spoonable no-calorie sweetener (or another natural brand about twice as sweet as sugar)

¼ cup whipped butter, room temperature

¼ cup unsweetened vanilla almond milk

2 teaspoons vanilla extract

½ cup raisins, chopped

¹⁄₁₂th of recipe (1 muffin): 128 calories, 2.5g total fat (1g sat fat), 222mg sodium, 26g carbs, 4g fiber, 6g sugars, 4g protein

You'll Need: 12-cup muffin pan, foil baking cups (or nonstick spray), large bowl, medium-large bowl, whisk

Prep: 20 minutes • **Cook:** 20 minutes

1. Preheat oven to 350 degrees. Line a 12-cup muffin pan with foil baking cups, or spray it with nonstick spray.

2. In a large bowl, combine flour, oats, cinnamon, baking powder, baking soda, nutmeg, and salt. Mix well.

3. In a medium-large bowl, combine all remaining ingredients *except* raisins. Whisk until uniform.

4. Add contents of the medium-large bowl to the large bowl, and mix until uniform. (Batter will be thick.)

5. Fold in ¾th of the chopped raisins. Evenly fill muffin pan with batter, and smooth out the tops.

6. Sprinkle with remaining chopped raisins, and lightly press to adhere. Bake until a toothpick inserted into the center of a muffin comes out clean, 18 to 20 minutes.

MAKES 12 SERVINGS

Chew on This . . .

The average store-bought muffin clocks in with over 400 calories.
So unnecessary!

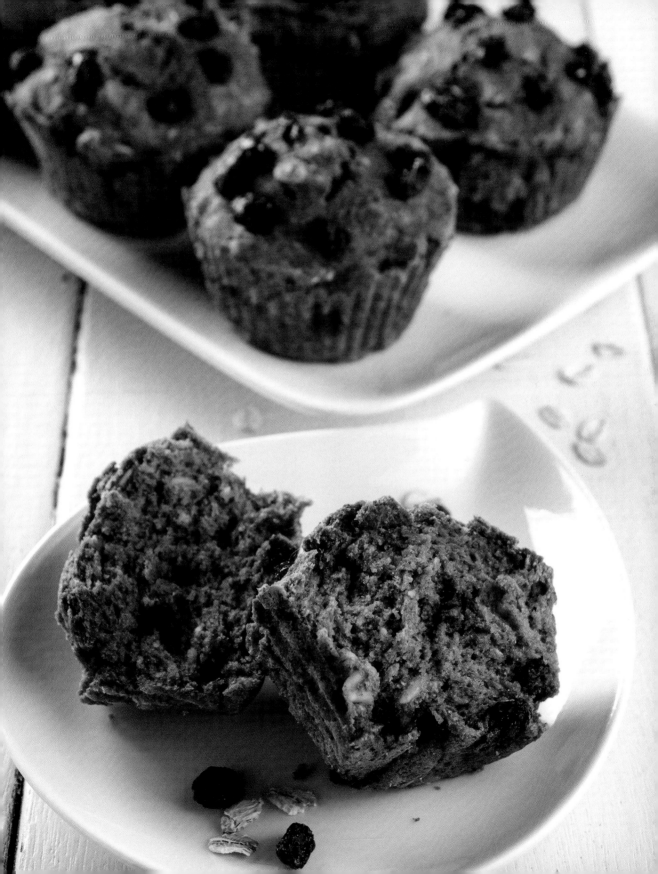

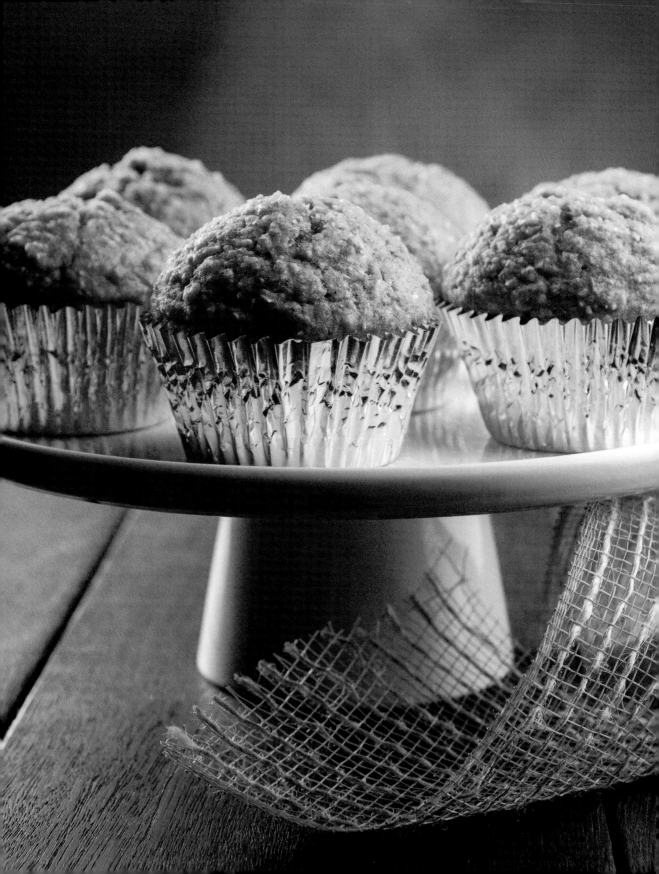

Crazy for Corn Muffins

 Great texture, and the perfect amount of sweetness!

1½ cups frozen sweet corn kernels, thawed

¾ cup fat-free plain Greek yogurt

1 cup whole-wheat flour

¾ cup yellow cornmeal

3½ tablespoons Truvia spoonable no-calorie sweetener (or another natural brand about twice as sweet as sugar)

2¼ teaspoons baking powder

½ teaspoon salt

¾ cup egg whites (about 6 large eggs' worth)

½ cup unsweetened vanilla almond milk

2 teaspoons vanilla extract

Chew on This...

Several US states have an official state muffin. Massachusetts' is the corn muffin!

1/12th of recipe (1 muffin): 101 calories, 0.5g total fat (0g sat fat), 232mg sodium, 21g carbs, 2.5g fiber, 1.5g sugars, 5.5g protein

You'll Need: 12-cup muffin pan, foil baking cups (or nonstick spray), small blender or food processor, large bowl, medium-large bowl, whisk

Prep: 15 minutes • **Cook:** 20 minutes

1. Preheat oven to 375 degrees. Line a 12-cup muffin pan with foil baking cups, or spray it with nonstick spray.

2. In a small blender or food processor, combine thawed corn with yogurt. Pulse until blended to the consistency of creamed corn.

3. In a large bowl, combine flour, cornmeal, sweetener, baking powder, and salt. Mix well.

4. In a medium-large bowl, combine corn-yogurt mixture, egg whites, almond milk, and vanilla extract. Whisk until uniform.

5. Transfer contents of the medium-large bowl to the large bowl, and mix until uniform.

6. Evenly fill muffin pan with batter, and smooth out the tops.

7. Bake until a toothpick inserted into the center of a muffin comes out clean, 15 to 17 minutes.

MAKES 12 SERVINGS

Freeze It: Muffin Edition

To Freeze: Tightly wrap each cooled muffin in foil or plastic wrap. Place wrapped muffins in a sealable container or bag, seal, and store in the freezer.

To Thaw: Unwrap, and place on a microwave-safe plate. Microwave at 50 percent power for 1 minute, or until it reaches your desired temperature. Or just refrigerate overnight!

Chocolate Chocolate Donuts

155 cal

V Obsession confession: It took SEVEN tries to get this recipe just right. The dark cocoa is key . . . It gives the donuts their intensely rich, fudgy flavor!

DONUTS

1 cup whole-wheat flour

⅓ cup unsweetened dark cocoa powder

2½ tablespoons Truvia spoonable no-calorie sweetener (or another natural brand about twice as sweet as sugar)

½ teaspoon baking powder

⅛ teaspoon baking soda

⅛ teaspoon salt

½ cup unsweetened vanilla almond milk

½ cup fat-free plain Greek yogurt

¼ cup egg whites (about 2 large eggs' worth)

¼ cup canned pure pumpkin

½ teaspoon vanilla extract

2½ tablespoons mini (or chopped) semi-sweet chocolate chips

TOPPING

1½ tablespoons mini (or chopped) semi-sweet chocolate chips

2 teaspoons unsweetened vanilla almond milk

⅙th of recipe (1 donut): 155 calories, 4g total fat (2g sat fat), 198mg sodium, 30g carbs, 4.5g fiber, 6.5g sugars, 7g protein

You'll Need: standard 6-cavity donut pan, nonstick spray, large bowl, medium bowl, whisk, baking sheet, very small microwave-safe bowl

Prep: 15 minutes • **Cook:** 15 minutes • **Cool:** 25 minutes

1. Preheat oven to 375 degrees. Spray a standard 6-cavity donut pan with nonstick spray.

2. In a large bowl, combine flour, cocoa powder, sweetener, baking powder, baking soda, and salt. Mix well.

3. In a medium bowl, combine all remaining donut ingredients *except* chocolate chips. Whisk until uniform.

4. Add contents of the medium bowl to the large bowl, and stir until smooth and uniform. (Batter will be thick.)

5. Fold in chocolate chips. Evenly fill donut pan with batter, and smooth out the tops.

6. Bake until a toothpick inserted into a donut comes out mostly clean, about 10 minutes.

7. Let donuts cool completely, about 10 minutes in the pan and 15 minutes out of the pan.

8. In a very small microwave-safe bowl, combine topping ingredients. Microwave at 50 percent power for 25 seconds.

9. Stir topping until smooth and uniform. Drizzle or spread over donuts.

MAKES 6 SERVINGS

Chew on This . . .

Sources say over 10 billion donuts are consumed in the US every year!

HG Donut Tip!

For extra-beautiful donuts, fill the donut cavities using a DIY piping bag. Just transfer the batter to a plastic bag, and squeeze it down toward a bottom corner. Snip off the corner with scissors, creating a small hole for piping.

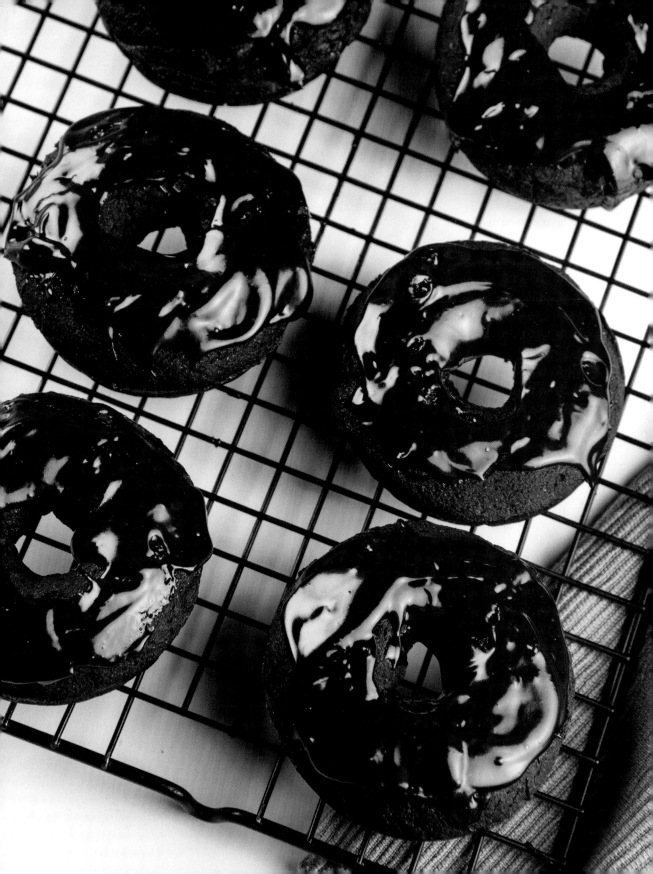

Apple Crumb Yum Donuts

122 cal

V   These will quickly become a staple in your life. Apple enthusiasts: Don't miss the Tumbly Crumbly Spiced Apple Bake (page 313) and Pump Up the Pecan Apple Streusel Bars (page 317)!

TOPPING

⅓ cup old-fashioned oats

1½ tablespoons whole-wheat flour

1½ tablespoons whipped butter, room temperature

1 teaspoon Truvia spoonable no-calorie sweetener (or another natural brand about twice as sweet as sugar)

¼ teaspoon cinnamon

Dash salt

DONUTS

¾ cup whole-wheat flour

2½ tablespoons Truvia spoonable no-calorie sweetener (or another natural brand about twice as sweet as sugar)

2 teaspoons cinnamon

½ teaspoon baking powder

¼ teaspoon pumpkin pie spice

¼ teaspoon ground nutmeg

⅛ teaspoon baking soda

⅛ teaspoon salt

⅓ cup unsweetened vanilla almond milk

⅓ cup fat-free plain Greek yogurt

¼ cup egg whites (about 2 large eggs' worth)

3 tablespoons canned pure pumpkin

2 teaspoons vanilla extract

½ cup peeled and finely chopped Granny Smith apple

⅙th of recipe (1 donut): 122 calories, 2.5g total fat (1g sat fat), 187mg sodium, 25g carbs, 3.5g fiber, 2.5g sugars, 5.5g protein

You'll Need: standard 6-cavity donut pan, nonstick spray, 2 medium bowls, large bowl, whisk

Prep: 20 minutes • **Cook:** 10 minutes • **Cool:** 25 minutes

1. Preheat oven to 375 degrees. Spray a standard 6-cavity donut pan with nonstick spray.

2. In a medium bowl, combine topping ingredients. Mash and stir until uniform and crumbly.

3. To make the donuts, in a large bowl, combine flour, sweetener, cinnamon, baking powder, pumpkin pie spice, nutmeg, baking soda, and salt. Mix well.

4. In a second medium bowl, combine all remaining donut ingredients *except* apple. Whisk until uniform.

5. Add contents of the second medium bowl to the large bowl, and stir until smooth and uniform. (Batter will be thick.)

6. Fold in apple. Evenly fill donut pan with batter, and smooth out the tops.

7. Sprinkle with topping, and lightly press to adhere.

8. Bake until a toothpick inserted into a donut comes out mostly clean, about 10 minutes.

9. Let donuts cool completely, about 10 minutes in the pan and 15 minutes out of the pan.

MAKES 6 SERVINGS

Chew on This . . .

Apparently, there are 15 people in the US with the first name "Donut." Yes, really.

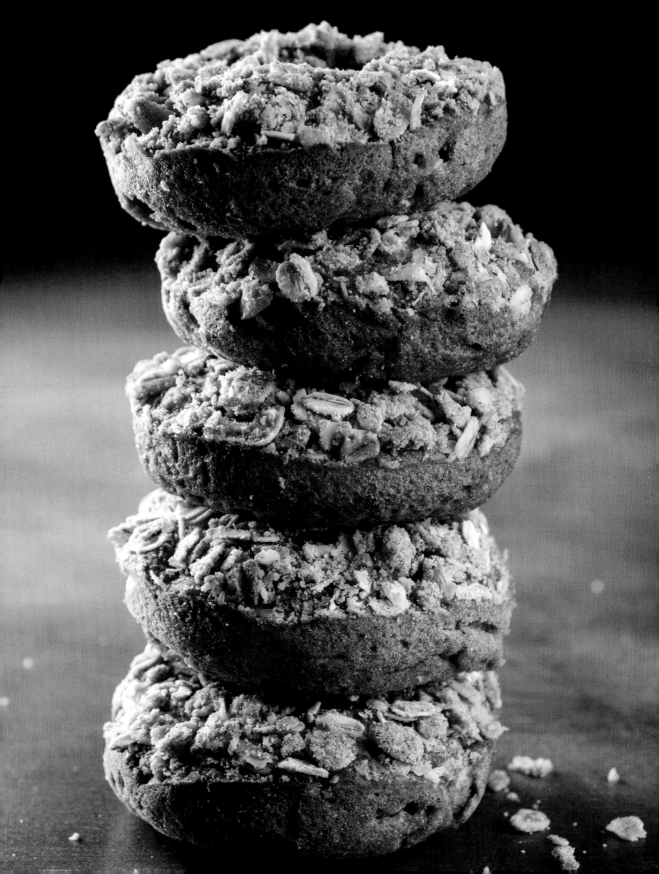

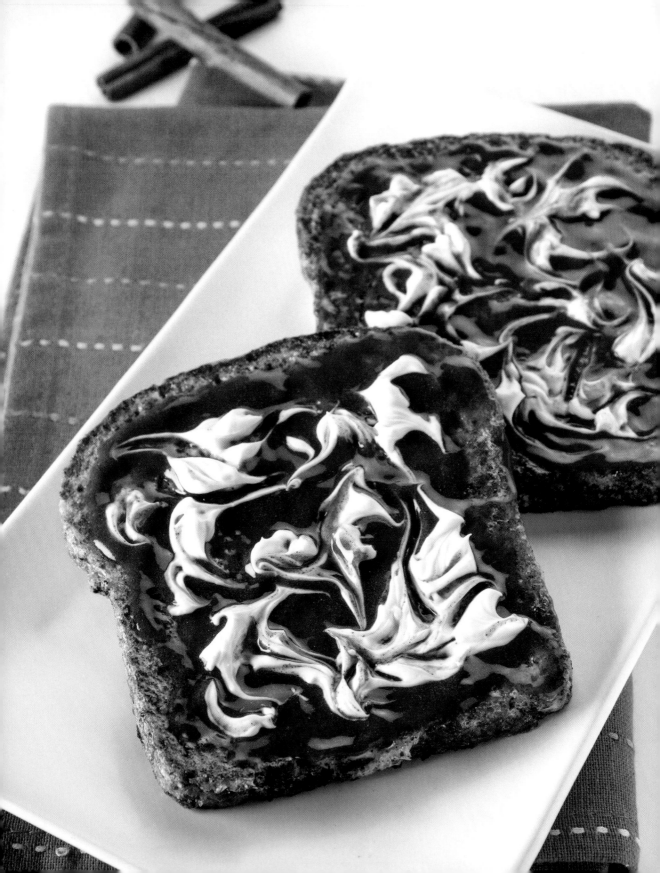

Hey, Honey! Cinnamon Roll French Toast

271 cal

  This sweetly spiced French toast is decadent yet light. Perfection!

FRENCH TOAST

⅓ cup egg whites (about 3 large eggs' worth)

1 packet natural no-calorie sweetener

½ teaspoon cinnamon

¼ teaspoon vanilla extract

2 slices whole-grain bread with 60 to 80 calories per slice

CINNAMON GLAZE

2 teaspoons honey

¼ teaspoon cinnamon

ICING

1 tablespoon light/reduced-fat cream cheese

Half a packet natural no-calorie sweetener

Drop vanilla extract

Entire recipe: 271 calories, 4.5g total fat (1.5g sat fat), 417mg sodium, 43.5g carbs, 6g fiber, 16.5g sugars, 16g protein

You'll Need: wide bowl, whisk, large skillet, nonstick spray, 2 small bowls (1 microwave-safe)

Prep: 10 minutes • **Cook:** 5 minutes

1. In a wide bowl, combine all French toast ingredients *except* bread. Whisk thoroughly.

2. Bring a large skillet sprayed with nonstick spray to medium-high heat. Coat bread with egg mixture. Cook until golden brown, 1 to 2 minutes per side.

3. In a small bowl, mix cinnamon glaze ingredients.

4. Combine icing ingredients in a small microwave-safe bowl. Add 1 teaspoon water, and mix well. Microwave for 10 seconds, or until melted.

5. Drizzle cinnamon glaze onto French toast, and top with icing.

MAKES 1 SERVING

Tropical Tiki French Toast

320 cal

15m **V** The mango topping is beyond-words amazing. Make extra, and put it on EVERYTHING. (You'll thank me later!)

FRENCH TOAST

⅓ cup egg whites (about 3 large eggs' worth)

1 packet natural no-calorie sweetener

¼ teaspoon cinnamon

¼ teaspoon coconut extract

⅛ teaspoon vanilla extract

1½ teaspoons whipped butter

2 slices whole-grain bread with 60 to 80 calories per slice

TOPPING

½ cup chopped mango

1 teaspoon arrowroot powder

1 packet natural no-calorie sweetener

¼ teaspoon coconut extract

1 tablespoon unsweetened shredded coconut

Entire recipe: 320 calories, 8.5g total fat (4.5g sat fat), 377mg sodium, 46.5g carbs, 7.5g fiber, 15.5g sugars, 15.5g protein

You'll Need: wide bowl, whisk, large skillet, nonstick spray, small blender or food processor, small microwave-safe bowl

Prep: 10 minutes • **Cook:** 5 minutes

1. In a wide bowl, combine all French toast ingredients *except* butter and bread. Whisk thoroughly.

2. Bring a large skillet sprayed with nonstick spray to medium-high heat. Add butter, and let it coat the bottom. Coat bread with egg mixture. Cook until golden brown, 1 to 2 minutes per side.

3. Place all topping ingredients *except* shredded coconut in a small blender or food processor. Add 1 tablespoon water, and puree until smooth.

4. Transfer topping mixture to a small microwave-safe bowl. Cover and microwave for 45 seconds.

5. Spoon mango topping over French toast (or serve on the side), and sprinkle French toast with shredded coconut.

MAKES 1 SERVING

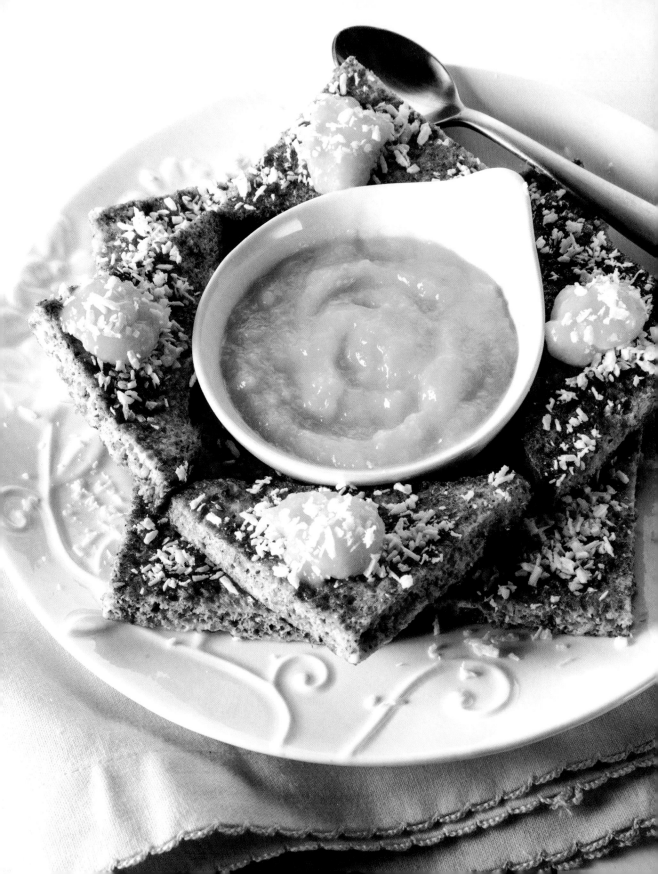

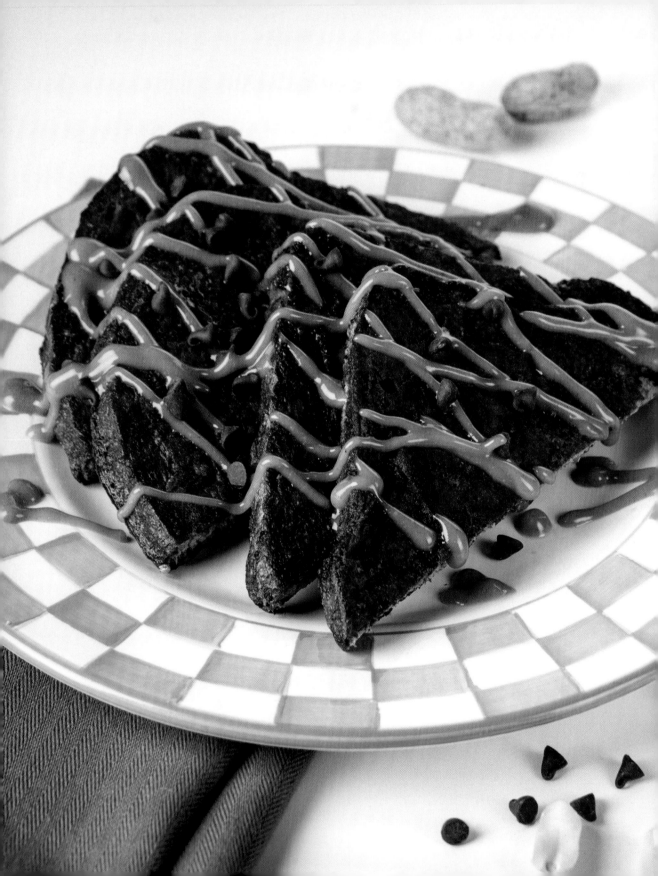

Peanut Butter Cup French Toast

It's like a bag of Reese's exploded all over your breakfast! If peanut butter is one of your obsessions, flip to page 363 for more PB deliciousness!

FRENCH TOAST

⅓ cup egg whites (about 3 large eggs' worth)

1 tablespoon unsweetened cocoa powder

2 teaspoons powdered peanut butter or defatted peanut flour

1 packet natural no-calorie sweetener

¼ teaspoon vanilla extract

¼ teaspoon cinnamon

1½ teaspoons whipped butter

2 slices whole-grain bread with 60 to 80 calories per slice

TOPPING

1 tablespoon powdered peanut butter or defatted peanut flour

1 tablespoon unsweetened vanilla almond milk

1½ teaspoons honey

1½ teaspoons mini (or chopped) semi-sweet chocolate chips

Entire recipe: 346 calories, 9.5g total fat (3.5g sat fat), 414mg sodium, 48.5g carbs, 9g fiber, 17.5g sugars, 21g protein

You'll Need: wide bowl, whisk, large skillet, nonstick spray, small bowl

Prep: 5 minutes • **Cook:** 5 minutes

1. In a wide bowl, combine all French toast ingredients *except* butter and bread. Whisk thoroughly.

2. Bring a large skillet sprayed with nonstick spray to medium-high heat. Add butter, and let it coat the bottom. Coat bread with egg mixture. Cook until golden brown, 1 to 2 minutes per side.

3. In a small bowl, combine all topping ingredients *except* chocolate chips. Mix until uniform.

4. Drizzle PB topping over French toast, and top with chocolate chips.

MAKES 1 SERVING

Perfect Pumpkin Pie Pancakes

230 cal

  These flapjacks are light, healthy, and (of course!) utterly crave-worthy . . .

TOPPING

3 tablespoons fat-free plain Greek yogurt

1 tablespoon canned pure pumpkin

Half a packet natural no-calorie sweetener

¼ teaspoon cinnamon

⅛ teaspoon vanilla extract

PANCAKES

¼ cup egg whites (about 2 large eggs' worth)

¼ cup oat bran

2 tablespoons canned pure pumpkin

2 tablespoons unsweetened applesauce

1 tablespoon whole-wheat flour

1 packet natural no-calorie sweetener

½ teaspoon baking powder

½ teaspoon cinnamon

¼ teaspoon pumpkin pie spice

⅛ teaspoon vanilla extract

Dash salt

Entire recipe: 230 calories, 2g total fat (<0.5g sat fat), 519mg sodium, 35g carbs, 8.5g fiber, 6.5g sugars, 17.5g protein

You'll Need: 2 medium bowls, skillet, nonstick spray, plate
Prep: 10 minutes • **Cook:** 10 minutes

1. In a medium bowl, mix topping ingredients until smooth and uniform. Cover and refrigerate.

2. In another medium bowl, mix pancake ingredients until uniform.

3. Bring a skillet sprayed with nonstick spray to medium heat. Add half of the batter to form a large pancake. Cook until it begins to bubble and is solid enough to flip, 1 to 2 minutes.

4. Gently flip, and cook until both sides are lightly browned and inside is cooked through, about 1 minute.

5. Plate pancake. Remove skillet from heat, re-spray, and return to medium heat. Repeat with remaining batter to make a second pancake.

6. Spoon topping over pancakes (or serve on the side).

MAKES 1 SERVING

Pancake Tip!

The first pancake generally takes longer to cook, so keep an eye on that second one; it'll cook faster.

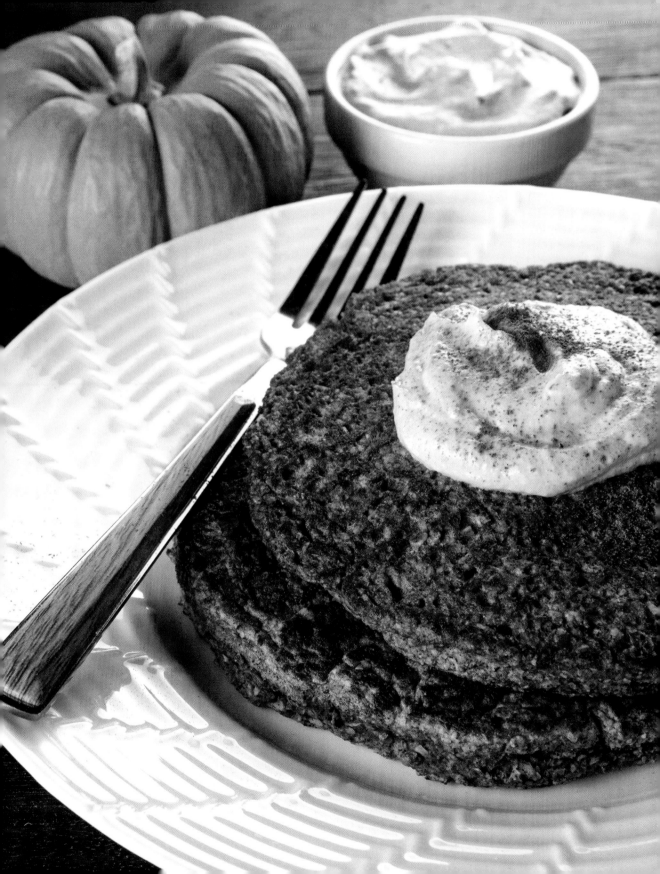

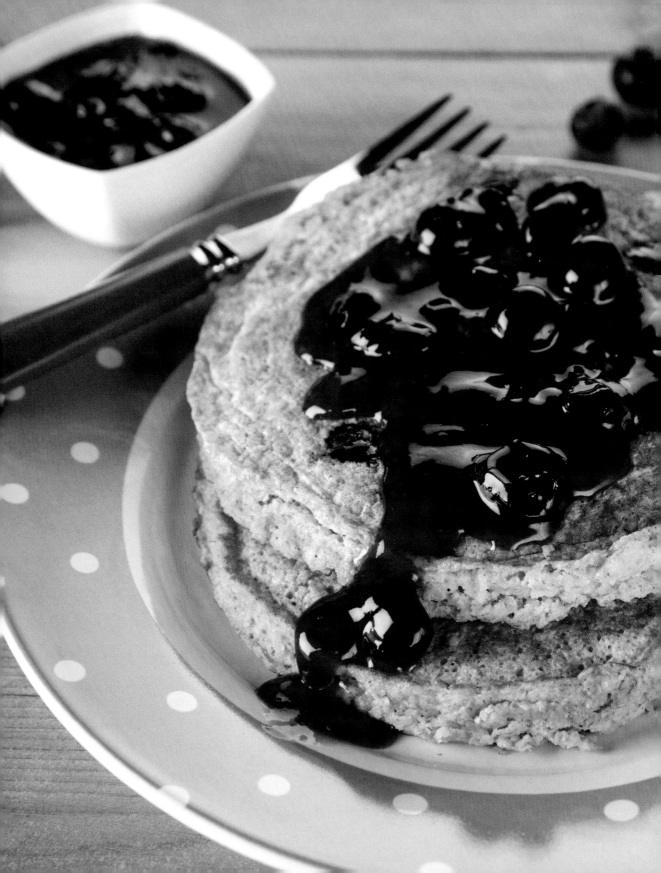

Out of the Blueberry Pancakes

247 cal

 V These p-cakes have blueberries inside 'em *and* a gooey blueberry topping. How great is that?!

PANCAKES

¼ cup egg whites (about 2 large eggs' worth)

¼ cup unsweetened applesauce

¼ cup oat bran

1 tablespoon whole-wheat flour

1 packet natural no-calorie sweetener

½ teaspoon baking powder

⅛ teaspoon vanilla extract

⅛ teaspoon salt

Dash cinnamon

¼ cup blueberries (fresh or thawed from frozen and drained)

TOPPING

1 teaspoon arrowroot powder

¼ cup blueberries (fresh or thawed from frozen and drained)

1 packet natural no-calorie sweetener

Dash cinnamon

Dash salt

Entire recipe: 247 calories, 2.5g total fat (<0.5g sat fat), 792mg sodium, 45g carbs, 8g fiber, 13.5g sugars, 13g protein

You'll Need: 2 medium bowls (1 microwave-safe), skillet, nonstick spray, plate

Prep: 10 minutes • **Cook:** 10 minutes

1. In a medium bowl, combine all pancake ingredients *except* blueberries. Mix until uniform.

2. Fold blueberries into batter.

3. Bring a skillet sprayed with nonstick spray to medium heat. Add half of the batter to form a large pancake. Cook until it begins to bubble and is solid enough to flip, 1 to 2 minutes.

4. Gently flip, and cook until both sides are lightly browned and inside is cooked through, about 1 minute.

5. Plate pancake. Remove skillet from heat, re-spray, and return to medium heat. Repeat with remaining batter to make a second pancake.

6. In a medium microwave-safe bowl, combine arrowroot powder with 3 tablespoons cold water; stir to dissolve. Add remaining topping ingredients, and mix well. Cover and microwave until hot and thickened, about 1 minute.

7. Mix well, and spoon topping over pancakes (or serve on the side).

MAKES 1 SERVING

Chew on This . . .

September 26th is National Pancake Day. I do NOT recommend restricting consumption of these pancakes to that day alone!

Choco Monkey Overnight Oats

323 cal

Ⓥ ⒼⒻ Obsession confession: This no-cook creation was inspired by one of the most popular HG recipes ever . . . and it's even better than the original!

1½ tablespoons unsweetened cocoa powder

½ cup unsweetened vanilla almond milk

½ cup mashed banana

⅓ cup old-fashioned oats

1 packet natural no-calorie sweetener

¼ teaspoon vanilla extract

⅛ teaspoon cinnamon

Dash salt

¼ ounce (about 1 tablespoon) chopped walnuts

1 teaspoon mini (or chopped) semi-sweet chocolate chips

Entire recipe: 323 calories, 10.5g total fat (2g sat fat), 245mg sodium, 54g carbs, 9.5g fiber, 17.5g sugars, 8g protein

You'll Need: medium bowl or jar

Prep: 5 minutes • **Chill:** 6 hours

1. In a medium bowl or jar, combine cocoa powder with 2 tablespoons hot water. Stir to dissolve.

2. Add all remaining ingredients *except* walnuts and chocolate chips. Mix well.

3. Cover and refrigerate for at least 6 hours, until oats are soft and have absorbed most of the liquid.

4. Top with walnuts and chocolate chips.

MAKES 1 SERVING

Chew on This . . .

A reported 75 percent of US households have oatmeal in their cupboard right now. (Including mine!)

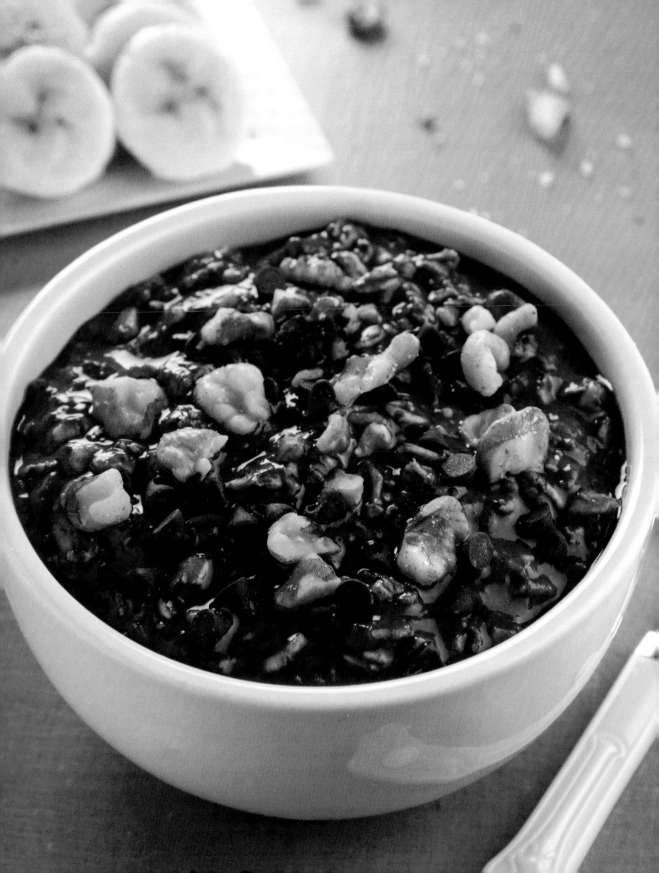

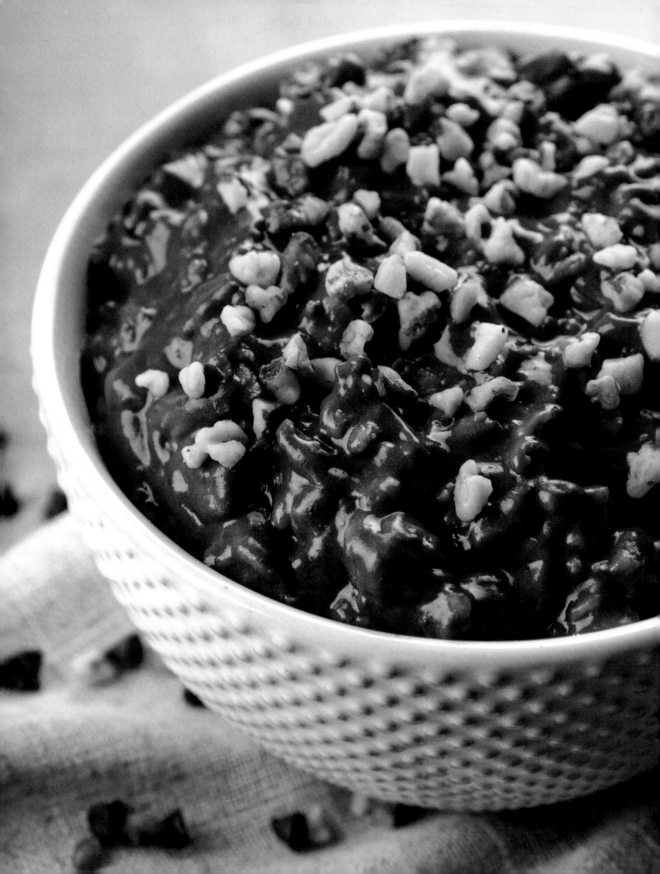

Brownie Batter Growing Oatmeal

292 cal

 Obsession confession: I used to lick brownie batter out of the mixing bowl when I was a kid! (I KNOW some of you did too!) With this recipe, there's no need to . . .

½ **cup old-fashioned oats**

1½ **tablespoons unsweetened cocoa powder**

¼ **teaspoon vanilla extract**

⅛ **teaspoon salt**

1 **cup unsweetened vanilla almond milk**

2 **packets natural no-calorie sweetener**

1 **teaspoon mini (or chopped) semi-sweet chocolate chips**

¼ **ounce (about 1 tablespoon) chopped walnuts**

Entire recipe: 292 calories, 12g total fat (2g sat fat), 469mg sodium, 39g carbs, 8g fiber, 4g sugars, 9g protein

You'll Need: nonstick pot, medium bowl

Prep: 5 minutes • **Cook:** 20 minutes • **Cool:** 10 minutes

1. In a nonstick pot, combine oats, cocoa powder, vanilla extract, and salt.
2. Add almond milk and 1 cup water. Bring to a boil.
3. Reduce to a simmer. Cook and stir until thick and creamy, 12 to 15 minutes.
4. Transfer to a medium bowl, and stir in sweetener and chocolate chips. Let cool until thickened, 5 to 10 minutes.
5. Gently stir, and top with walnuts.

MAKES 1 SERVING

HG FYI

Don't be alarmed by the amount of liquid. That's what makes this oatmeal GROW! It'll thicken up as it cools.

Crazy Carrot Cake Oatmeal Bake

249 cal

  This breakfast bake tastes exactly like carrot cake. I dare you to disagree!

3 cups old-fashioned oats

3 tablespoons plain protein powder with about 100 calories per serving

5 packets natural no-calorie sweetener

1½ tablespoons chia seeds

1 tablespoon cinnamon

2 teaspoons baking powder

½ teaspoon ground nutmeg

¼ teaspoon salt

1½ cups unsweetened vanilla almond milk

½ cup unsweetened applesauce

½ cup egg whites (about 4 large eggs' worth)

2 teaspoons vanilla extract

1 cup shredded carrots, finely chopped

½ cup canned crushed pineapple packed in juice, lightly drained

3 tablespoons raisins, chopped

⅙th of bake: 249 calories, 4.5g total fat (0.5g sat fat), 357mg sodium, 42g carbs, 7g fiber, 10g sugars, 10.5g protein

You'll Need: 8-inch by 8-inch baking pan, nonstick spray, large bowl, medium-large bowl

Prep: 15 minutes • **Cook:** 35 minutes

1. Preheat oven to 350 degrees. Spray an 8-inch by 8-inch baking pan with nonstick spray.

2. In a large bowl, combine oats, protein powder, sweetener, chia seeds, cinnamon, baking powder, nutmeg, and salt. Mix well.

3. In a medium-large bowl, combine almond milk, applesauce, egg whites, and vanilla extract. Mix until uniform.

4. Add mixture in the medium-large bowl to the large bowl. Stir until uniform.

5. Fold in chopped carrots, lightly drained pineapple, and chopped raisins. Transfer to the baking pan, and smooth out the top.

6. Bake until light golden brown and cooked through, about 35 minutes.

MAKES 6 SERVINGS

Chew on This...

When asked what they consumed for breakfast, a reported 90 percent of those surveyed said they'd eaten oatmeal within the past two weeks. Wow!

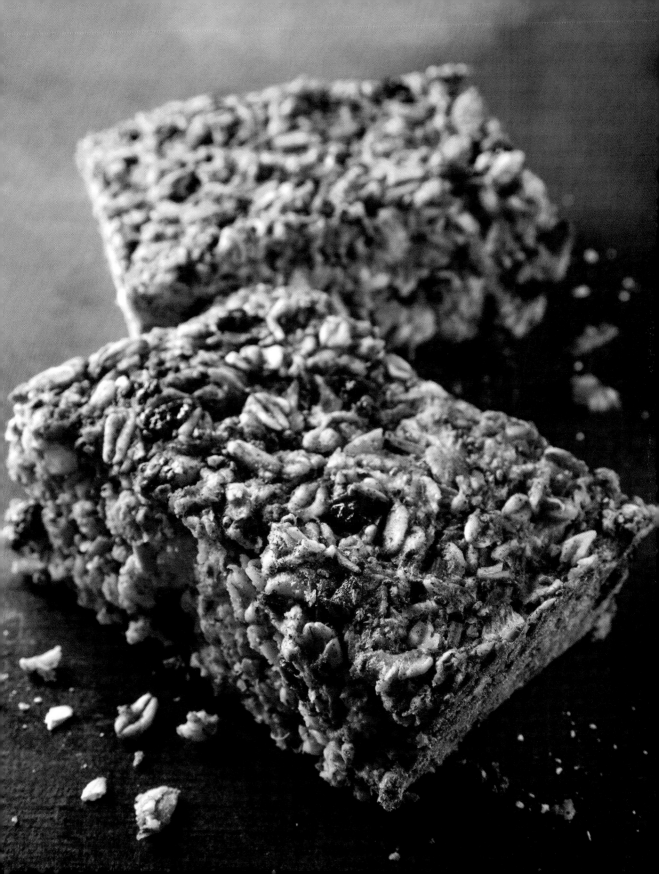

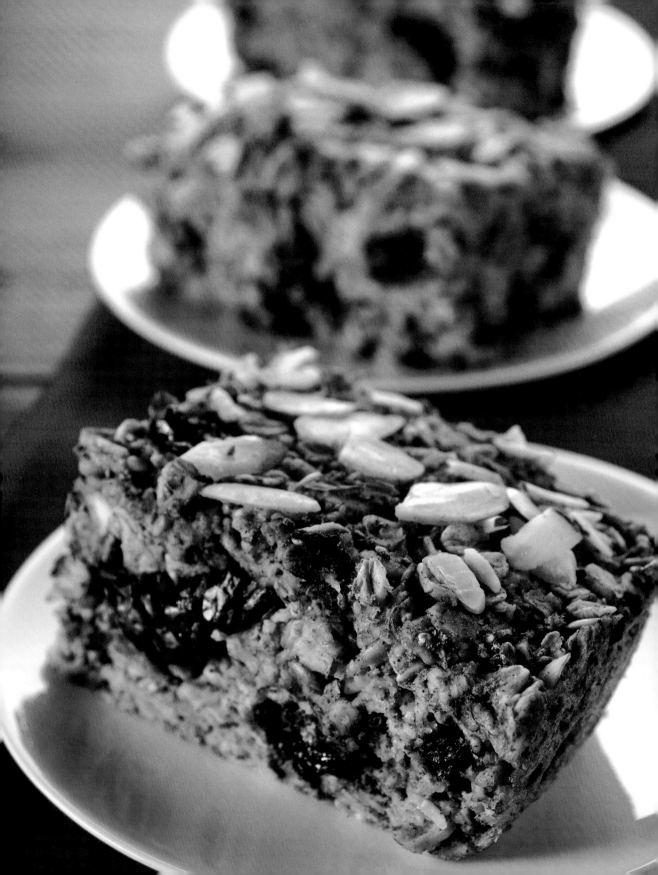

Oh My Cherry Pie Oatmeal Bake

241 cal

V **GF**   Best. Thing. Ever. Don't be surprised if this becomes a brand-new obsession for you! (It's one of mine!)

3 cups old-fashioned oats

5 packets natural no-calorie sweetener

1½ tablespoons chia seeds

2 teaspoons cinnamon

2 teaspoons baking powder

¼ teaspoon salt

1½ cups unsweetened vanilla almond milk

½ cup unsweetened applesauce

½ cup egg whites (about 4 large eggs' worth)

2 teaspoons vanilla extract

¼ teaspoon almond extract

1 cup frozen unsweetened pitted dark sweet cherries, thawed, drained, chopped

¾ ounce (about 3 tablespoons) sliced almonds

⅙th of bake: 241 calories, 6g total fat (0.5g sat fat), 336mg sodium, 37.5g carbs, 7g fiber, 6.5g sugars, 9.5g protein

You'll need: 8-inch by 8-inch baking pan, nonstick spray, large bowl, medium-large bowl
Prep: 10 minutes • **Cook:** 35 minutes

1. Preheat oven to 350 degrees. Spray an 8-inch by 8-inch baking pan with nonstick spray.

2. In a large bowl, combine oats, sweetener, chia seeds, cinnamon, baking powder, and salt. Mix well.

3. In a medium-large bowl, combine almond milk, applesauce, egg whites, vanilla extract, and almond extract. Mix until uniform.

4. Add mixture in the medium-large bowl to the large bowl. Stir until uniform.

5. Gently fold in cherries. Transfer to the baking pan, and smooth out the top.

6. Sprinkle with almonds, and lightly press to adhere.

7. Bake until light golden brown and cooked through, about 35 minutes.

MAKES 6 SERVINGS

Freeze It: Oatmeal Bake Edition

To Freeze: Once cool, tightly wrap each serving in foil or plastic wrap. Put individually wrapped pieces in a sealable container or bag, seal, and place in the freezer.

To Thaw: Unwrap one piece, and place on a microwave-safe plate. For a just-baked texture, cover or wrap it loosely in a paper towel. Microwave for 1½ minutes, or until it reaches your desired temperature.

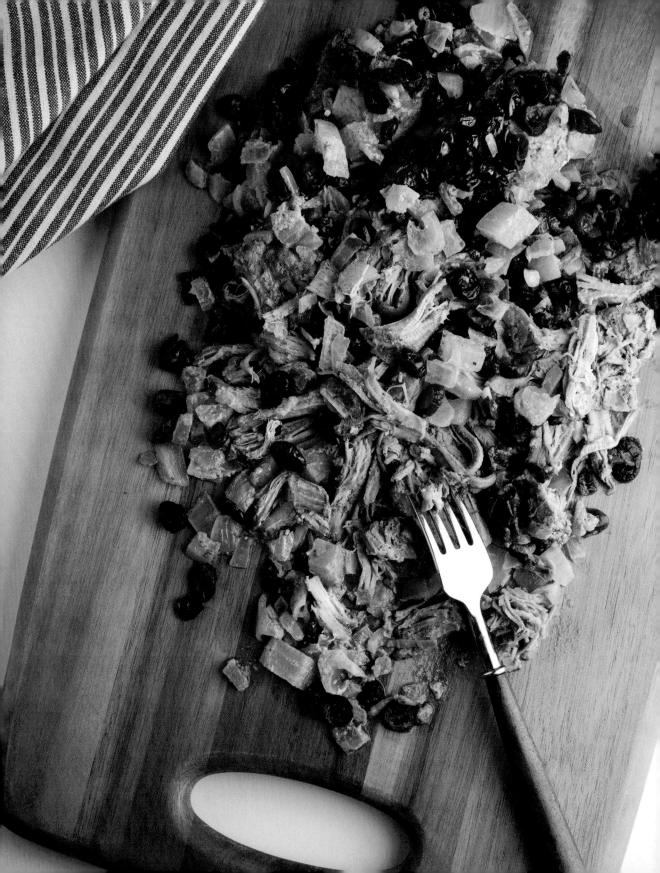

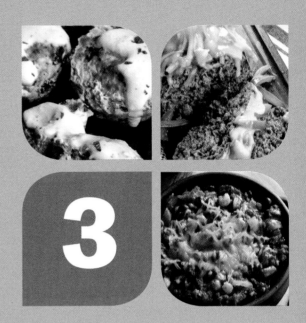

3

Mom's the Word!

Who doesn't CRAVE comfort food? Exactly. Sadly, those family classics are generally calorie catastrophes. Enter these slimmed-down spins! From meatloaf to mashies, this chapter has you covered . . .

Love Me Tender Pot Roast

272 cal

GF Technically, this is a pan roast, since it's baked in a pan, not cooked in a pot. Call it whatever you want: The taste and texture are PERFECTION.

2 pounds raw boneless chuck beef roast, trimmed of excess fat

6 peeled garlic cloves

1 teaspoon each salt and black pepper

3 cups carrots cut into ½-inch coins

2 cups beef broth

1½ cups sliced mushrooms

1½ cups sweet onions cut into ½-inch chunks

1 cup celery cut into ½-inch pieces

2 fresh thyme sprigs

2 bay leaves

⅙th of recipe (about 3½ ounces meat with 1 cup veggies and broth): 272 calories, 9.5g total fat (4g sat fat), 819mg sodium, 13g carbs, 3g fiber, 5.5g sugars, 35g protein

You'll Need: 9-inch by 13-inch baking pan, nonstick spray, large skillet, foil

Prep: 25 minutes • **Cook:** 3 hours and 10 minutes

1. Preheat oven to 325 degrees. Spray a 9-inch by 13-inch baking pan with nonstick spray.

2. Cut six deep slits into the top of the roast, evenly spaced. Insert a garlic clove into each slit. Season roast with ¼ teaspoon each salt and pepper.

3. Bring a large skillet sprayed with nonstick spray to high heat. Rotating occasionally, cook roast until browned on all sides, about 5 minutes.

4. Transfer to the baking pan. Add remaining ingredients, including remaining ¾ teaspoon each salt and black pepper.

5. Cover pan with foil. Bake for 3 hours, or until meat is tender and veggies are soft.

6. Remove and discard thyme sprigs and bay leaves.

MAKES 6 SERVINGS

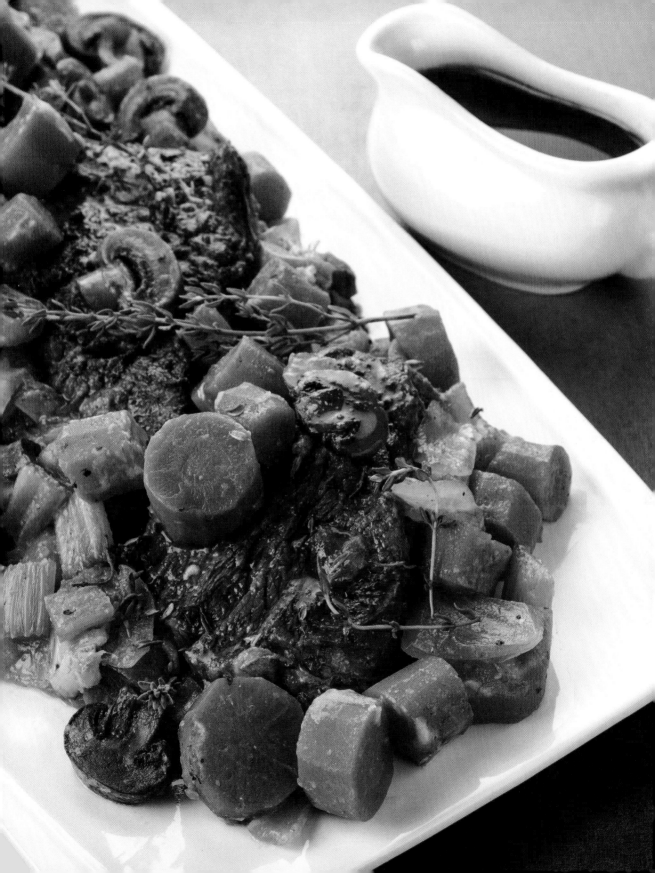

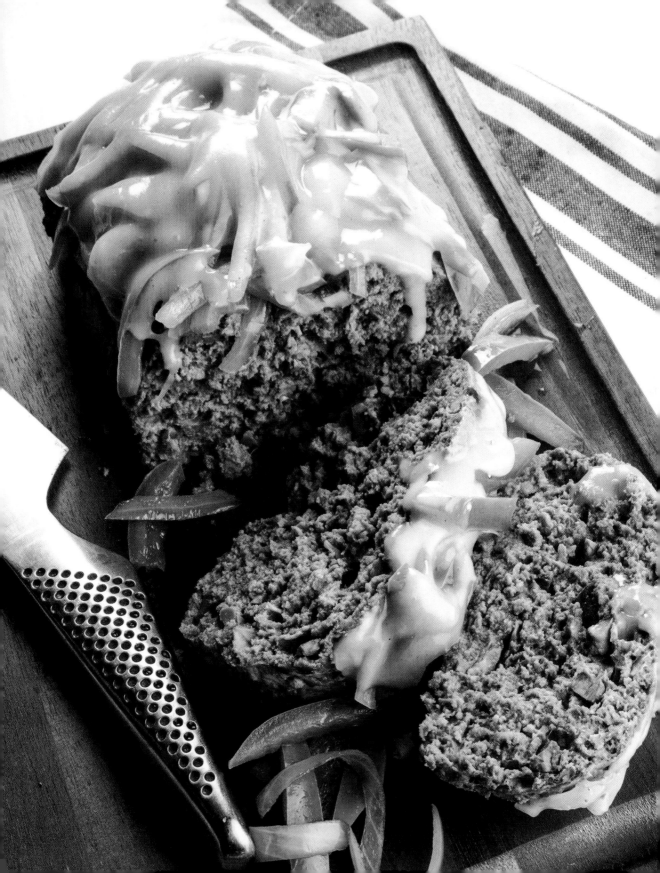

Philly You Up Cheesesteak Meatloaf

198 cal

Food mashup! It doesn't get much better than a cheesesteak-inspired meatloaf, people . . .

MEATLOAF

1 pound raw extra-lean ground beef (4% fat or less)

2 cups finely chopped brown mushrooms

¼ cup whole-wheat panko breadcrumbs

¼ cup egg whites (about 2 large eggs' worth)

½ teaspoon onion powder

½ teaspoon garlic powder

½ teaspoon each salt and black pepper

TOPPING

1½ cups sliced onions

1½ cups sliced green bell peppers

⅛ teaspoon each salt and black pepper

3 slices reduced-fat provolone cheese

⅕th of loaf: 198 calories, 6.5g total fat (3g sat fat), 464mg sodium, 9g carbs, 2g fiber, 3g sugars, 25.5g protein

You'll Need: 9-inch by 5-inch loaf pan, nonstick spray, large bowl, large skillet, foil

Prep: 15 minutes • **Cook:** 1 hour

1. Preheat oven to 400 degrees. Spray a 9-inch by 5-inch loaf pan with nonstick spray.

2. In a large bowl, thoroughly mix meatloaf ingredients. Transfer to the loaf pan, and smooth out the top.

3. To make the topping, bring a large skillet sprayed with nonstick spray to medium-high heat. Add veggies, and sprinkle with seasonings. Cook and stir until slightly softened and lightly browned, 5 to 7 minutes.

4. Top meatloaf with cooked veggies, and gently press to adhere.

5. Cover pan with foil. Bake for 45 minutes, or until cooked through.

6. Uncover pan. Tear cheese slices in half, and place over meatloaf. Bake until melted, about 5 minutes.

MAKES 5 SERVINGS

Chew on This . . .

The Philadelphia Eagles once set the world record for longest cheesesteak with a sandwich longer than a football field. That's over 360 feet of deliciousness!

Pizza-fied Meatloaf

225 cal

The entire Hungry Girl staff FLIPPED when they first laid forks on this delicious creation! Pizza lovers: Don't miss Chapter 4, a.k.a. You Wanna Pizza Me?

½ cup canned crushed tomatoes

1 teaspoon garlic powder

1 teaspoon onion powder

1 teaspoon Italian seasoning

1 pound raw extra-lean ground beef (4% fat or less)

1 cup finely chopped onion

1 cup finely chopped green bell pepper

1 cup finely chopped mushrooms

¼ cup whole-wheat panko breadcrumbs

¼ cup egg whites (about 2 large eggs' worth)

½ teaspoon each salt and black pepper

¾ cup shredded part-skim mozzarella cheese

1 tablespoon grated Parmesan cheese

⅕th of loaf: 225 calories, 7.5g total fat (4g sat fat), 509mg sodium, 10.5g carbs, 2g fiber, 3.5g sugars, 27.5g protein

You'll Need: 9-inch by 5-inch loaf pan, nonstick spray, medium bowl, large bowl

Prep: 15 minutes • **Cook:** 50 minutes

1. Preheat oven to 400 degrees. Spray a 9-inch by 5-inch loaf pan with nonstick spray.

2. In a medium bowl, combine crushed tomatoes with ½ teaspoon each garlic powder, onion powder, and Italian seasoning. Mix well.

3. In a large bowl, combine remaining ½ teaspoon each garlic powder, onion powder, and Italian seasoning. Add all remaining ingredients *except* mozzarella and Parm.

4. Add half of the seasoned tomatoes to the large bowl, and mix thoroughly. Transfer to the loaf pan, and smooth out the top.

5. Top with remaining seasoned tomatoes.

6. Bake until cooked through, about 45 minutes.

7. Top with mozzarella and Parm. Bake until melted, about 5 minutes.

MAKES 5 SERVINGS

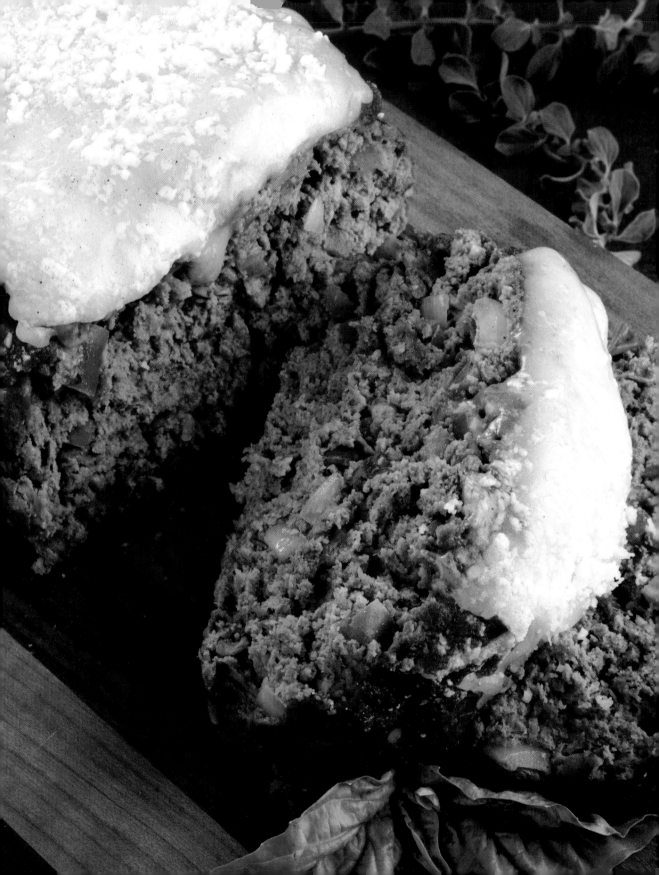

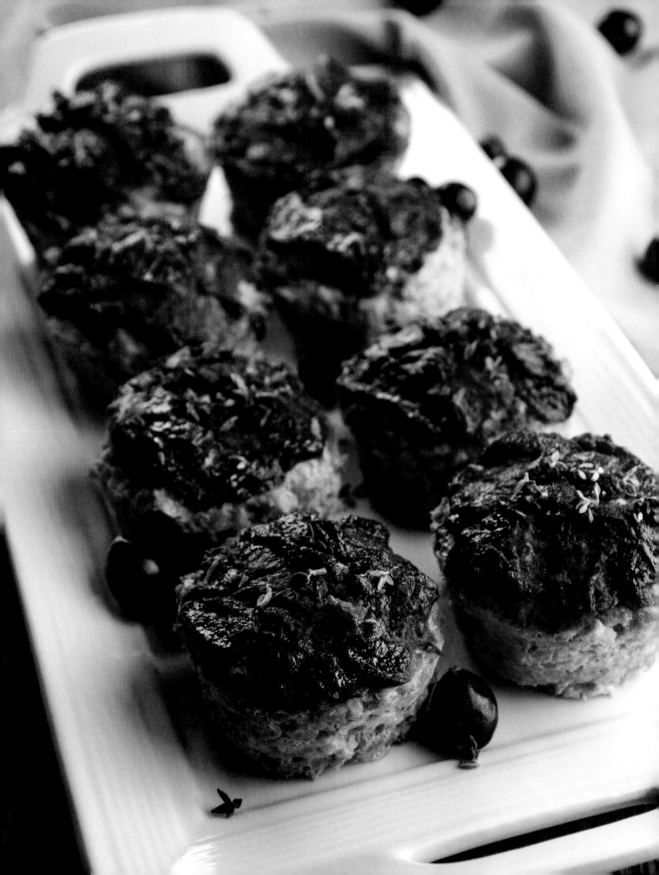

Thanksgiving Meatloaf Minis

203 cal

Enjoy the flavors of Turkey Day without all the calories by whipping up these tasty mini meatloaves. The texture is out of this world.

⅓ cup sweetened dried cranberries, chopped

5 cups cauliflower rice/ crumbles

½ cup finely chopped celery

½ cup finely chopped onion

1 teaspoon chopped garlic

1 pound raw lean ground turkey (7% fat or less)

⅓ cup egg whites (about 3 large eggs' worth)

¼ cup whole-wheat panko breadcrumbs

¼ teaspoon ground sage

¼ teaspoon ground thyme

¼ teaspoon each salt and black pepper

½ cup Clean & Hungry Ketchup (recipe and store-bought alternatives on page 343)

Optional topping: fresh thyme

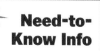

Need-to-Know Info

Use store-bought cauliflower crumbles/ rice, or DIY! See page 346 for the 411.

⅙th of recipe (2 meatloaves): 203 calories, 5.5g total fat (2g sat fat), 346mg sodium, 20g carbs, 4g fiber, 11g sugars, 20g protein

You'll Need: 12-cup muffin pan, nonstick spray, small bowl, large skillet with a lid, large bowl

Prep: 15 minutes • **Cook:** 45 minutes

1. Preheat oven to 375 degrees. Spray a 12-cup muffin pan with nonstick spray.

2. In a small bowl, cover chopped cranberries with warm water to soften.

3. Bring a large skillet sprayed with nonstick spray to medium-high heat. Add cauliflower rice/crumbles, celery, and onion. Cover and cook for 5 minutes, or until mostly softened.

4. Add garlic to the skillet, and cook and stir until fragrant, about 1 minute.

5. Transfer skillet contents to a large bowl. Add all remaining ingredients *except* ketchup.

6. Drain cranberries, and pat dry. Add half of the cranberries to the large bowl. Mix thoroughly.

7. Evenly fill muffin pan with meatloaf mixture, and smooth out the tops. (Cups will be very full.)

8. Add ketchup to the remaining cranberries, and mix well. Spread over meatloaves.

9. Bake until firm with lightly browned edges, about 35 minutes.

MAKES 6 SERVINGS

Chew on This...

The average American consumes around 4,500 calories on Thanksgiving Day. 4,500!

The Great Greek Mini Meatloaves

121 cal

The sauce takes this dish to the next level. Feel free to have two (or more!) of these at a time. Pssst . . . Check out the Cutie-Pie Greek Eggplant Pizzas on page 113!

SAUCE

⅓ cup fat-free plain Greek yogurt

¼ cup chopped and seeded cucumber, patted dry

1 tablespoon white wine vinegar

1 teaspoon chopped garlic

1 teaspoon lemon juice

¼ teaspoon each salt and black pepper

MEATLOAVES

½ cup finely chopped onion

1½ teaspoons chopped garlic

4 cups chopped spinach leaves

1 pound raw lean ground turkey (7% fat or less)

¾ cup crumbled feta cheese

¼ cup egg whites (about 2 large eggs' worth)

¼ cup whole-wheat panko breadcrumbs

½ teaspoon dried basil

½ teaspoon dried oregano

¼ teaspoon each salt and black pepper

Optional topping: fresh chopped basil

⅑th of recipe (1 meatloaf with about 2 teaspoons sauce): 121 calories, 5.5g total fat (2.5g sat fat), 312mg sodium, 4g carbs, 0.5g fiber, 1g sugars, 14g protein

You'll Need: 12-cup muffin pan, nonstick spray, small blender or food processor, large skillet, large bowl

Prep: 20 minutes • **Cook:** 40 minutes

1. Preheat oven to 375 degrees. Spray 9 cups of a 12-cup muffin pan with nonstick spray.

2. Combine sauce ingredients in small blender or food processor. Pulse until smooth and uniform. Cover and refrigerate.

3. Bring a large skillet sprayed with nonstick spray to medium-high heat. Add onion and garlic. Cook and stir until fragrant and slightly softened, about 2 minutes.

4. Add spinach to the skillet. Cook and stir until spinach has wilted and excess moisture has evaporated, about 1 minute.

5. Transfer to a large bowl, and pat dry. Add remaining meatloaf ingredients, and thoroughly mix.

6. Evenly fill the 9 cups of the muffin pan with meatloaf mixture, and smooth out the tops.

7. Bake until firm with lightly browned edges, about 35 minutes.

8. Just before serving, spoon sauce over meatloaves, about 2 teaspoons each.

MAKES 9 SERVINGS

Chew on This . . .

Meatloaf can reportedly be traced back to the fourth or fifth century, where it first appeared in a Roman cookbook. And the world has been enjoying it ever since!

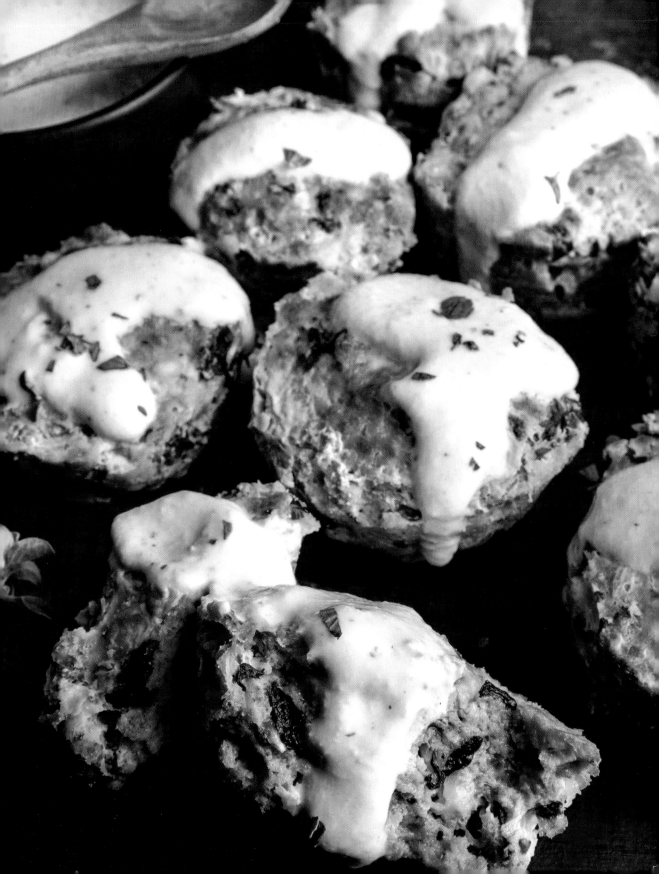

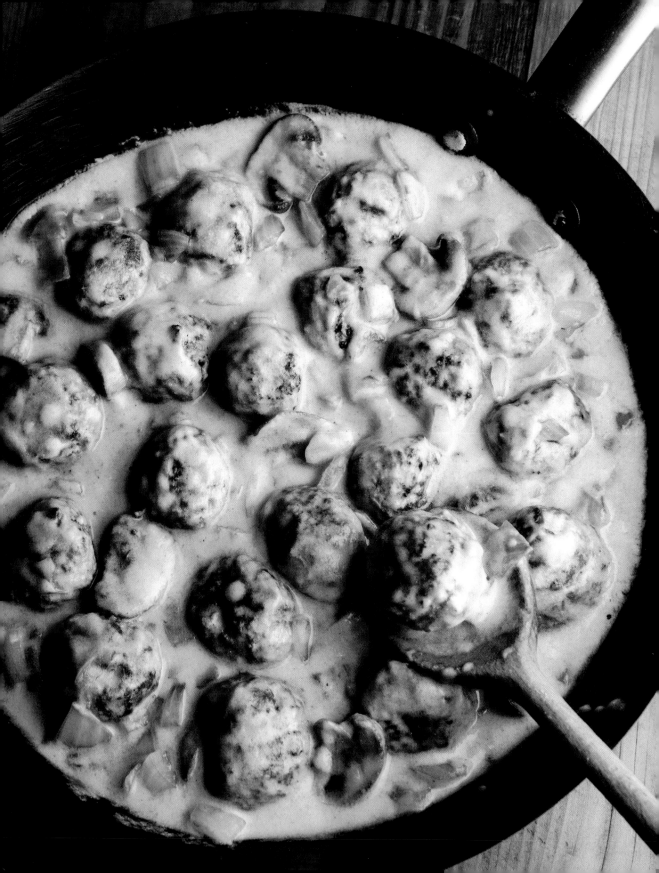

Skillet Swedish Meatball Madness

244 cal

This sauce is LIFE-CHANGING. For more meatball goodness, flip to page 277 for my Party-Time Pineapple BBQ Meatballs!

SAUCE

2 cups reduced-sodium chicken broth

2 tablespoons whole-wheat flour

1 tablespoon Dijon mustard

1 tablespoon white wine vinegar

1 cup chopped onion

1 cup sliced mushrooms

2 tablespoons light/reduced-fat cream cheese

2 teaspoons whipped butter

MEATBALLS

1 pound raw extra-lean ground beef (4% fat or less)

¼ cup whole-wheat panko breadcrumbs

⅓ cup egg whites (about 3 large eggs' worth)

½ teaspoon garlic powder

¼ teaspoon each salt and black pepper

⅛ teaspoon ground nutmeg

¼th of recipe (5 meatballs with sauce): 244 calories, 7.5g total fat (3.5g sat fat), 654mg sodium, 12g carbs, 2g fiber, 3g sugars, 29g protein

You'll Need: 2 large bowls, whisk, extra-large skillet with a lid, nonstick spray

Prep: 20 minutes • **Cook:** 25 minutes

1. To make the sauce, in a large bowl, combine broth, flour, mustard, and vinegar. Whisk until uniform.

2. Bring an extra-large skillet sprayed with nonstick spray to medium-high heat. Add onion and mushrooms. Cook and stir until slightly softened, about 4 minutes.

3. Carefully add broth mixture, cream cheese, and butter to the skillet. Cook and stir until cream cheese and butter have melted and mixture is uniform, about 3 minutes. Transfer to the large bowl.

4. In a second large bowl, thoroughly mix meatball ingredients. Firmly and evenly form into 20 meatballs.

5. Clean skillet, if needed. Re-spray, and return to medium-high heat. Place meatballs in the skillet. Cook and rotate until browned on all sides, about 5 minutes.

6. Reduce heat to medium low. Carefully add sauce, coating the meatballs. Cover and cook for 10 minutes, or until meatballs are cooked through.

MAKES 4 SERVINGS

Chew on This...

In America, Swedish meatballs were very popular in the early 1900s and again in the '50s and '60s. Time for a renaissance!

Crushin' on Cranberry Pulled Pork

5i **GF** By combining two cuts of meat (one marbled and one lean), you get juicy pulled pork with an impressively low calorie count. P.S. Check out all the slow-cooker recipes on page 366!

¼ cup spicy brown mustard

½ teaspoon garlic powder

12 ounces raw lean boneless pork tenderloin, trimmed of excess fat

12 ounces raw boneless pork shoulder (the leanest piece you can find), trimmed of excess fat

¼ teaspoon each salt and black pepper

2 cups roughly chopped onions

1 cup sweetened dried cranberries

⅙th of recipe (about ⅔ cup): 234 calories, 4.5g total fat (1.5g sat fat), 287mg sodium, 23g carbs, 2g fiber, 17g sugars, 23g protein

You'll Need: small bowl, slow cooker, large bowl

Prep: 20 minutes • **Cook:** 3 to 4 hours or 7 to 8 hours

1. In a small bowl, combine mustard with garlic powder. Add 2 teaspoons water, and mix well.

2. Add both kinds of pork to the slow cooker, and season with salt and pepper. Top with onions, cranberries, and mustard mixture.

3. Cover and cook on high for 3 to 4 hours or on low for 7 to 8 hours, until pork is cooked through.

4. Transfer pork to a large bowl. Shred with two forks.

5. Return shredded pork to the slow cooker, and mix well.

MAKES 6 SERVINGS

Chew on This...

How can you tell if a cranberry is fresh and ripe? If it bounces, you've got yourself a keeper! (This recipe calls for the dried fruit, so don't expect any bouncing berries.)

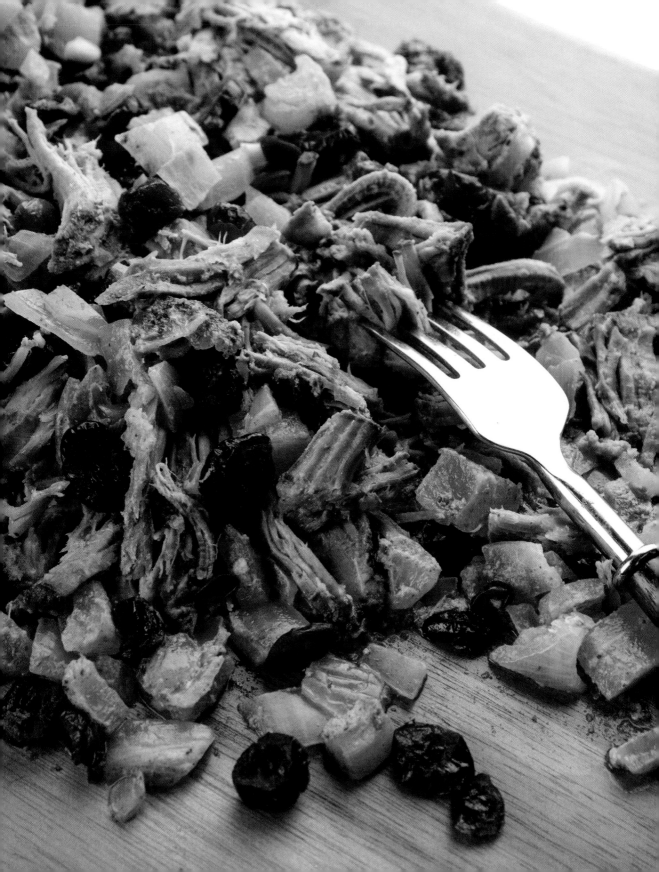

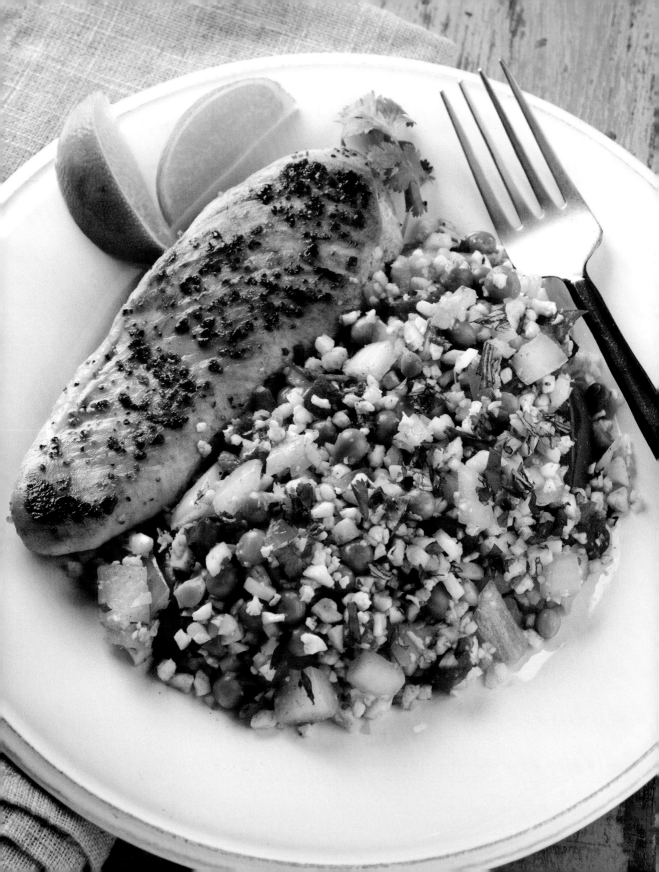

Arroz Con Pollo, Por Favor

 240 cal

 GF Amazing flavor in this cauliflower-rice rock star! And the serving size? HUGE.

3 cups cauliflower rice/crumbles

½ teaspoon oregano

¼ teaspoon turmeric

⅛ teaspoon cayenne pepper

Four 4-ounce raw boneless skinless chicken breast cutlets

¼ teaspoon black pepper

⅛ teaspoon paprika

¾ teaspoon salt

1½ cups sliced red bell pepper

1 cup chopped onion

2 cups seeded and chopped tomatoes

½ cup chopped fresh cilantro

1 tablespoon chopped garlic

1 cup frozen peas

¾ cup chicken broth

2 bay leaves

Optional seasonings: additional salt and black pepper

Optional topping: additional chopped fresh cilantro

Need-to-Know Info

Use store-bought cauliflower crumbles/rice, or DIY! See page 346 for the 411.

¼th of recipe (1 chicken cutlet with about 1¼ cups veggies): 240 calories, 3.5g total fat (0.5g sat fat), 714mg sodium, 21g carbs, 6.5g fiber, 9.5g sugars, 31.5g protein

You'll Need: large bowl, meat mallet, large pot with a lid, nonstick spray, plate

Prep: 30 minutes • **Cook:** 35 minutes

1. Place cauliflower rice/crumbles in a large bowl. Sprinkle with oregano, turmeric, and cayenne pepper. Mix well.

2. Pound chicken to ½-inch thickness. Season with black pepper, paprika, and ¼ teaspoon salt. Bring a large pot sprayed with nonstick spray to medium heat. Cook chicken for about 4 minutes per side, until cooked through. Transfer chicken to a plate, and cover to keep warm.

3. Remove pot from heat; clean, if needed. Re-spray, and bring to medium-high heat. Add bell pepper and onion. Cook and stir until mostly softened, 6 to 8 minutes.

4. Add tomatoes, cilantro, garlic, and remaining ½ teaspoon salt. Cook and stir until tomatoes have softened, about 3 minutes.

5. Add seasoned cauliflower rice/crumbles, peas, broth, and bay leaves. Bring to a boil.

6. Reduce to a simmer. Cover and cook for 6 minutes.

7. Uncover pot. Cook and stir until cauliflower rice is tender, about 4 minutes.

8. Remove and discard bay leaves. Serve chicken with cauliflower rice.

MAKES 4 SERVINGS

Chew on This...

There are more than 40,000 varieties of rice . . . not counting my favorite, cauliflower rice!

Tuna Zoodle Casserole

229 cal

This super-satisfying calorie-slashed recipe is made with zucchini noodles and panko breadcrumbs. More veggie-noodle recipes await on page 362 . . .

1 cup chopped onion

1 cup sliced brown mushrooms

½ cup frozen peas

1½ pounds spiralized zucchini (about 3 medium zucchini)

One 5-ounce can albacore tuna packed in water, thoroughly drained

⅓ cup light mayonnaise

2 tablespoons light sour cream

2 tablespoons fat-free milk

2 tablespoons grated Parmesan cheese

1 teaspoon garlic powder

¼ teaspoon each salt and black pepper

¼ cup whole-wheat panko breadcrumbs

⅓ cup shredded reduced-fat cheddar cheese

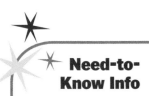

Need-to-Know Info

It's super easy to spiralize zucchini. Get the 411 on page 349!

¼th of casserole: 229 calories, 10.5g total fat (3g sat fat), 565mg sodium, 19.5g carbs, 4g fiber, 9g sugars, 15.5g protein

You'll Need: 8-inch by 8-inch baking pan, nonstick spray, extra-large skillet, strainer, large bowl, medium bowl

Prep: 15 minutes • **Cook:** 35 minutes

1. Preheat oven to 375 degrees. Spray an 8-inch by 8-inch baking pan with nonstick spray.

2. Bring an extra-large skillet sprayed with nonstick spray to medium-high heat. Add onion, mushrooms, and peas. Cook and stir until fresh veggies have slightly softened and peas have thawed, about 4 minutes.

3. Add zucchini to the skillet. Cook and stir until hot and slightly softened, about 3 minutes.

4. Transfer skillet contents to a strainer, and drain excess liquid. Place in a large bowl.

5. Add tuna, mayo, sour cream, milk, 1 tablespoon Parm, ½ teaspoon garlic powder, and ⅛ teaspoon each salt and pepper. Thoroughly mix.

6. Transfer mixture to the baking pan, and smooth out the top.

7. In a medium bowl, combine breadcrumbs with remaining 1 tablespoon Parm, ½ teaspoon garlic powder, and ⅛ teaspoon each salt and pepper. Stir in cheddar.

8. Sprinkle breadcrumb mixture over contents of the pan. Bake until hot and bubbly, about 25 minutes.

MAKES 4 SERVINGS

Chew on This . . .

Traditional tuna casseroles are often made with egg noodles and topped with potato chips or fried onions, causing calorie and fat counts to skyrocket!

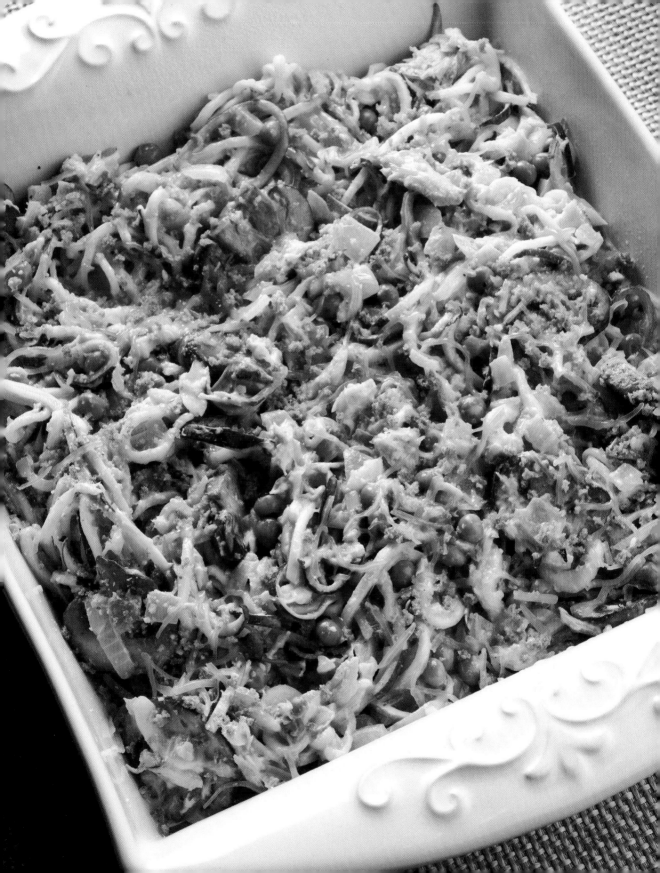

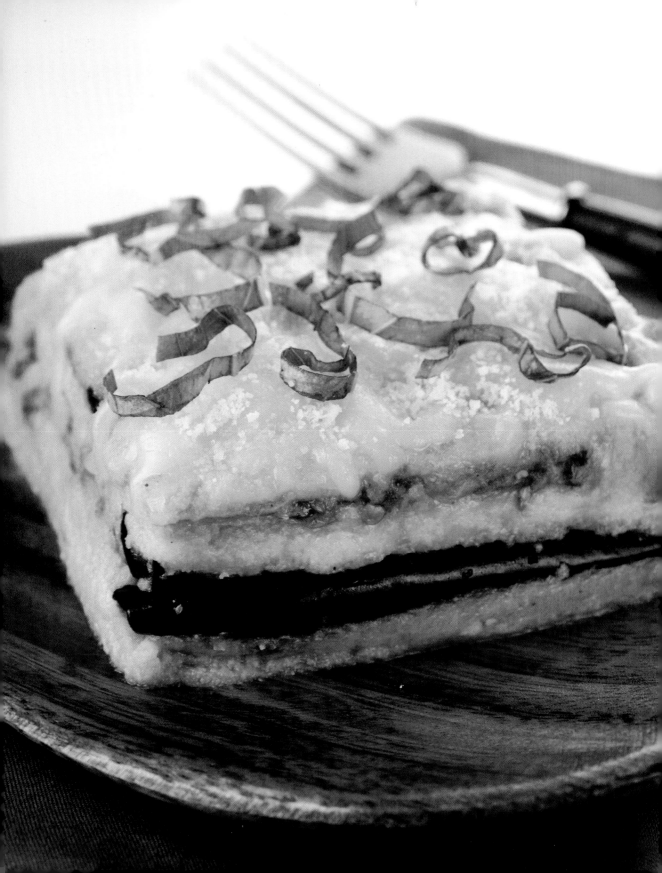

White Eggplant Parm Casserole

199 cal

V **GF** This dish is one of the best possible ways to enjoy eggplant. If it were available at a restaurant, I'd go there EVERY day just to order it!

CASEROLE

1 large eggplant (about 20 ounces)

¼ teaspoon onion powder

¼ teaspoon garlic powder

¼ teaspoon salt

⅛ teaspoon black pepper

1 cup shredded part-skim mozzarella cheese

¼ cup grated Parmesan cheese

SAUCE

2½ cups roughly chopped cauliflower

¼ cup fat-free milk

2 tablespoons grated Parmesan cheese

1 teaspoon chopped garlic

¼ teaspoon salt

⅛ teaspoon black pepper

Optional topping: chopped fresh basil

¼th of casserole: 199 calories, 9.5g total fat (5.5g sat fat), 729mg sodium, 14.5g carbs, 6g fiber, 7.5g sugars, 16.5g protein

You'll Need: baking sheet, 8-inch by 8-inch baking pan, nonstick spray, medium-large microwave safe bowl, blender or food processor, foil

Prep: 20 minutes • **Cook:** 1 hour and 5 minutes • **Cool:** 10 minutes

1. Preheat oven to 400 degrees. Spray a baking sheet and an 8-inch by 8-inch baking pan with nonstick spray.

2. Slice off and discard eggplant ends. Cut eggplant lengthwise into ½-inch slices. Sprinkle with seasonings.

3. Evenly lay eggplant on the baking sheet. Bake for 20 minutes.

4. Flip eggplant. Bake until slightly softened and lightly browned, about 10 more minutes.

5. Meanwhile, make the sauce. Place cauliflower in a medium-large microwave-safe bowl. Add 3 tablespoons water. Cover and microwave for 4 minutes, or until soft.

6. Drain excess liquid from cauliflower, and transfer to a blender or food processor. Add remaining sauce ingredients and 1½ tablespoons warm water. Blend on high speed until smooth and uniform.

7. Remove sheet from oven, but leave oven on.

8. Evenly layer the following ingredients in the baking pan: ¼th of sauce (about ¼ cup), half of the eggplant slices, ¼th of sauce (about ¼ cup), ½ cup mozzarella, 2 tablespoons Parm, and ¼th of sauce (about ¼ cup).

9. Continue layering with remaining eggplant slices, sauce, ½ cup mozzarella, and 2 tablespoons Parm.

10. Cover pan with foil. Bake for 30 minutes, or until hot and bubbly.

11. Uncover and bake until cheese has melted and lightly browned, about 5 minutes.

12. Let cool for 10 minutes before slicing.

MAKES 4 SERVINGS

Classic Cheesy Mac Casserole

V This take on classic mac 'n cheese delivers plenty of cheesy goodness without overdoing it on the calorie front. So creamy! And don't miss the Beefed-Up Cheesy Mac on page 140.

5 ounces (about 1½ cups) uncooked whole-grain elbow macaroni

4 cups roughly chopped cauliflower

⅔ cup shredded reduced-fat cheddar cheese

⅓ cup light/reduced-fat cream cheese

¼ cup fat-free milk

2 teaspoons Dijon mustard

2 teaspoons chopped garlic

1 tablespoon whipped butter

½ cup whole-wheat panko breadcrumbs

½ teaspoon onion powder

½ teaspoon garlic powder

½ teaspoon each salt and black pepper

2 tablespoons grated Parmesan cheese

¼th of recipe (about 1¼ cups): 339 calories, 12g total fat (6.5g sat fat), 715mg sodium, 41g carbs, 7g fiber, 5.5g sugars, 17.5g protein

You'll Need: 8-inch by 8-inch baking pan, nonstick spray, large pot, strainer, large bowl, 2 medium microwave-safe bowls

Prep: 15 minutes • **Cook:** 45 minutes

1. Preheat oven to 375 degrees. Spray an 8-inch by 8-inch baking pan with nonstick spray.

2. Bring a large pot of water to a boil. Add pasta and cauliflower. Cook per pasta package instructions, about 8 minutes.

3. Drain pasta and cauliflower in a strainer. Transfer to a large bowl.

4. In a medium microwave-safe bowl, combine cheddar, cream cheese, milk, mustard, and chopped garlic. Mix well. Microwave for 1 minute, or until cheddar has melted. Mix until smooth.

5. Add cheese mixture to the large bowl, and stir to coat. Transfer mixture to the baking pan, and smooth out the top.

6. In a second medium microwave-safe bowl, microwave butter for 20 seconds, or until melted. Add breadcrumbs and seasonings, and mix well.

7. Evenly distribute breadcrumb mixture over the contents of the baking pan. Sprinkle with Parm.

8. Bake until lightly browned, 25 to 30 minutes.

MAKES 4 SERVINGS

Chew on This . . .

Sources say that since 1970, the average American has gone from eating eight pounds of cheese per year to over 30 pounds annually!

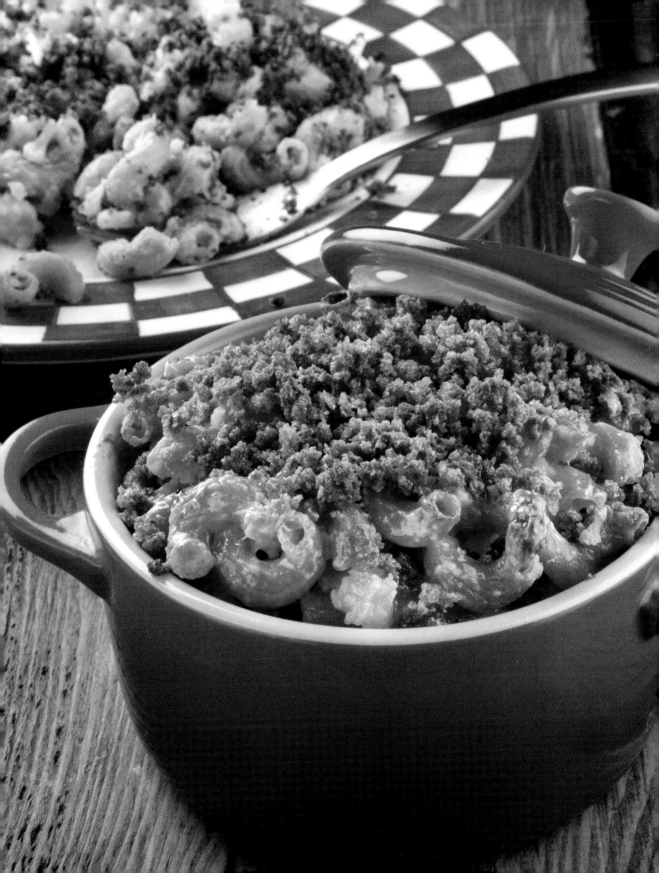

Oh, Wow! Chicken & Waffles

353 cal

If you didn't think I could come up with a Clean & Hungry version of crispy fried chicken and waffles, you don't know Hungry Girl! For more "faux-frys," flip to page 363.

CHICKEN

¼ cup whole-wheat panko breadcrumbs

¼ teaspoon onion powder

⅛ teaspoon paprika

⅛ teaspoon each salt and black pepper

Two 4-ounce raw boneless skinless chicken breast cutlets

¼ cup egg whites (about 2 large eggs' worth)

Optional seasoning: additional salt

WAFFLES

¼ cup egg whites (about 2 large eggs' worth)

1 tablespoon whipped butter

½ cup whole-wheat flour

¼ cup unsweetened vanilla almond milk

1 packet natural no-calorie sweetener

1 teaspoon baking powder

1 teaspoon vanilla extract

¼ teaspoon cinnamon

⅛ teaspoon salt

Optional topping: maple syrup

½ of recipe (1 waffle with 1 chicken cutlet): 353 calories, 7.5g total fat (2.5g sat fat), 751mg sodium, 31.5g carbs, 4.5g fiber, 1.5g sugars, 37g protein

You'll Need: baking sheet, nonstick spray, 2 wide bowls, meat mallet, medium bowl, electric mixer, large microwave-safe bowl, whisk, standard round waffle maker, plate

Prep: 15 minutes • **Cook:** 30 minutes

1. Preheat oven to 375 degrees. Spray a baking sheet with nonstick spray.

2. In a wide bowl, mix breadcrumbs with seasonings.

3. Pound chicken to ½-inch thickness. Place in a second wide bowl, top with egg whites, and flip to coat.

4. One at a time, shake chicken cutlets to remove excess egg, and coat with seasoned crumbs.

5. Evenly lay on the baking sheet. Bake for 10 minutes.

6. Flip chicken. Bake until cooked through and crispy, 10 to 12 minutes.

7. Meanwhile, make the waffles. Place egg whites in a medium bowl. With an electric mixer set to medium speed, beat until fluffy, 1 to 2 minutes.

8. In a large microwave-safe bowl, microwave butter for 30 seconds, or until melted. Add remaining waffle ingredients (excluding whipped egg whites) and ⅓ cup water. Whisk until smooth and uniform.

9. Gently but thoroughly fold egg whites into batter. Stir until just mixed and uniform.

10. Spray a standard round waffle maker with nonstick spray, and set heat to medium. Once hot, add half of the batter. Close and cook for 4 minutes, or until golden brown and crispy.

11. Plate waffle. Repeat with remaining batter, re-spraying waffle maker if needed.

12. Top waffles with chicken.

MAKES 2 SERVINGS

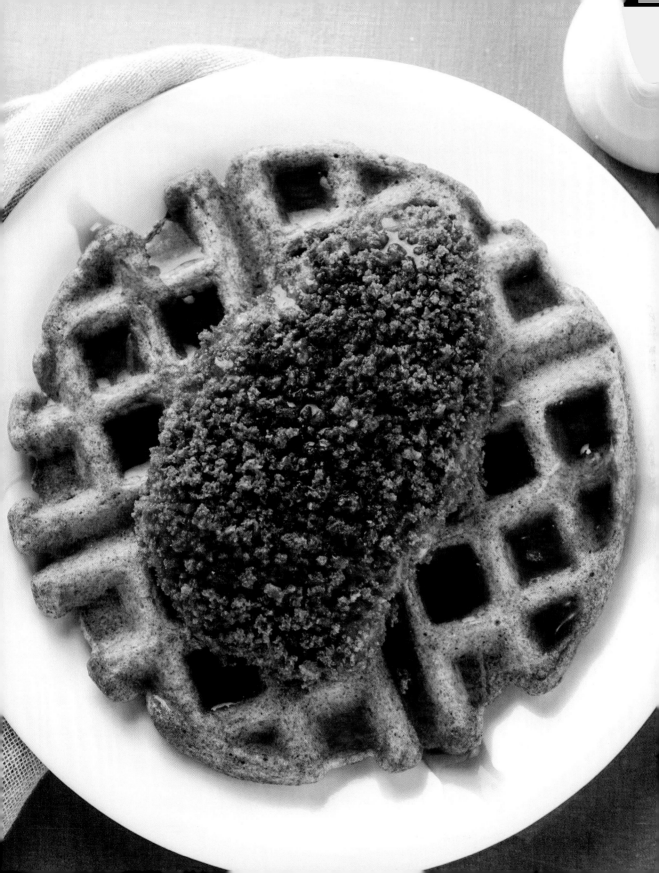

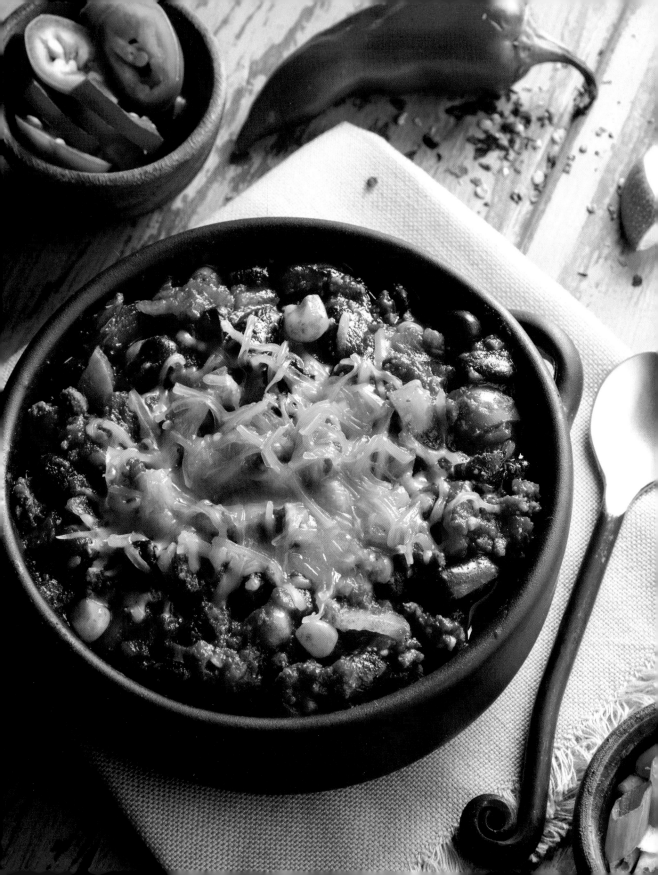

Fully Loaded Dan-Good Chili

257 cal

GF The original Dan-Good Chili was created by my wonderful husband, Dan Schneider. This just may be the best Hungry Girl chili ever. And it's so simple to make!

1 pound raw extra-lean ground beef (4% fat or less)

¼ teaspoon black pepper

¾ teaspoon salt

4 cups canned crushed tomatoes

1¼ cups chopped carrots

1¼ cups chopped onions

1¼ cups chopped portabella mushrooms

1¼ cups chopped red bell pepper

1¼ cups chopped green bell pepper

1 cup frozen sweet corn kernels

1 cup canned diced tomatoes with green chiles (not drained)

¾ cup canned black beans, drained and rinsed

¾ cup canned red kidney beans, drained and rinsed

¼ cup seeded and chopped jalapeño peppers

1 tablespoon chili powder

1½ teaspoons crushed garlic

¾ teaspoon ground cumin

1 cup shredded reduced-fat cheddar cheese

Optional seasonings: additional salt and black pepper

Optional toppings: sliced jalapeño peppers, chopped scallions

⅛th of recipe (about 1 cup): 257 calories, 6g total fat (3g sat fat), 826mg sodium, 29.5g carbs, 8g fiber, 10g sugars, 22g protein

You'll Need: extra-large pot with a lid, nonstick spray

Prep: 25 minutes • **Cook:** 1 hour and 30 minutes

1. Bring an extra-large pot sprayed with nonstick spray to medium-high heat. Add beef, and season with black pepper and ¼ teaspoon salt. Cook and crumble for about 5 minutes, until fully cooked.

2. Add remaining ½ teaspoon salt and all remaining ingredients *except* cheese. Mix thoroughly. Bring to a boil.

3. Reduce to a simmer. Cover and cook for 1 hour and 20 minutes, or until veggies are tender, uncovering occasionally to stir.

4. Top each serving with 2 tablespoons cheese.

MAKES 8 SERVINGS

Chew on This . . .

Cool job title alert: Chili Queen. That's what chili-selling women at a San Antonio market in the late 1800s and early 1900s went by.

Overflowing with Chili Acorn Squash

V **GF**   I could LIVE on this dish. It's that good! Acorn squash is seriously underrated . . .

Two 20-ounce acorn squash, halved, seeds removed

½ cup chopped portabella mushrooms

⅓ cup chopped onion

⅓ cup chopped bell pepper

2 tablespoons seeded and chopped jalapeño pepper

¾ cup seeded and chopped tomato

1½ cups canned crushed tomatoes

½ cup canned black beans, drained and rinsed

1½ teaspoons chopped garlic

1½ teaspoons chili powder

¾ teaspoon ground cumin

¼ cup shredded reduced-fat Mexican-blend cheese

¼th of recipe (1 stuffed squash half): 199 calories, 2g total fat (1g sat fat), 327mg sodium, 42g carbs, 8.5g fiber, 6g sugars, 8g protein

You'll Need: baking sheet, nonstick spray, medium pot

Prep: 15 minutes • **Cook:** 30 minutes

1. Preheat oven to 400 degrees. Spray a baking sheet with nonstick spray.

2. Place squash halves on the baking sheet, cut sides down. Bake until soft, 25 to 30 minutes.

3. Meanwhile, make the chili. Bring a medium pot sprayed with nonstick spray to medium heat. Add mushrooms, onion, bell pepper, and jalapeño pepper. Cook and stir until partially softened, about 3 minutes.

4. Add chopped tomato to the pot. Cook and stir until mostly softened, about 2 minutes.

5. Add all remaining ingredients *except* cheese to the pot. Cook and stir until hot and well mixed, about 1 minute. Remove from heat.

6. Flip squash halves. Fill with chili, and sprinkle with cheese.

MAKES 4 SERVINGS

Chew on This . . .

Chili: beans or no beans? That very question is rumored to have caused a heated debate, resulting in the first-ever chili cook-off known as the Great Chili Confrontation. Oddly, a judge claimed he was poisoned and no winner was named.

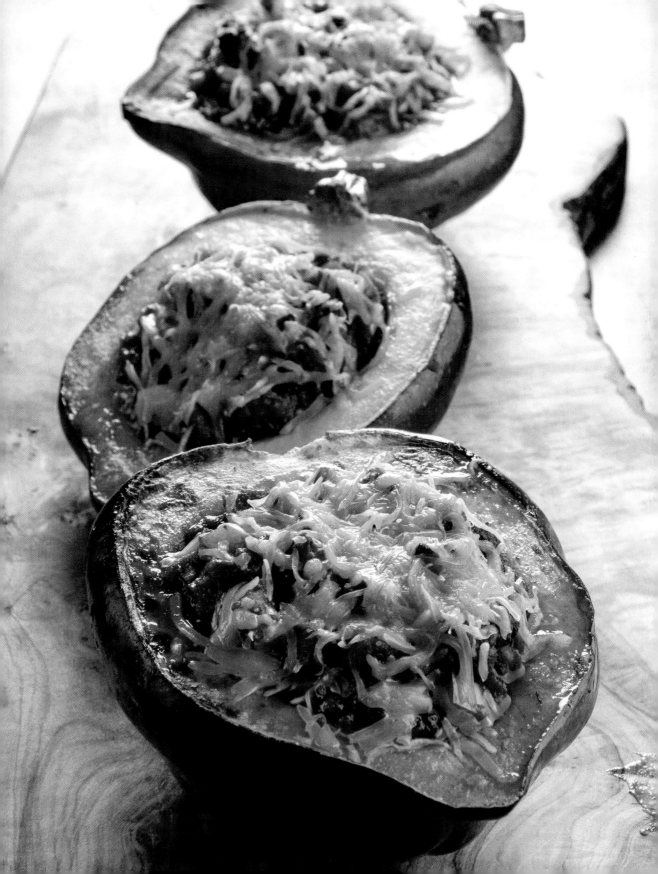

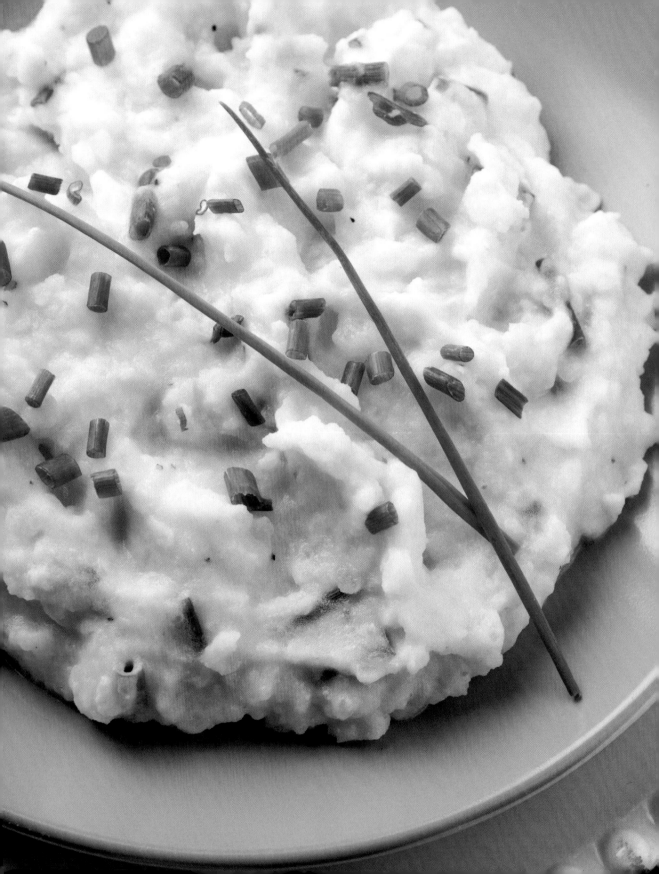

Sour Cream & Chive Mashies

115 cal

   This recipe is creamy, flavorful, and all-around amazing!

12 ounces (about 1 medium) russet potato

3 cups cauliflower florets

¼ cup light sour cream

¼ cup light/reduced-fat cream cheese

¾ teaspoon onion powder

½ teaspoon garlic powder

½ teaspoon salt

⅛ teaspoon black pepper

¼ cup plus 5 tablespoons chopped chives

⅕th of recipe (about ⅔ cup): 115 calories, 3.5g total fat (2g sat fat), 321mg sodium, 18g carbs, 2.5g fiber, 3.5g sugars, 4g protein

You'll Need: medium pot, strainer, large bowl, potato masher
Prep: 10 minutes • **Cook:** 30 minutes

1. Bring a medium pot of water to a boil. Peel and cube potato.

2. Add potato and cauliflower. Once returned to a boil, reduce heat to medium. Cook until very tender, 15 to 20 minutes.

3. Drain potato and cauliflower in a strainer. Transfer to a large bowl.

4. Add all remaining ingredients *except* chives. Thoroughly mash and mix.

5. Fold in ¼ cup chives.

6. Top each serving with 1 tablespoon of remaining chives.

MAKES 5 SERVINGS

Mashie Mania!

How do you make a starchy side dish even higher in calories? Mash in high-fat dairy! Clearly, classic mashed potatoes could use a makeover. These recipes use cauliflower to bulk up the serving sizes without adding a lot of calories. Reduced-fat add-ins keep things nice and light. HG tip: For extra-creamy mashies, use a blender or food processor to smooth 'em out before stirring in any extras.

Caramelized Onion Mashies

143 cal

V **GF** Sweet buttery onions + fluffy mashies = one freakishly delicious side dish! If you like this, you'll love my Caramelized Onion Cauli-Crust Pizza (page 110), Caramelized Onion Chickpea Burgers (page 157), and OMG! Caramelized Onion Dip (page 274).

1 tablespoon whipped butter

4 cups chopped sweet onions

12 ounces (about 1 medium) russet potato

3 cups cauliflower florets

¼ cup fat-free plain Greek yogurt

½ teaspoon garlic powder

½ teaspoon onion powder

½ teaspoon salt

⅛ teaspoon black pepper

2 teaspoons Dijon mustard

⅕th of recipe (about ¾ cup): 143 calories, 1.5g total fat (1g sat fat), 315mg sodium, 28.5g carbs, 4.5g fiber, 8g sugars, 5g protein

You'll Need: large skillet, medium pot, strainer, large bowl, potato masher

Prep: 20 minutes • **Cook:** 50 minutes

1. Melt butter in a large skillet over medium-high heat. Cook and stir onions for 10 minutes.

2. Reduce heat to medium low. Stirring often, cook until caramelized, 35 to 40 minutes.

3. Meanwhile, make mashies. Bring a medium pot of water to a boil. Peel and cube potato.

4. Add potato and cauliflower to the pot. Once returned to a boil, reduce heat to medium. Cook until very tender, 15 to 20 minutes.

5. Drain potato and cauliflower in a strainer. Transfer to a large bowl.

6. Add all remaining ingredients *except* mustard to the bowl. Thoroughly mash and mix.

7. Stir mustard into onions, and stir onions into the mashies.

MAKES 5 SERVINGS

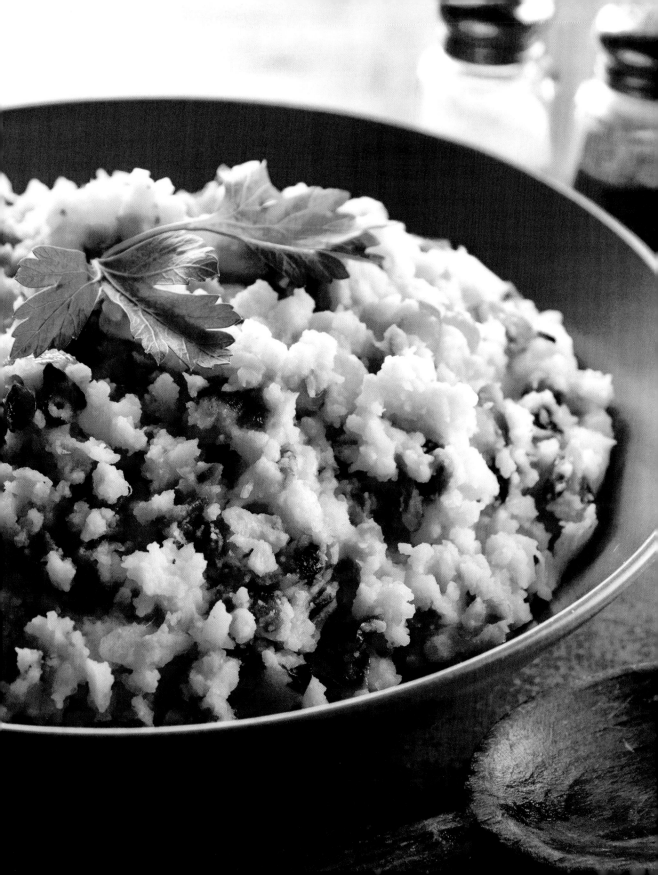

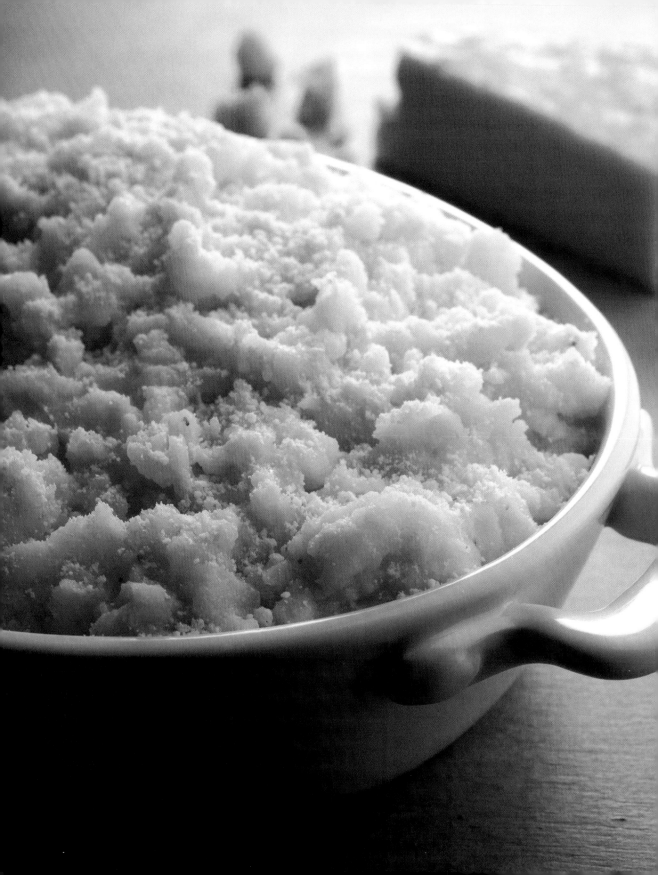

Three-Cheese Mashies

V **GF** Not one, not two, but THREE cheeses in these yummy mashies! The ricotta adds sooooo much creaminess . . . You won't believe your taste buds.

12 ounces (about 1 medium) russet potato

3 cups cauliflower florets

¼ cup light/low-fat ricotta cheese

1 tablespoon whipped butter

½ teaspoon garlic powder

¼ teaspoon salt

⅛ teaspoon black pepper

½ cup shredded reduced-fat cheddar cheese

5 teaspoons grated Parmesan cheese

⅕th of recipe (about ⅔ cup): 141 calories, 5.5g total fat (3g sat fat), 296mg sodium, 16.5g carbs, 2g fiber, 2.5g sugars, 8g protein

You'll Need: medium pot, strainer, large bowl, potato masher

Prep: 15 minutes • **Cook:** 30 minutes

1. Bring a medium pot of water to a boil. Peel and cube potato.

2. Add potato and cauliflower. Once returned to a boil, reduce heat to medium. Cook until very tender, 15 to 20 minutes.

3. Drain potato and cauliflower in a strainer. Transfer to a large bowl.

4. Add all remaining ingredients *except* cheddar and Parm. Thoroughly mash and mix.

5. Fold in cheddar. Top each serving with 1 teaspoon Parm.

MAKES 5 SERVINGS

Chew on This . . .

Mashed potato recipes date all the way back to 1747. Bet they didn't think to mix in cauliflower back then!

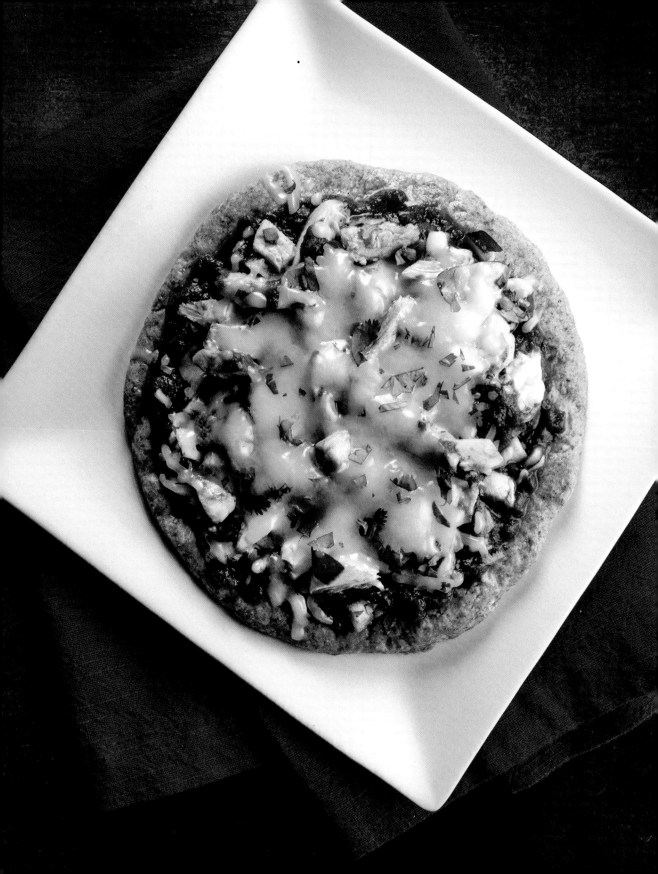

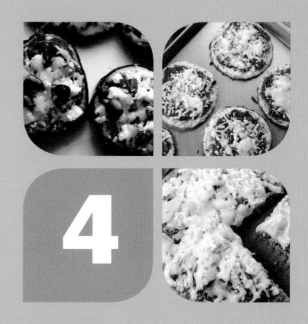

You Wanna
Pizza Me?

Word has it, Americans eat about 350 slices of pizza per second . . . And a reported 93 percent of us have eaten it in the last month! Safe to say we're obsessed with the cheesy, saucy favorite! Good news, hungry humans: I've got nine amazing, calorie-slashed creations for your chewing pleasure!

Squash-Crust Cheese Pizza

277 cal

 Future classic! The pizza crust is shockingly easy to make, and the entire thing is super flavorful.

CRUST

1¾ pounds (about 4 medium) yellow squash

¼ cup egg whites (about 2 large eggs' worth)

¼ cup shredded part-skim mozzarella cheese

2 tablespoons grated Parmesan cheese

1 teaspoon Italian seasoning

⅛ teaspoon each salt and black pepper

TOPPING

½ cup canned crushed tomatoes

½ teaspoon garlic powder

½ teaspoon onion powder

½ teaspoon Italian seasoning

½ cup shredded part-skim mozzarella cheese

2 tablespoons finely chopped fresh basil

½ of recipe (1 pizza): 277 calories, 11.5g total fat (7g sat fat), 755mg sodium, 22.5g carbs, 5.5g fiber, 14.5g sugars, 23.5g protein

You'll Need: baking sheet, parchment paper, box or hand grater, large microwave-safe bowl, fine-mesh strainer, clean dish towel (or paper towels), medium bowl

Prep: 20 minutes • **Cook:** 45 minutes • **Cool:** 10 minutes

1. Preheat oven to 400 degrees. Line a baking sheet with parchment paper.

2. Using the shredder side of a box or hand grater (the one with larger holes), shred squash into a large microwave-safe bowl. Cover and microwave for 3 minutes.

3. Uncover and stir. Re-cover and microwave for another 3 minutes, or until hot and soft.

4. Transfer squash to a fine-mesh strainer to drain. Let cool for 10 minutes, or until cool enough to handle.

5. Using a clean dish towel (or paper towels), firmly press out as much liquid as possible—there will be a lot.

6. Return squash to the large bowl, and add remaining crust ingredients. Mix thoroughly.

7. Divide crust mixture into two circles on the baking sheet, each about ¼ inch thick and 7 inches in diameter.

8. Bake until the tops have browned, about 30 minutes.

9. Meanwhile, in a medium bowl, stir seasonings into crushed tomatoes.

10. Spread seasoned tomatoes over the crusts, leaving ½-inch borders. Top with mozzarella and basil.

11. Bake until cheese has melted and crust is crispy, 5 to 7 minutes.

MAKES 2 SERVINGS

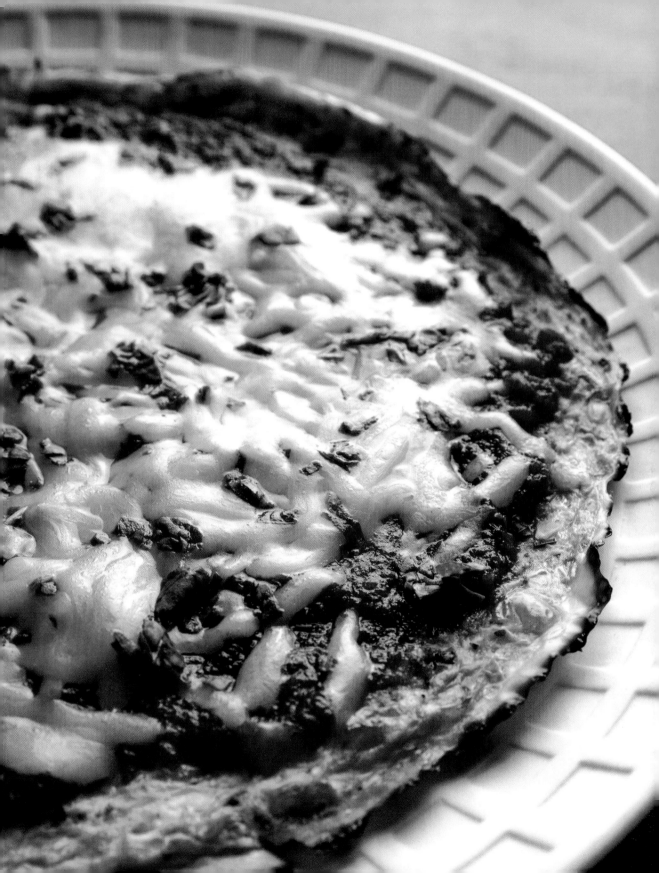

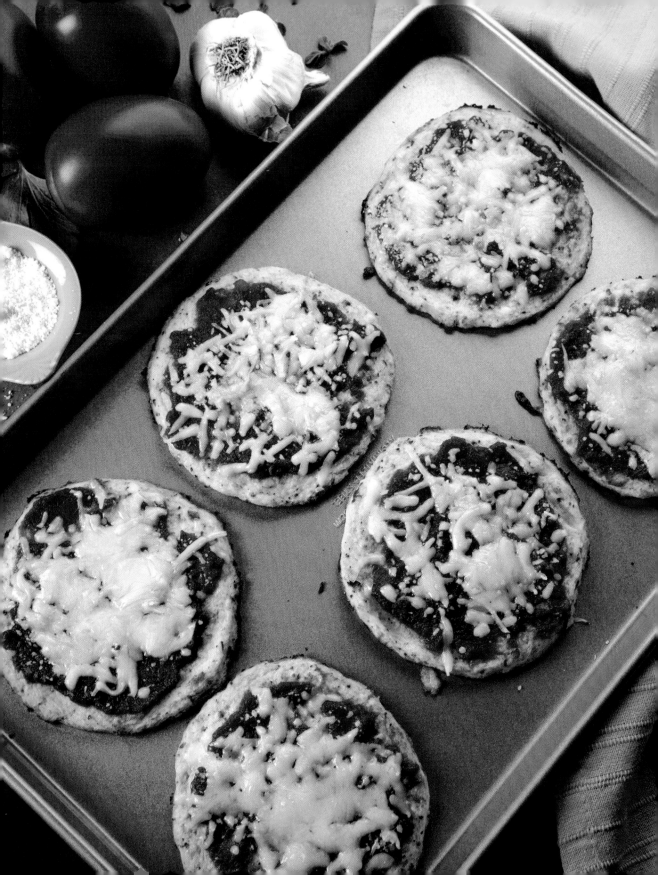

Cutie-Pie Cauliflower-Crust Pizzas

173 cal

5i **V** **GF** Seriously, how cute are these miniature pizzas!?! The only thing more impressive than their adorableness is their deliciousness . . .

CRUST

5 cups roughly chopped cauliflower (about 1 medium head)

¼ cup egg whites (about 2 large eggs' worth)

¼ cup shredded part-skim mozzarella cheese

2 tablespoons grated Parmesan cheese

1 teaspoon Italian seasoning

¼ teaspoon black pepper

⅛ teaspoon salt

TOPPING

⅓ cup canned crushed tomatoes

¼ teaspoon garlic powder

¼ teaspoon onion powder

¼ teaspoon Italian seasoning

½ cup shredded part-skim mozzarella cheese

⅓rd of recipe (2 mini pizzas): 173 calories, 7g total fat (4.5g sat fat), 524mg sodium, 12.5g carbs, 4.5g fiber, 5.5g sugars, 16g protein

You'll Need: baking sheet, parchment paper, food processor, large microwave-safe bowl, fine-mesh strainer, clean dish towel (or paper towels), medium bowl

Prep: 20 minutes • **Cook:** 40 minutes • **Cool:** 10 minutes

1. Preheat oven to 400 degrees. Line a baking sheet with parchment paper.

2. Pulse cauliflower in a food processor until reduced to the consistency of coarse breadcrumbs, working in batches as needed.

3. Transfer to a large microwave-safe bowl; cover and microwave for 3½ minutes.

4. Uncover and stir. Re-cover and microwave for another 3½ minutes, or until hot and soft.

5. Transfer to a fine-mesh strainer to drain. Let cool for 10 minutes, or until cool enough to handle.

6. Using a clean dish towel (or paper towels), press out as much moisture as possible—there will be a lot of excess liquid.

7. Return cauliflower to the bowl, and add remaining crust ingredients. Mix thoroughly.

8. Evenly distribute crust mixture into six circles on the baking sheet, each about ¼ inch thick and 3½ inches in diameter. Bake until the tops have browned, about 28 minutes.

9. Meanwhile, in a medium bowl, add all topping ingredients *except* mozzarella. Mix well.

10. Spread seasoned tomatoes on the crusts, leaving ½-inch borders. Sprinkle with mozzarella.

11. Bake until cheese has melted and crusts are crispy, about 5 minutes.

MAKES 3 SERVINGS

Caramelized Onion Cauli-Crust Pizza

316 cal

V **GF** Life-changing pizza recipe! Try it ASAP and see. And don't miss the Caramelized Onion Mashies (page 100), Caramelized Onion Chickpea Burgers (page 157), and OMG! Caramelized Onion Dip (page 274).

CRUST

5 cups roughly chopped cauliflower

¼ cup egg whites (about 2 large eggs' worth)

¼ cup shredded part-skim mozzarella cheese

2 tablespoons grated Parmesan cheese

1 teaspoon Italian seasoning

¼ teaspoon black pepper

⅛ teaspoon salt

TOPPING

2 teaspoons whipped butter

2½ cups thinly sliced sweet onions

⅛ teaspoon salt

1 cup chopped brown mushrooms

2 cups spinach leaves

1 tablespoon chopped garlic

⅓ cup shredded part-skim mozzarella cheese

½ of recipe (1 pizza): 316 calories, 12g total fat (7g sat fat), 837mg sodium, 32.5g carbs, 9g fiber, 12.5g sugars, 24.5g protein

You'll Need: baking sheet, parchment paper, food processor, large microwave-safe bowl, fine-mesh strainer, clean dish towel (or paper towels), skillet

Prep: 25 minutes • **Cook:** 50 minutes • **Cool:** 10 minutes

1. Preheat oven to 400 degrees. Line a baking sheet with parchment paper.

2. Working in batches as needed, pulse cauliflower in a food processor until reduced to the consistency of coarse breadcrumbs.

3. Transfer cauliflower crumbs to a large microwave-safe bowl; cover and microwave for 3½ minutes.

4. Uncover and stir. Re-cover and microwave for another 3½ minutes, or until hot and soft.

5. Transfer cauliflower crumbs to a fine-mesh strainer to drain. Let cool for 10 minutes, or until cool enough to handle.

6. Using a clean dish towel (or paper towels), firmly press out as much liquid as possible—there will be a lot.

7. Return cauliflower to the bowl, and add remaining crust ingredients. Mix thoroughly.

8. Divide crust mixture into two circles on the baking sheet, each about ¼ inch thick and 7 inches in diameter.

9. Bake until the tops have browned, about 35 minutes.

10. Meanwhile, make the topping. Melt butter in a skillet over medium-high heat. Add onions, and sprinkle with salt. Stirring often, cook until softened and lightly browned, about 6 minutes.

11. Reduce heat to medium low. Add mushrooms. Stirring occasionally, cook until browned and caramelized, about 15 minutes.

12. Increase heat to medium high. Add spinach and garlic. Cook and stir until spinach has wilted, 1 to 2 minutes.

13. Divide topping mixture between the crusts. Top with mozzarella.

14. Bake until cheese has melted and crusts are crispy, 5 to 7 minutes.

MAKES 2 SERVINGS

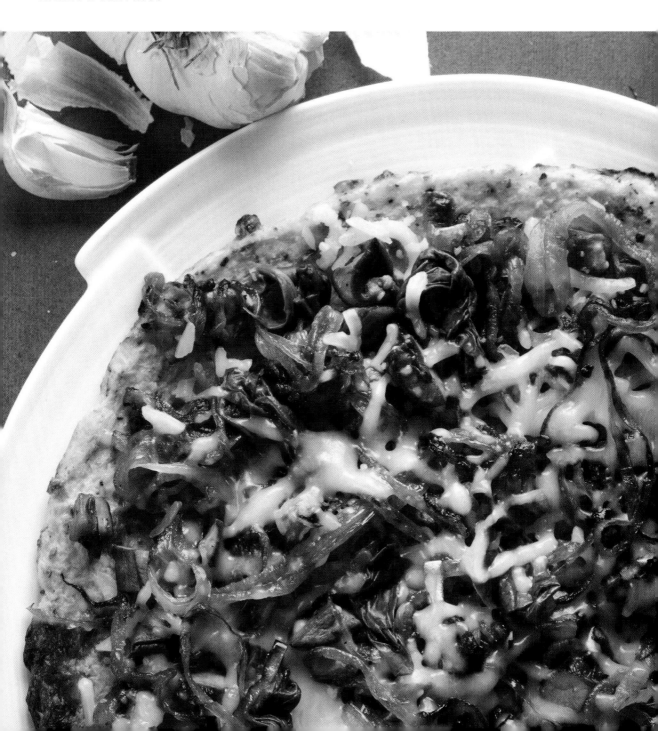

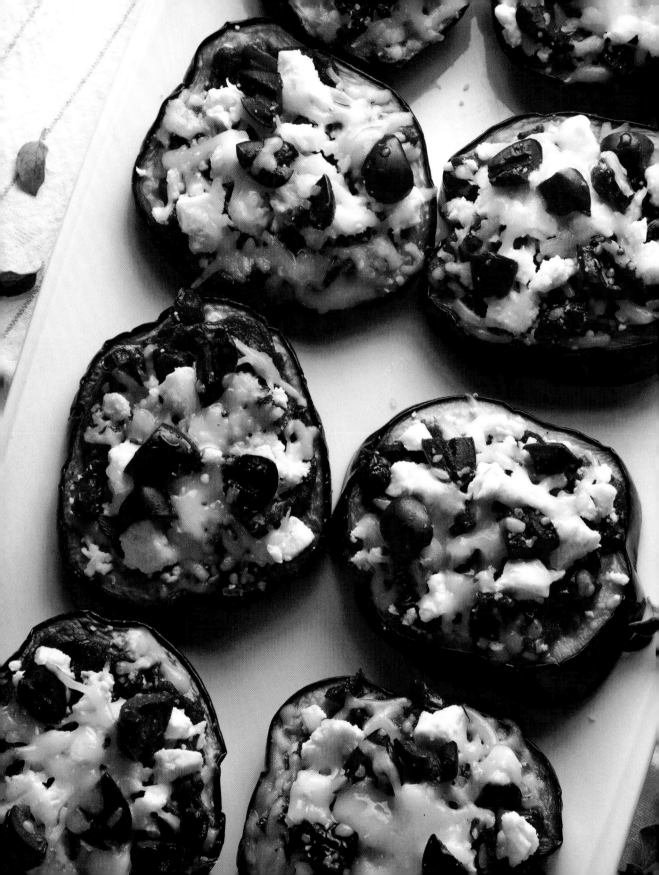

Cutie-Pie Greek Eggplant Pizzas

206 cal

V **GF** These li'l pizza pies are beyond-words delicious. I still can't believe they have only 103 calories each!

Eight ¾-inch-thick eggplant slices (cut widthwise from the center of a wide eggplant), patted dry

½ teaspoon each salt and black pepper

½ cup canned crushed tomatoes

½ teaspoon garlic powder

½ teaspoon onion powder

½ teaspoon Italian seasoning

¾ cup shredded part-skim mozzarella cheese

½ cup crumbled feta cheese

½ cup chopped red onion

⅓ cup bagged sun-dried tomatoes (not packed in oil), chopped

¼ cup sliced kalamata or black olives

¼th of recipe (2 mini pizzas): 206 calories, 8.5g total fat (4.5g sat fat), 777mg sodium, 22g carbs, 7.5g fiber, 11.5g sugars, 11g protein

You'll Need: baking sheet, nonstick spray, medium bowl
Prep: 20 minutes • **Cook:** 35 minutes

1. Preheat oven to 375 degrees. Spray a baking sheet with nonstick spray.

2. Sprinkle eggplant with salt and pepper, and lay on the baking sheet. Bake for 10 minutes.

3. Flip eggplant. Bake until softened, about 10 more minutes.

4. Meanwhile, in a medium bowl, stir seasonings into crushed tomatoes.

5. Spread seasoned tomatoes over eggplant, leaving ¼-inch borders. Top with remaining ingredients.

6. Bake until hot and lightly browned, 10 to 12 minutes.

MAKES 4 SERVINGS

Chew on This . . .

The largest pizza, named Ottavia (because you have to name your pizza), had a surface area of 13,580.28 ft^2. And oddly, it was 100 percent gluten-free.

Meatza Pizza

232 cal

Yup; this pizza crust is made of ground beef! Come on, it's not the weirdest thing to happen to pizza. I once saw one topped with BANANA. (Ewww . . .)

CRUST

1 pound raw extra-lean ground beef (4% fat or less)

2 tablespoons egg whites (about 1 large egg's worth)

2 tablespoons grated Parmesan cheese

1 teaspoon Italian seasoning

¾ teaspoon salt

½ teaspoon onion powder

½ teaspoon garlic powder

¼ teaspoon black pepper

TOPPING

⅓ cup chopped mushrooms

¼ cup chopped onion

¼ cup chopped bell pepper

½ cup canned crushed tomatoes

½ teaspoon Italian seasoning

½ teaspoon onion powder

½ teaspoon garlic powder

½ cup shredded part-skim mozzarella cheese

Optional topping: fresh basil

¼th of pizza: 232 calories, 9g total fat (4.5g sat fat), 751mg sodium, 5.5g carbs, 1g fiber, 2.5g sugars, 31g protein

You'll Need: baking sheet, parchment paper, large bowl, skillet, nonstick spray, medium bowl

Prep: 10 minutes • **Cook:** 20 minutes

1. Preheat oven to 350 degrees. Line a baking sheet with parchment paper.

2. Thoroughly mix crust ingredients in a large bowl. Shape into a circle on the baking sheet, about ¼ inch thick and 10 inches in diameter.

3. Bake until cooked through, about 15 minutes.

4. Meanwhile, make the topping. Bring a skillet sprayed with nonstick spray to medium heat. Add mushrooms, onion, and bell pepper. Cook and stir until mostly softened and lightly browned, about 4 minutes.

5. In a medium bowl, stir seasonings into crushed tomatoes.

6. Carefully drain excess liquid from baking sheet, and thoroughly blot crust dry.

7. Spread crust with seasoned tomatoes, leaving a ½-inch border. Top with cooked veggies and mozzarella.

8. Bake until cheese has melted, about 5 minutes.

MAKES 4 SERVINGS

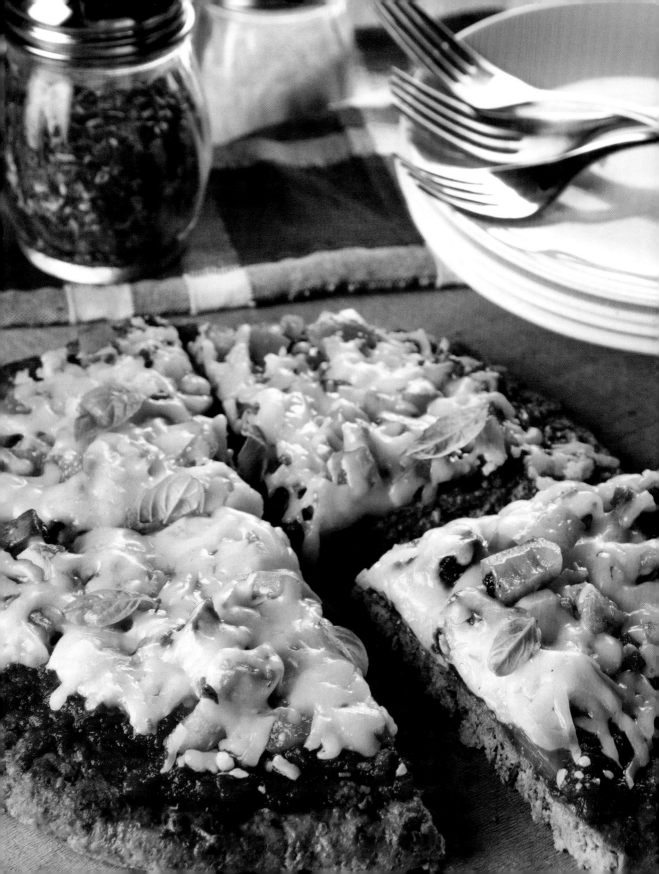

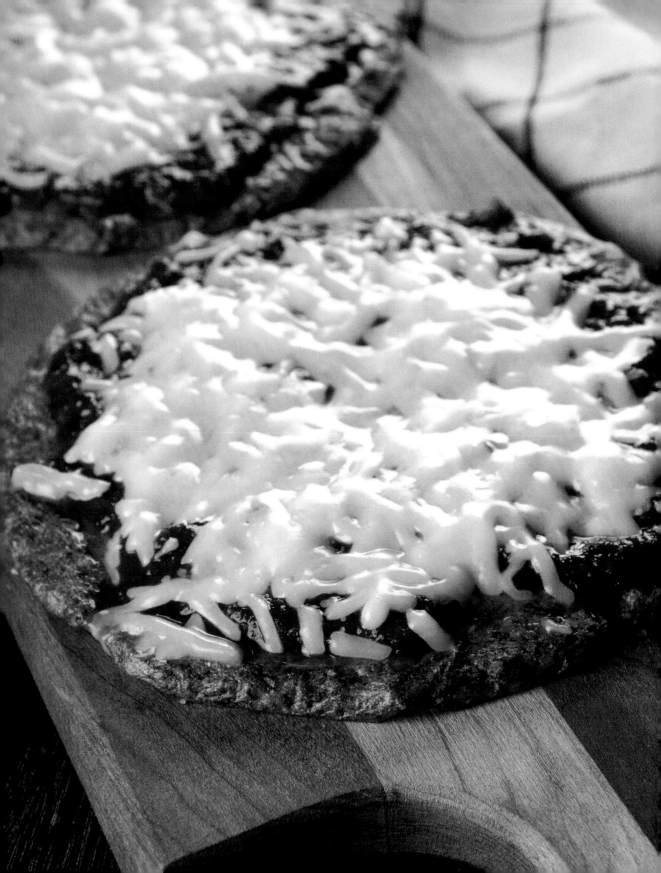

Popeye's Pizza

267 cal

V You won't believe how perfectly crispy this pizza crust is. Must-try recipe, people!

CRUST

2 cups spinach leaves

¼ cup egg whites (about 2 large eggs' worth)

2 tablespoons shredded part-skim mozzarella cheese

2 tablespoons whole-wheat flour

1 tablespoon grated Parmesan cheese

¼ teaspoon Italian seasoning

⅛ teaspoon onion powder

⅛ teaspoon garlic powder

TOPPING

¼ cup canned crushed tomatoes

¼ teaspoon Italian seasoning

¼ teaspoon onion powder

¼ teaspoon garlic powder

3 tablespoons shredded part-skim mozzarella cheese

Entire recipe: 267 calories, 9.5g total fat (5.5g sat fat), 663mg sodium, 21g carbs, 4.5g fiber, 3.5g sugars, 24.5g protein

You'll Need: baking sheet, parchment paper, food processor, medium bowl

Prep: 10 minutes • **Cook:** 30 minutes

1. Preheat oven to 400 degrees. Line a baking sheet with parchment paper.

2. Place crust ingredients in a food processor. Puree until uniform.

3. Pour onto the center of the baking sheet. Using a spatula, shape into a circle, about ¼ inch thick and 6 inches in diameter.

4. Bake until top has browned and edges are slightly crispy, about 20 minutes.

5. Meanwhile, make the topping. In a medium bowl, stir seasonings into crushed tomatoes.

6. Spread seasoned tomatoes over the crust, leaving a ½-inch border. Top with mozzarella.

7. Bake until cheese has melted and crust is mostly crispy, 8 to 10 minutes.

MAKES 1 SERVING

Chew on This . . .

I've heard that in the '30s, Popeye's love for spinach helped boost sales of the leafy green by 33 percent. Well, blow me down!

No-Joke Spinach & Artichoke Pizza

307 cal

30m **V** Food mashup alert! This recipe combines gooey spinach & artichoke dip with crispy pizza. No joke! Of course, if you'd prefer to dig into the dip itself, flip fast to page 273 . . .

CRUST

3 tablespoons old-fashioned oats

3 tablespoons whole-wheat flour

½ teaspoon Italian seasoning

½ teaspoon onion powder

½ teaspoon garlic powder

⅛ teaspoon baking powder

⅛ teaspoon baking soda

Dash salt

¼ cup egg whites (about 2 large eggs' worth)

TOPPING

3 tablespoons light/low-fat ricotta cheese

¼ teaspoon chopped garlic

⅛ teaspoon onion powder

⅛ teaspoon Italian seasoning

¼ cup chopped spinach leaves

3 tablespoons shredded part-skim mozzarella cheese

2 tablespoons finely chopped artichoke hearts (previously packed in water)

1 teaspoon grated Parmesan cheese

Entire recipe: 307 calories, 8.5g total fat (4.5g sat fat), 832mg sodium, 35.5g carbs, 5.5g fiber, 4.5g sugars, 24g protein

You'll Need: baking sheet, parchment paper, small blender or food processor, 2 medium bowls

Prep: 15 minutes • **Cook:** 15 minutes

1. Preheat oven to 400 degrees. Line a baking sheet with parchment paper.

2. In a small blender or food processor, grind oats to the consistency of coarse flour. Transfer to a medium bowl.

3. Add all remaining crust ingredients *except* egg whites. Mix until uniform. Add egg whites, and stir until it reaches a dough-like consistency.

4. Shape crust into a circle on the baking sheet, about ¼ inch thick and 6 inches in diameter.

5. Bake until top has browned and edges are slightly crispy, about 10 minutes.

6. Meanwhile, make the topping. In a second medium bowl, combine ricotta, garlic, onion powder, and Italian seasoning. Mix well. Stir in 1 tablespoon spinach and 1 tablespoon mozzarella.

7. Spread topping mixture over the crust, leaving a ½-inch border. Top with remaining 3 tablespoons spinach, chopped artichoke hearts, and remaining 2 tablespoons mozzarella.

8. Bake until cheese has melted and crust is crispy, about 5 minutes.

9. Sprinkle with Parm.

MAKES 1 SERVING

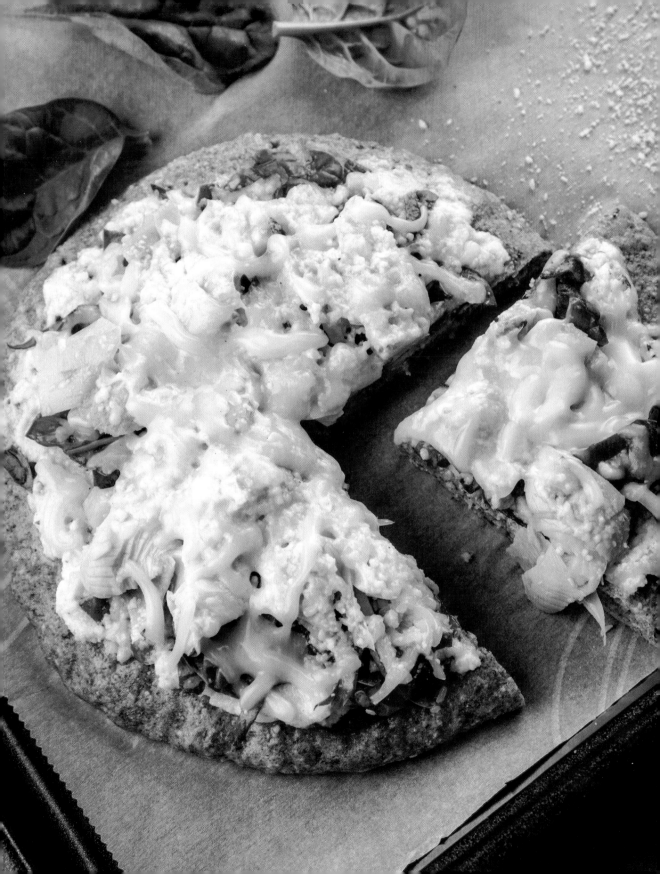

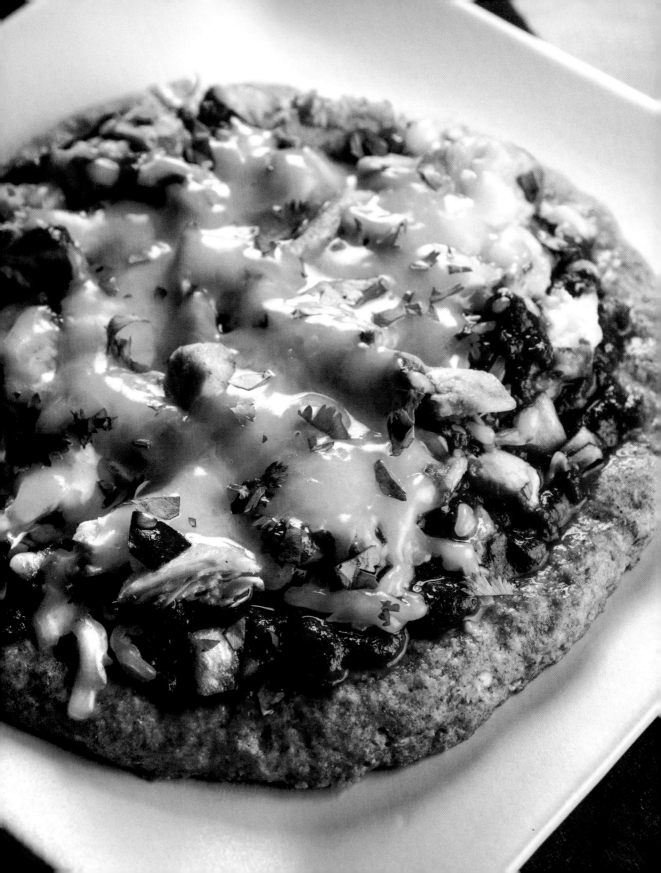

Crispy Crunchy BBQ Chicken Pizza

368 cal

30m DIY whole-wheat crust is easier to make than you might think! And it's SO good topped with BBQ chicken. For more BBQ deliciousness, check out the Tiki Time BBQ Chicken Tacos (page 188) and Party-Time Pineapple BBQ Meatballs (page 277)!

CRUST

3 tablespoons old-fashioned oats

3 tablespoons whole-wheat flour

½ teaspoon Italian seasoning

½ teaspoon onion powder

½ teaspoon garlic powder

⅛ teaspoon baking powder

⅛ teaspoon baking soda

Dash salt

¼ cup egg whites (about 2 large eggs' worth)

TOPPING

One 3-ounce raw boneless skinless chicken breast cutlet

⅛ teaspoon garlic powder

⅛ teaspoon onion powder

1½ tablespoons Clean & Hungry BBQ Sauce (recipe and store-bought alternatives on page 335)

1 tablespoon finely chopped red onion

3 tablespoons shredded part-skim mozzarella cheese

1 tablespoon finely chopped fresh cilantro

Entire recipe: 368 calories, 7.5g total fat (3g sat fat), 769mg sodium, 36g carbs, 5g fiber, 5.5g sugars, 37g protein

You'll Need: baking sheet, parchment paper, small blender or food processor, medium bowl, meat mallet, skillet, nonstick spray

Prep: 15 minutes • **Cook:** 15 minutes

1. Preheat oven to 400 degrees. Line a baking sheet with parchment paper.

2. In a small blender or food processor, grind oats to the consistency of coarse flour. Transfer to a medium bowl.

3. Add all remaining crust ingredients *except* egg whites. Mix until uniform. Add egg whites, and stir until it reaches a dough-like consistency.

4. Shape dough into a circle on the baking sheet, about ¼ inch thick and 6 inches in diameter.

5. Bake until top has browned and edges are slightly crispy, about 10 minutes.

6. Meanwhile, pound chicken to ½-inch thickness, and sprinkle with seasonings. Bring a skillet sprayed with nonstick spray to medium heat. Cook chicken for about 4 minutes per side, until cooked through.

7. Spread 1 tablespoon BBQ sauce over crust, leaving a ½-inch border.

8. Chop chicken. Top pizza with chicken and onion, and drizzle with remaining ½ tablespoon BBQ sauce.

9. Top with mozzarella. Bake until cheese has melted and crust is crispy, about 5 minutes.

10. Top with cilantro.

MAKES 1 SERVING

Messy Mexican Skillet Pizza

298 cal

   Don't worry . . . It's only messy if you try to eat it with your hands. (This one's more of a fork 'n knife pizza.)

¼ **cup chickpea flour**

2 **tablespoons egg whites (about 1 large egg's worth)**

Dash salt

¼ **cup chopped bell pepper**

¼ **cup chopped onion**

½ **cup canned crushed tomatoes**

½ **teaspoon garlic powder**

½ **teaspoon chili powder**

¼ **teaspoon ground cumin**

¼ **cup shredded reduced-fat Mexican-blend cheese**

1 **tablespoon sliced black olives**

HG FYI

The chickpea flour is a must, and is definitely worth seeking out. Look for it in the ethnic foods aisle, or order it online. Bob's Red Mill is my go-to brand.

Entire recipe: 298 calories, 9g total fat (3.5g sat fat), 760mg sodium, 36g carbs, 9.5g fiber, 10.5g sugars, 19.5g protein

You'll Need: 2 medium bowls, whisk, 10-inch skillet with a lid, nonstick spray, small bowl, offset spatula or flexible rubber spatula

Prep: 15 minutes • **Cook:** 10 minutes

1. To make the crust, in a medium bowl, combine chickpea flour, egg whites, and salt. Add ¼ cup water, and whisk until smooth and uniform. Let thicken for 10 minutes.

2. Meanwhile, bring a 10-inch skillet sprayed with nonstick spray to medium heat. Add pepper and onion. Cook and stir until mostly softened, about 3 minutes. Transfer to a second medium bowl, and cover to keep warm.

3. In a small bowl, stir seasonings into crushed tomatoes.

4. Remove skillet from heat; clean, if needed. Re-spray, and return to medium heat. Pour crust mixture into the skillet, quickly tilting the skillet in all directions to evenly coat the bottom. Cook until lightly browned and cooked through, about 2 minutes per side, flipping carefully with an offset spatula or flexible rubber spatula.

5. Still in the skillet, top crust with seasoned tomatoes, leaving a ¼-inch border. Sprinkle with cheese, and top with cooked veggies and olives.

6. Cover and cook until cheese has melted, about 2 minutes.

MAKES 1 SERVING

Hungry for More?

Don't miss the Pizza-fied Meatloaf (page 74), White Pizza-fied Grilled Cheese (page 172), or Zucchini-Bottomed Pizza Bites (page 278) . . .

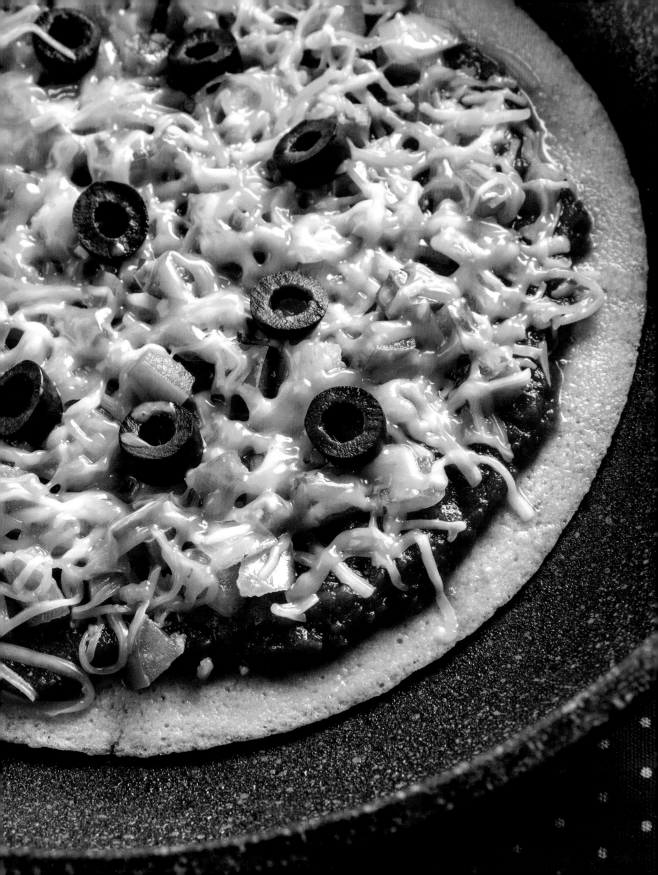

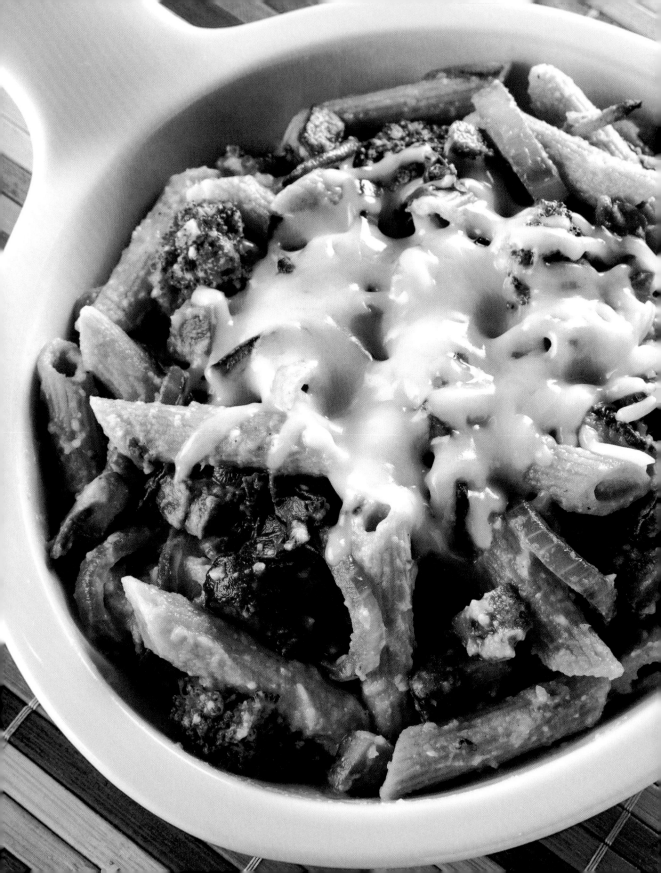

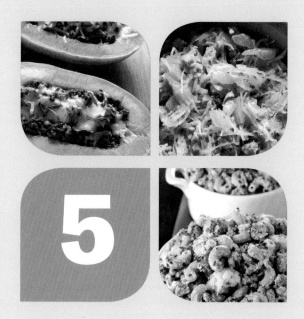

Noodle This!

The average American eats nearly 20 pounds of pasta a year. That's a whole lot of noodles: almost 15,000 calories' worth! (FYI: In Italy, they eat THREE TIMES as much.) Of course, there's nothing wrong with enjoying noodles in moderation. This chapter serves up pasta dishes super-sized with veggies, plus magical pasta swaps. Eggplant, zucchini, spaghetti squash . . . The gang's all here!

Mad About Eggplant Manicotti

264 cal

V GF Obsession confession: I love this stuff so much I sometimes eat it for breakfast! Eggplant plays the part of pasta here . . . and it does a fantastic job!

Four ½-inch-thick eggplant slices (cut lengthwise from the center of a medium eggplant)

1 teaspoon Italian seasoning

½ teaspoon garlic powder

¼ teaspoon salt

½ cup canned crushed tomatoes

½ cup finely chopped onion

¾ cup light/low-fat ricotta cheese

¼ cup chopped fresh basil

2 tablespoons grated Parmesan cheese

½ teaspoon chopped garlic

⅛ teaspoon black pepper

⅓ cup shredded part-skim mozzarella cheese

Optional topping: additional chopped fresh basil

Chew on This . . .

Here's a head scratcher. Eggplants aren't really vegetables; they're berries! CRAZY.

½ of recipe (2 manicotti): 264 calories, 10.5g total fat (6.5g sat fat), 816mg sodium, 24.5g carbs, 7.5g fiber, 14.5g sugars, 20.5g protein

You'll Need: baking sheet, 8-inch by 8-inch baking pan, nonstick spray, 2 medium bowls, skillet

Prep: 15 minutes • **Cook:** 45 minutes

1. Preheat oven to 400 degrees. Spray a baking sheet and an 8-inch by 8-inch baking pan with nonstick spray.

2. Sprinkle eggplant with ¼ teaspoon Italian seasoning, ¼ teaspoon garlic powder, and ⅛ teaspoon salt.

3. Lay eggplant on the baking sheet. Bake for 10 minutes.

4. Flip eggplant. Bake until slightly softened and lightly browned, about 10 more minutes.

5. Meanwhile, in a medium bowl, combine canned crushed tomatoes with ½ teaspoon Italian seasoning and remaining ¼ teaspoon garlic powder. Mix well.

6. Reduce oven temperature to 350 degrees.

7. Thoroughly blot eggplant dry, and set aside.

8. Bring a skillet sprayed with nonstick spray to medium-high heat. Cook and stir onion until slightly softened and lightly browned, about 2 minutes.

9. Transfer onion to a second medium bowl. Add ricotta, basil, Parm, chopped garlic, pepper, remaining ¼ teaspoon Italian seasoning, and remaining ⅛ teaspoon salt. Mix until uniform.

10. Spoon ¼th of the ricotta mixture (about ¼ cup) onto the bottom of an eggplant slice. Roll up eggplant, and place in the baking pan, seam side down.

11. Repeat to make 3 more manicotti.

12. Evenly top with seasoned tomatoes. Bake until hot and bubbly, about 20 minutes.

13. Top with mozzarella. Bake until melted, about 3 minutes.

MAKES 2 SERVINGS

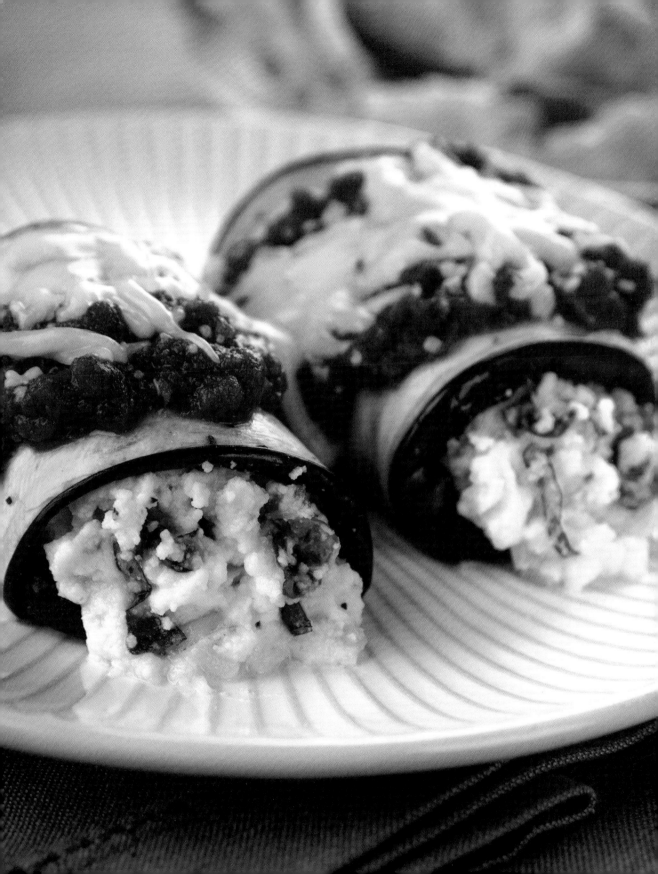

Love at First Bite Lasagna

318 cal

In this recipe, zucchini slices act as lasagna sheets, so you only use half the amount of actual pasta. Brilliant! P.S. Don't miss page 136's Lasagna-Stuffed Spaghetti Squash.

1¼ pounds (2 to 3 medium) zucchini

½ teaspoon garlic powder

½ teaspoon onion powder

½ teaspoon each salt and black pepper

8 ounces raw extra-lean ground beef (4% fat or less)

½ teaspoon Italian seasoning

1 cup Clean & Hungry Marinara Sauce (recipe and store-bought alternatives on page 336)

1 cup light/low-fat ricotta cheese

¼ cup egg whites (about 2 large eggs' worth)

½ teaspoon chopped garlic

⅛ teaspoon ground nutmeg

4 whole-grain oven-ready lasagna sheets

½ cup shredded part-skim mozzarella cheese

2 tablespoons grated Parmesan cheese

Chew on This . . .

Humans aren't the only ones infatuated with lasagna. Garfield creator Jim Davis jokingly gave his fictional cat a lasagna obsession but claims people constantly tell him their cats love the saucy pasta dish!

¼th of lasagna: 318 calories, 10g total fat (5g sat fat), 790mg sodium, 28g carbs, 5g fiber, 10g sugars, 30.5g protein

You'll Need: baking sheet, 8-inch by 8-inch baking pan, nonstick spray, large skillet, medium bowl, foil

Prep: 25 minutes • **Cook:** 1 hour and 10 minutes • **Cool:** 10 minutes

1. Preheat oven to 375 degrees. Spray a baking sheet and an 8-inch by 8-inch baking pan with nonstick spray.

2. Slice off and discard zucchini ends. Cut zucchini in half widthwise, and cut each half lengthwise into ¼-inch-thick strips.

3. Sprinkle with ¼ teaspoon garlic powder, ¼ teaspoon onion powder, and ⅛ teaspoon each salt and pepper.

4. Evenly lay zucchini on the baking sheet, overlapping if needed. Bake for 10 minutes.

5. Meanwhile, bring a large skillet sprayed with nonstick spray to medium-high heat. Add beef, and sprinkle with Italian seasoning, ¼ teaspoon each salt and pepper, remaining ¼ teaspoon garlic powder, and remaining ¼ teaspoon onion powder. Cook and crumble for about 5 minutes, until fully cooked.

6. Remove skillet from heat. Add marinara sauce, and mix well.

7. Flip zucchini. Bake until softened, about 10 more minutes.

8. Meanwhile, in a medium bowl, combine ricotta, egg whites, chopped garlic, nutmeg, and remaining ⅛ teaspoon each salt and pepper. Mix until smooth and uniform.

9. Remove sheet from oven, but leave oven on. Thoroughly blot zucchini dry.

10. If needed, break lasagna sheets to fit the baking pan.

11. Evenly layer the following in the baking pan: ⅓rd of the zucchini, half (about ½ cup) of the seasoned ricotta, 2 lasagna sheets, and ⅓rd (about ½ cup) of the meat sauce.

12. Repeat layering process. Evenly top with remaining zucchini and meat sauce. Sprinkle with mozzarella and Parm.

13. Cover pan with foil. Bake for 40 minutes.

14. Uncover and bake until lasagna sheets are cooked through and cheese has lightly browned, about 8 minutes.

15. Let cool for 10 minutes before slicing.

MAKES 4 SERVINGS

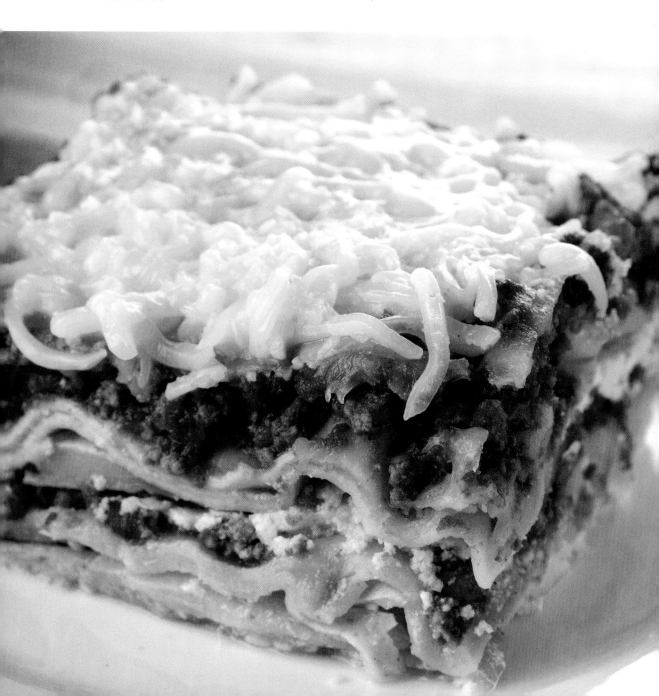

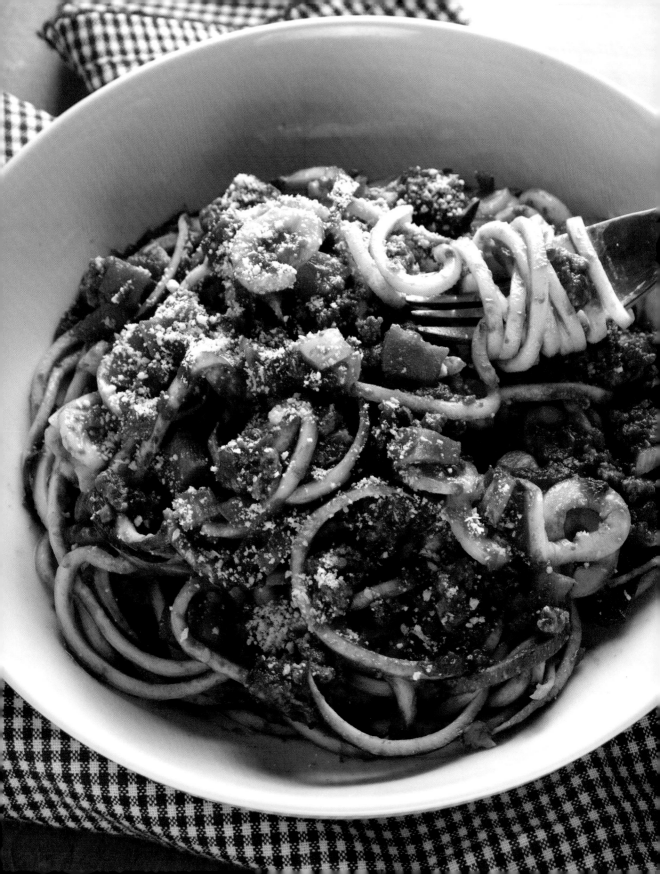

Z'paghetti Bolognese

181 cal

30m **GF** Obsession confession: I've been known to have TWO servings of this recipe at once . . . It's one of my absolute favorites, and the calorie count is so low!

2 pounds spiralized zucchini (about 4 medium zucchini)

1¾ cups canned crushed tomatoes

2 tablespoons tomato paste

1½ teaspoons white wine vinegar

½ teaspoon Italian seasoning

¾ teaspoon garlic powder

¾ teaspoon onion powder

1½ teaspoons olive oil

¼ cup chopped celery

¼ cup chopped onion

¼ cup chopped carrots

8 ounces raw extra-lean ground beef (4% fat or less)

½ teaspoon salt

⅛ teaspoon black pepper

Optional topping: grated Parmesan cheese

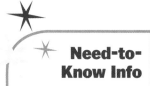

Need-to-Know Info

It's super easy to spiralize zucchini. Get the 411 on page 349!

¼th of recipe (about 1¾ cups): 181 calories, 5g total fat (1.5g sat fat), 579mg sodium, 18.5g carbs, 5g fiber, 11g sugars, 17g protein

You'll Need: extra-large skillet, nonstick spray, strainer, medium-large bowl

Prep: 15 minutes • **Cook:** 15 minutes

1. Bring an extra-large skillet sprayed with nonstick spray to medium-high heat. Cook and stir zucchini until hot and slightly softened, about 3 minutes.

2. Transfer zucchini to a strainer, and thoroughly drain excess liquid.

3. In a medium-large bowl, combine crushed tomatoes, tomato paste, vinegar, and Italian seasoning. Add ½ teaspoon each garlic powder and onion powder, and mix well.

4. Drizzle oil in the skillet, and return to medium-high heat. Add celery, onion, and carrots. Cook and stir until slightly softened, about 2 minutes.

5. Reduce heat to medium. Add beef, and season with salt, pepper, and remaining ¼ teaspoon each garlic powder and onion powder. Cook, stir, and crumble until veggies have softened and beef is fully cooked, about 5 minutes.

6. Add tomato mixture to the skillet. Cook and stir until hot and well mixed, about 1 minute.

7. Add drained zucchini, and cook and stir until hot and well mixed, about 2 minutes.

MAKES 4 SERVINGS

Chew on This . . .

Move over, bananas. A zucchini actually has MORE potassium than a banana!

Z'paghetti with Red Clam Sauce

174 cal

30m GF   This clam-happy dish is a little on the spicy side . . . I LOVE the hit of heat, but if you're not a fan of spicy stuff, leave out the red pepper flakes!

1 cup canned crushed tomatoes

2 tablespoons tomato paste

1 teaspoon Italian seasoning

¾ teaspoon garlic powder

¾ teaspoon onion powder

¼ teaspoon red pepper flakes

1 pound spiralized zucchini (about 2 medium zucchini)

½ cup chopped onion

One 6.5-ounce can chopped clams in clam juice (not drained)

2 tablespoons chopped fresh basil

2 teaspoons grated Parmesan cheese

½ of recipe (about 1⅔ cups): 174 calories, 1.5g total fat (0.5g sat fat), 808mg sodium, 26.5g carbs, 6g fiber, 13.5g sugars, 16g protein

You'll Need: medium bowl, large skillet, nonstick spray, strainer

Prep: 10 minutes • **Cook:** 10 minutes

1. In a medium bowl, combine crushed tomatoes, tomato paste, and seasonings. Mix until uniform.

2. Bring a large skillet sprayed with nonstick spray to medium-high heat. Cook and stir zucchini until hot and slightly softened, about 2 minutes.

3. Transfer zucchini to a strainer, and thoroughly drain excess liquid.

4. Remove skillet from heat. Re-spray, and return to medium-high heat. Cook and stir onion until mostly softened, about 3 minutes.

5. Reduce heat to medium. Add drained zucchini, tomato mixture, clams (and juice), and basil. Cook and stir until hot and well mixed, about 2 minutes.

6. Serve topped with Parm.

MAKES 2 SERVINGS

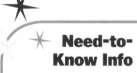

Need-to-Know Info

It's super easy to spiralize zucchini. Get the 411 on page 349!

Chew on This . . .

Giant clams can be as large as four feet across. I'm all for big portions, but I'll stick to standard-sized clams in this dish!

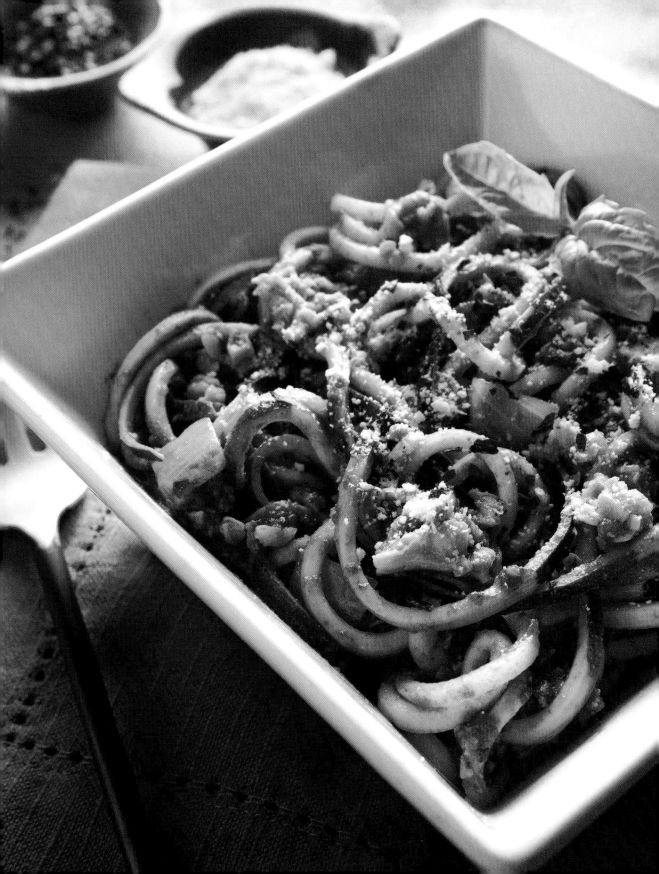

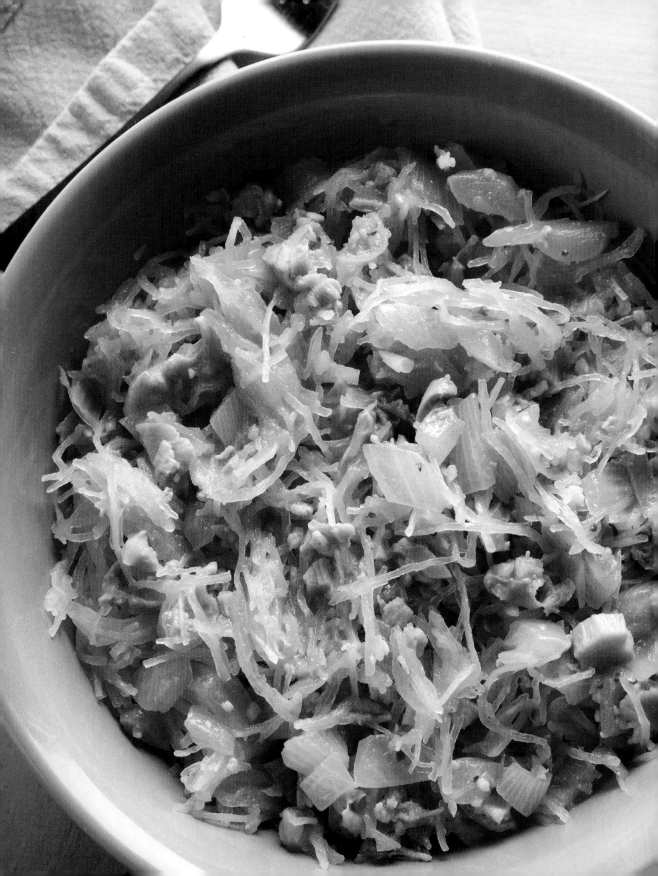

Surprise Spaghetti with White Clam Sauce

204 cal

30m **GF** Surprise! The spaghetti in this dish is actually spaghetti squash. It *totally* works with buttery sauce . . .

1 cup chopped onion

2 teaspoons chopped garlic

One 6.5-ounce can chopped clams in clam juice (not drained)

2 tablespoons whipped butter

2 teaspoons lemon juice

¼ teaspoon red pepper flakes

¼ teaspoon dried oregano

3 cups cooked spaghetti squash, drained of excess moisture

Optional seasonings: salt, black pepper

Optional topping: grated Parmesan cheese

½ of recipe (about 1½ cups): 204 calories, 7g total fat (4g sat fat), 572mg sodium, 26.5g carbs, 4.5g fiber, 9.5g sugars, 11.5g protein

You'll Need: large skillet, nonstick spray

Prep: 10 minutes • **Cook:** 10 minutes

Plus prep and cook times for spaghetti squash (page 350) if not made in advance.

1. Bring a large skillet sprayed with nonstick spray to medium-high heat. Cook and stir onion for 3 minutes.

2. Add garlic. Cook and stir until onion has mostly softened and lightly browned and garlic is fragrant, about 2 minutes.

3. Reduce heat to medium. Add all remaining ingredients *except* squash. Cook and stir until hot and well mixed, about 1 minute.

4. If needed, add squash to the skillet to reheat; cook and stir until hot and well mixed, about 2 minutes. Otherwise, pour skillet contents over spaghetti squash, and toss to mix.

MAKES 2 SERVINGS

Chew on This . . .

Sources say that 1 in 5,000 clams can form a pearl. It's unlikely any gems will appear in your grocery-store clams . . . which is probably a good thing!

Lasagna-Stuffed Spaghetti Squash

215 cal

GF This twist on the Italian classic is jaw-droppingly good! Lasagna lovers should also check out the Love at First Bite Lasagna on page 128.

1 spaghetti squash (about 4½ pounds)

¾ cup canned crushed tomatoes

¼ cup light/low-fat ricotta cheese

1½ teaspoons chopped garlic

¾ teaspoon onion powder

¾ teaspoon Italian seasoning

2 tablespoons chopped fresh basil

½ teaspoon salt

¼ teaspoon black pepper

12 ounces raw extra-lean ground beef (4% fat or less)

¼ cup shredded part-skim mozzarella cheese

¼th of recipe (¼ stuffed squash): 215 calories, 6g total fat (3g sat fat), 538mg sodium, 17.5g carbs, 3.5g fiber, 7.5g sugars, 23g protein

You'll Need: 1 to 2 large baking pans, medium bowl, skillet, nonstick spray

Prep: 10 minutes • **Cook:** 55 minutes

1. Preheat oven to 400 degrees.

2. Microwave squash for 6 minutes, until soft enough to cut. Halve lengthwise; scoop out and discard seeds.

3. Fill a large baking pan with ½ inch water. Add squash halves, cut sides down. (Use 2 pans, if needed.)

4. Bake until tender, about 40 minutes.

5. Meanwhile, in a medium bowl, combine crushed tomatoes, ricotta, garlic, onion powder, and Italian seasoning. Add 1 tablespoon basil, ¼ teaspoon salt, and ⅛ teaspoon pepper. Mix until uniform.

6. About 10 minutes before squash is done baking, bring a skillet sprayed with nonstick spray to medium-high heat. Add beef, and season with remaining ¼ teaspoon salt and ⅛ teaspoon pepper. Cook and crumble for about 5 minutes, until fully cooked.

7. Reduce heat to low. Add tomato mixture to the skillet. Cook and stir until hot and well mixed, about 1 minute.

8. Remove baking pan from the oven, but leave oven on. Remove squash halves, and blot away excess moisture.

9. Empty water from baking pan. Return squash halves, cut side up.

10. Fill squash halves with beef mixture. Top with mozzarella and remaining 1 tablespoon basil.

11. Bake until filling is hot and cheese has melted, about 5 minutes.

MAKES 4 SERVINGS

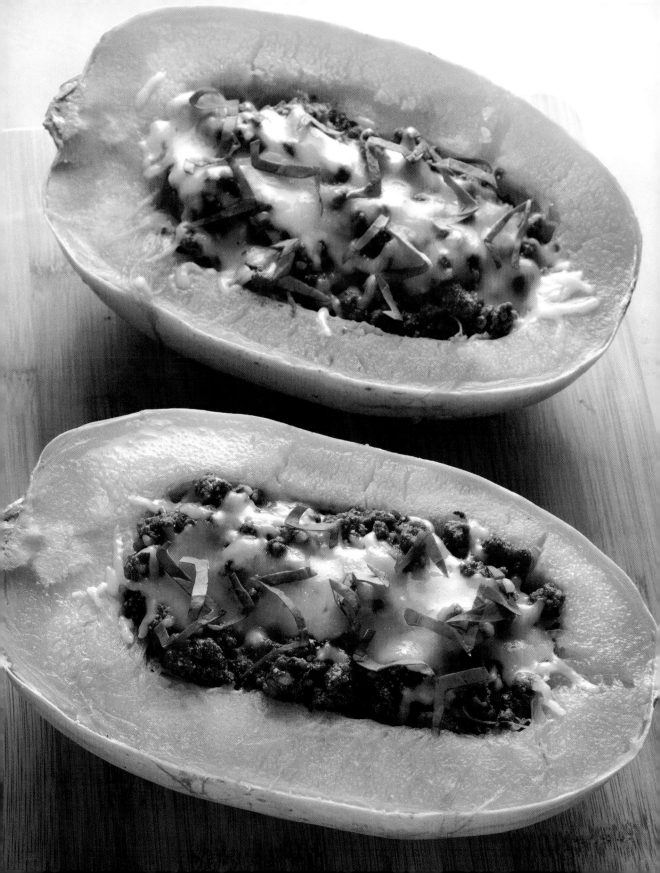

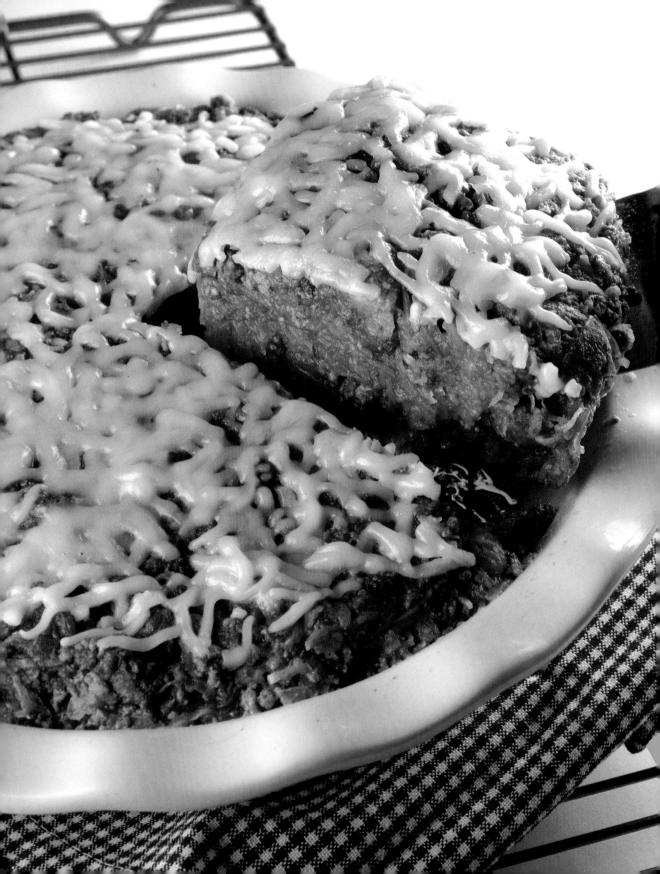

Spaghetti Squash Pie in the Sky

5i **GF** You'll be amazed once you taste this savory pie . . . and the serving size is tremendous!

5 cups cooked spaghetti squash, drained of excess moisture

1 pound raw extra-lean ground beef (4% fat or less)

¼ teaspoon salt

1½ teaspoons onion powder

1½ teaspoons garlic powder

2 cups canned crushed tomatoes

½ cup egg whites (about 4 large eggs' worth)

1 teaspoon Italian seasoning

½ cup shredded part-skim mozzarella cheese

¼th of pie: 300 calories, 8g total fat (4g sat fat), 645mg sodium, 22.5g carbs, 5g fiber, 9.5g sugars, 34g protein

You'll Need: large pie pan, nonstick spray, large bowl, large skillet

Prep: 10 minutes • **Cook:** 40 minutes • **Cool:** 10 minutes

Plus prep and cook times for spaghetti squash (page 350) if not made in advance.

1. Preheat oven to 400 degrees. Spray a large pie pan with nonstick spray.

2. Place spaghetti squash in a large bowl.

3. Bring a large skillet sprayed with nonstick spray to medium-high heat. Add beef, and season with salt, ½ teaspoon onion powder, and ½ teaspoon garlic powder. Cook and crumble for about 5 minutes, until fully cooked.

4. Add beef to the large bowl. Add canned crushed tomatoes, egg whites, Italian seasoning, and remaining 1 teaspoon each onion powder and garlic powder. Mix thoroughly.

5. Transfer to the pie pan, and smooth out the top. Bake until slightly firm, about 25 minutes.

6. Sprinkle with cheese. Bake until cheese has melted and lightly browned, about 10 minutes.

7. Let cool for 10 minutes before slicing.

MAKES 4 SERVINGS

Chew on This . . .

I've never seen one in the wild, but I've heard spaghetti squash grow on vines up to twenty feet long!

Beefed-Up Cheesy Mac

287 cal

5i My delicious beefed-up take on mac 'n cheese ditches excess calories, so you can feel good about indulging! And if you prefer your mac 'n cheese on the traditional side, look no further than page 90's Classic Cheesy Mac Casserole.

5 ounces (about 1½ cups) uncooked whole-grain elbow macaroni

5 cups chopped cauliflower

1 pound raw extra-lean ground beef (4% fat or less)

1 teaspoon garlic powder

1 teaspoon onion powder

¾ teaspoon salt

½ teaspoon black pepper

¾ cup light/reduced-fat cream cheese

3 tablespoons light sour cream

Optional seasonings: additional salt and black pepper

Optional topping: chopped fresh parsley

⅙th of recipe (about 1½ cups): 287 calories, 10.5g total fat (5.5g sat fat), 509mg sodium, 24.5g carbs, 4.5g fiber, 4.5g sugars, 23.5g protein

You'll Need: large pot, large microwave-safe bowl, strainer, large skillet, nonstick spray, medium bowl

Prep: 15 minutes • **Cook:** 30 minutes

1. Bring a large pot of water to a boil. Cook pasta per package instructions, about 8 minutes.

2. Meanwhile, place cauliflower in a large microwave-safe bowl. Add ¼ cup water. Cover and microwave for 6 minutes, or until soft.

3. Transfer pasta and cauliflower to a strainer to drain. Add both to the large bowl, and cover to keep warm.

4. Bring a large skillet sprayed with nonstick spray to medium-high heat. Add beef, and season with ½ teaspoon garlic powder, ½ teaspoon onion powder, ½ teaspoon salt, and ¼ teaspoon pepper. Cook and crumble for about 5 minutes, until fully cooked.

5. Add beef to the large bowl, and stir well. Re-cover to keep warm.

6. To make the sauce, in a medium bowl, combine cream cheese with sour cream. Add remaining ½ teaspoon garlic powder, ½ teaspoon onion powder, and ¼ teaspoon each salt and pepper. Mix well. Microwave for 45 seconds, or until hot. Stir until smooth and uniform.

7. Add sauce to the large bowl, and stir to coat.

MAKES 6 SERVINGS

Chew on This . . .

In a 12-week period, approximately one-third of the US population will eat mac 'n cheese at least once. Good thing you have this recipe . . .

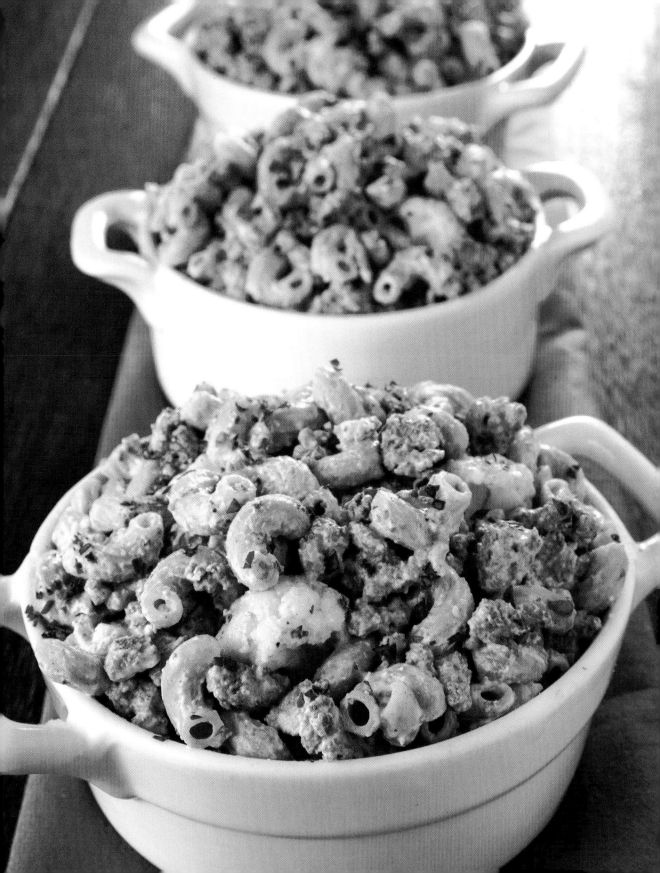

Hungry Girlfredo Ziti Bake

V "Hungry Girlfredo" refers to my calorie-slashed spin on decadent Alfredo sauce. You'd never guess this, but CAULIFLOWER is what makes it extra creamy. I love this recipe so much I could cry!

5 ounces (about 1½ cups) uncooked whole-grain ziti pasta

2 cups broccoli florets

2½ cups roughly chopped cauliflower

¼ cup fat-free milk

1 teaspoon chopped garlic

⅛ teaspoon black pepper

¼ cup grated Parmesan cheese

½ teaspoon salt

1 cup thinly sliced onion

1 cup chopped brown mushrooms

2 cups chopped spinach leaves

2 tablespoons chopped fresh basil

½ cup shredded part-skim mozzarella cheese

Optional seasoning: additional salt

HG Alternative

Can't find whole-grain ziti? Go for penne instead!

¼th of pan: 269 calories, 6.5g total fat (3.5g sat fat), 591mg sodium, 37g carbs, 7.5g fiber, 5g sugars, 17.5g protein

You'll Need: 8-inch by 8-inch baking pan, nonstick spray, large pot, medium-large microwave-safe bowl, strainer, large bowl, blender or food processor, extra-large skillet, foil

Prep: 20 minutes • **Cook:** 45 minutes • **Cool:** 10 minutes

1. Preheat oven to 425 degrees. Spray an 8-inch by 8-inch baking pan with nonstick spray.

2. Bring a large pot of water to a boil. Add pasta and broccoli. Cook both according to the instructions on the pasta package, about 8 minutes.

3. Meanwhile, place cauliflower in a medium-large microwave-safe bowl, and add 3 tablespoons water. Cover and microwave for 5 minutes, or until soft. Drain excess liquid.

4. Transfer pasta and broccoli to a strainer to drain. Place in a large bowl.

5. To make the sauce, in a blender or food processor, combine the cooked cauliflower, milk, and garlic. Add pepper, 2 tablespoons Parm, and ¼ teaspoon salt. Add 2 tablespoons warm water, and blend on high speed until smooth and uniform. Transfer to the large bowl.

6. Bring an extra-large skillet sprayed with nonstick spray to medium-high heat. Add onion and mushrooms. Cook and stir until slightly softened and lightly browned, about 4 minutes.

7. Add spinach and basil to the skillet. Cook and stir until spinach has wilted, about 1 minute.

8. Transfer skillet contents to the large bowl. Add remaining ¼ teaspoon salt, and mix well.

9. Transfer to the baking pan. Top with mozzarella and remaining 2 tablespoons Parm.

10. Cover pan with foil. Bake for 15 minutes, or until hot and bubbly.

11. Uncover and bake until cheese has melted and slightly browned, about 5 minutes.

12. Let cool for 10 minutes before serving.

MAKES 4 SERVINGS

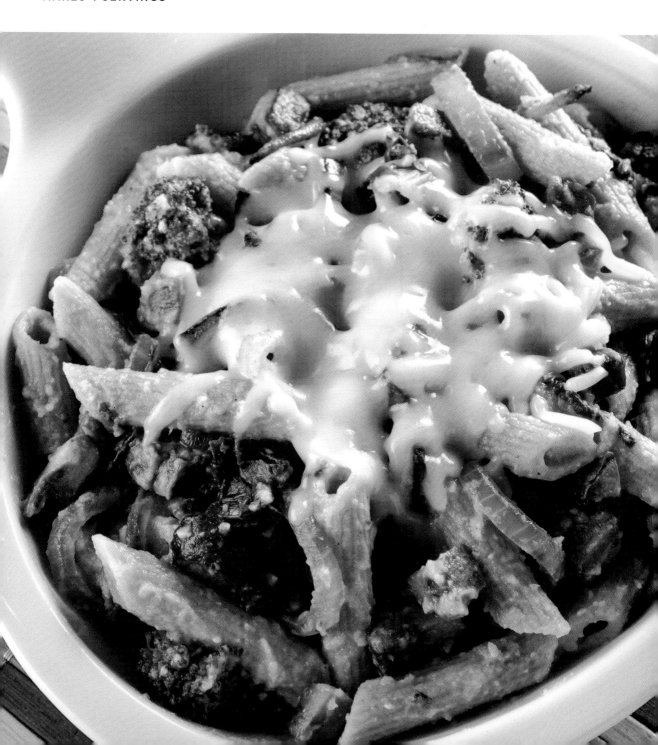

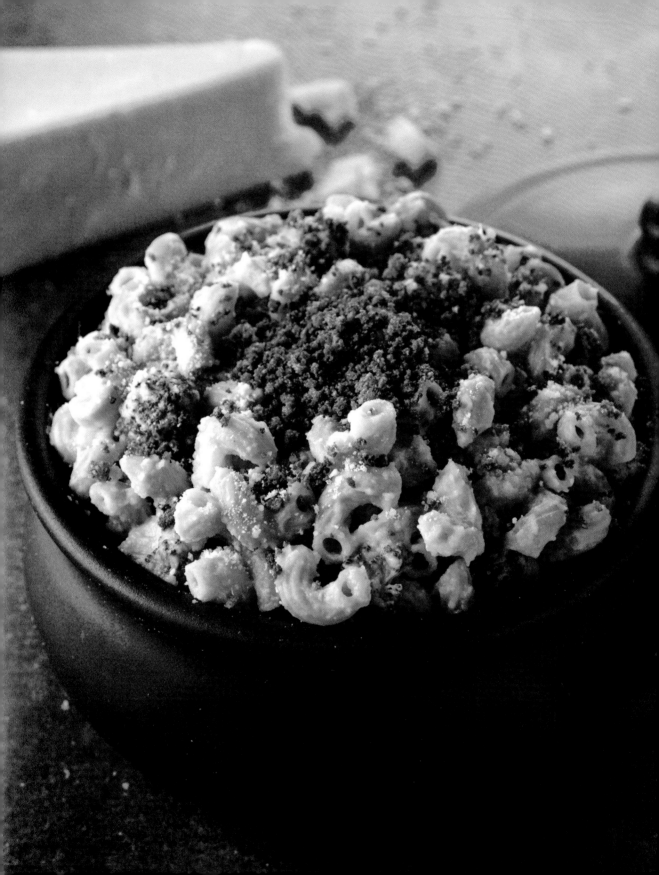

Hungry Girlfredo Mac 'n Broc Bake

192 cal

V You'll flip once you sink your teeth into this hearty noodle dish. Creamy, dreamy, macaroni madness!

4½ ounces (about 1¼ cups) uncooked whole-grain elbow macaroni

4 cups broccoli florets

6 cups roughly chopped cauliflower

2 teaspoons chopped garlic

¾ teaspoon salt

½ teaspoon black pepper

¾ cup fat-free milk

⅓ cup plus 2 tablespoons grated Parmesan cheese

¼ cup whole-wheat panko breadcrumbs

⅙th of pan: 192 calories, 4g total fat (2g sat fat), 548mg sodium, 29.5g carbs, 6g fiber, 6g sugars, 12.5g protein

You'll Need: 8-inch by 8-inch baking pan, nonstick spray, large pot, 2 large bowls (1 microwave-safe), strainer, blender or food processor

Prep: 15 minutes • **Cook:** 40 minutes • **Cool:** 10 minutes

1. Preheat oven to 375 degrees. Spray an 8-inch by 8-inch baking pan with nonstick spray.

2. Bring a large pot of water to a boil. Add pasta and broccoli. Cook both according to the instructions on the pasta package, about 8 minutes.

3. Meanwhile, place cauliflower in a large microwave-safe bowl. Add ⅓ cup water. Cover and microwave for 8 minutes, or until soft.

4. Transfer pasta and broccoli to a strainer to drain. Place in a large bowl.

5. To make the sauce, in a blender or food processor, combine cooked cauliflower, garlic, salt, and pepper. Add milk, ⅓ cup Parm, and ¼ cup water. Blend on high speed until smooth and uniform.

6. Add sauce to the large bowl, and stir to coat. Transfer to the baking pan, and smooth out the top.

7. Sprinkle with breadcrumbs and remaining 2 tablespoons Parm. Bake until top is golden brown and entire dish is hot and bubbly, 15 to 20 minutes.

8. Let cool for 10 minutes before serving.

MAKES 6 SERVINGS

Chew on This . . .

Look who's back! After four years of slow growth, a report by Google shows pasta is making a comeback, with a 26 percent rise in search results from 2015 to 2016.

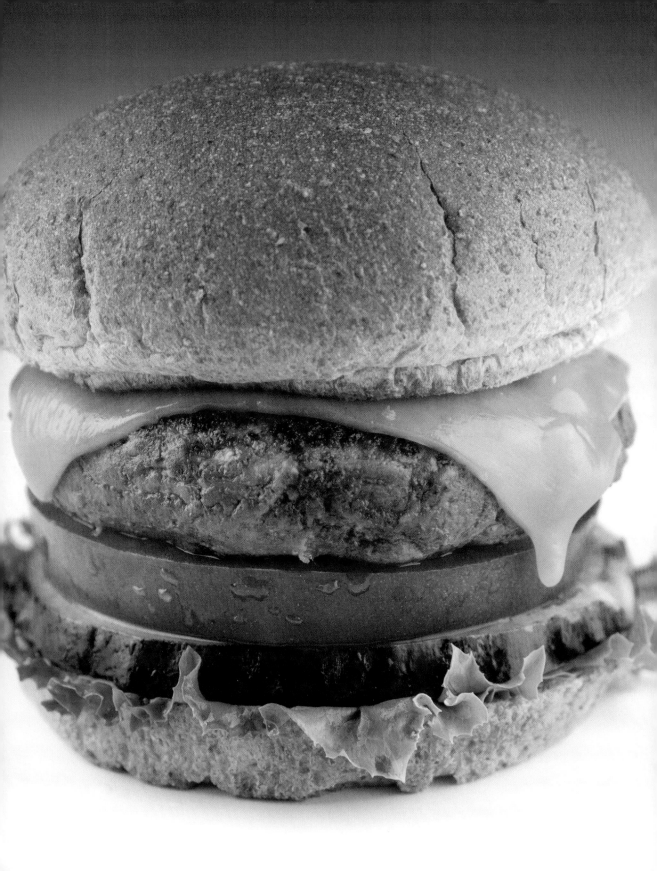

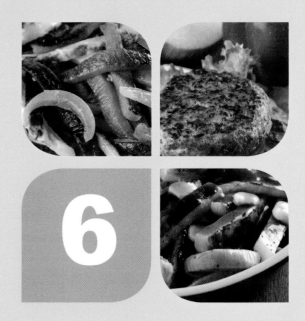

6

Welcome to Goodburger

Both burgers and fries top the list of the most craved foods in America. In fact, 40 percent of sandwiches sold in restaurants are said to be hamburgers! But considering the average fast-food meal contains over 800 calories, you might want to think twice before hitting the drive-thru. This chapter serves up some of the best burgers and fries to ever come out of the Hungryland kitchen, all of them guilt-free and mind-meltingly delicious!

Bread Swap 'Til You Drop!

On the next few pages, we're serving up recipes for perfect burger patties (toppings too!). How you want to transport that burger to your mouth, however, is entirely up to you. Add all the fresh veggies you like: tomatoes, onion, and more. Then grab a whole-grain bun, or try these calorie-saving swaps!

Lettuce at It! Easy and fresh with a satisfying crunch! Just use 4 large leaves of iceberg or butter lettuce: 2 for the bottom half of the "bun" and 2 for the top. Each lettuce bun has only around 15 calories, plus a gram of fiber. A sturdier option? Slice the sides off a round head of lettuce, and use those as your bun! For a fork 'n knife option, enjoy your burger over a bed of shredded lettuce.

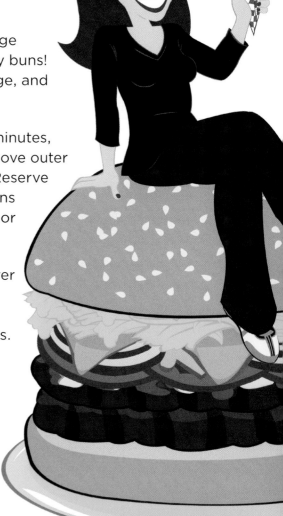

Cabbage-Patch It! Steamed or boiled cabbage leaves are another amazing alternative to carby buns! Start with half a medium head of green cabbage, and then pick your cooking method . . .

> **Nuke it:** Microwave in a bowl for about 4 minutes, until the leaves begin to loosen. Gently remove outer leaves, and place them back in the bowl. (Reserve the rest for another time.) Add 2 tablespoons water. Cover and microwave for 2 minutes, or until very soft.

> **Boil it:** Place in an extra-large pot, and cover with water. Bring to a boil. Cover and cook, rotating occasionally, until leaves soften, loosen, and fall off the head, 8 to 10 minutes. Drain, and gently remove outer leaves.

> **Slow cook it:** Place in a slow cooker with 1 cup water. Cover and cook on high for 1½ hours, or until soft. Gently remove outer leaves.

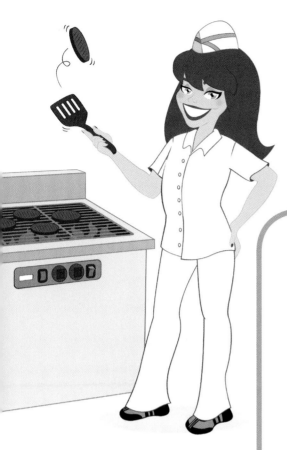

HG's Top Ate Burger Toppings

1. Clean & Hungry Special Sauce

2. Clean & Hungry Ketchup

3. Clean & Hungry BBQ Sauce

4. Yellow mustard

5. Clean & Hungry Chunky Blue Cheese Dressing

6. Clean & Hungry Creamy Fresh Sriracha

7. Clean & Hungry Ranch Dressing

8. Frank's RedHot Original Cayenne Pepper Sauce

Recipes and store-bought alternatives in Chapter 15: Clean & Hungry Staples (page 333)!

Say Cheeseburger

221 cal

   These perfectly seasoned burgers will become a staple in your life!

1 pound raw extra-lean ground beef (4% fat or less)

¼ cup egg whites (about 2 large eggs' worth)

1 tablespoon yellow mustard

1 teaspoon garlic powder

1 teaspoon onion powder

½ teaspoon each salt and black pepper

4 slices reduced-fat cheddar cheese

¼th of recipe (1 patty): 221 calories, 8.5g total fat (4.5g sat fat), 564mg sodium, 2g carbs, <0.5g fiber, 0.5g sugars, 31.5g protein

You'll Need: large bowl, grill pan (or large skillet), nonstick spray

Prep: 10 minutes • **Cook:** 10 minutes

1. In a large bowl, thoroughly mix all ingredients *except* cheese.

2. Evenly form into 4 patties, each about ½ inch thick.

3. Bring a grill pan (or large skillet) sprayed with nonstick spray to medium-high heat. Cook patties for about 4 minutes per side, until cooked to your preference. (Reduce cook time for rare; increase for well done.)

4. Reduce heat to low. Top patties with cheese. Cook until melted, about 1 minute.

MAKES 4 SERVINGS

Chew on This...

The largest recorded hamburger in history weighed over 2,000 pounds and was topped with 40 pounds of cheese! I love a nice big cheeseburger, but that's out of control...

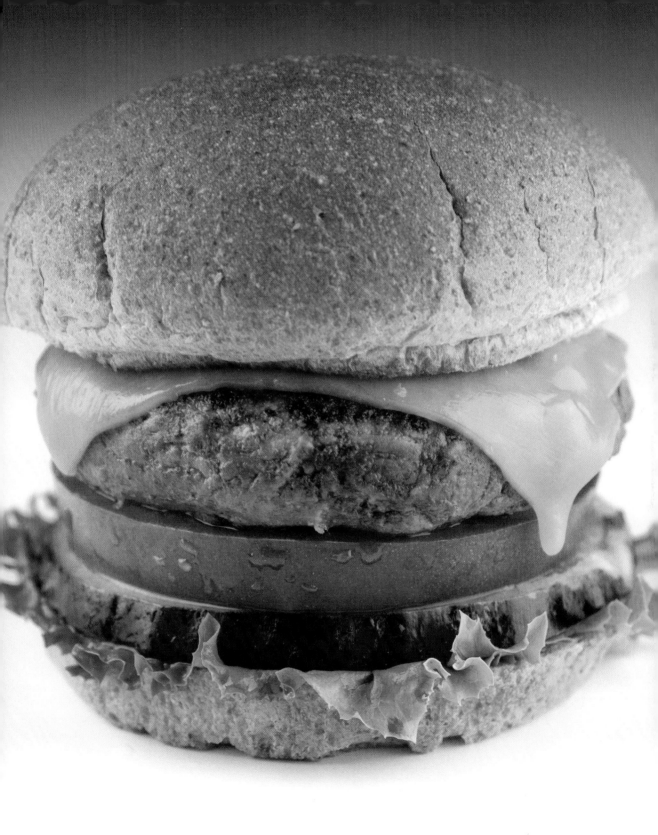

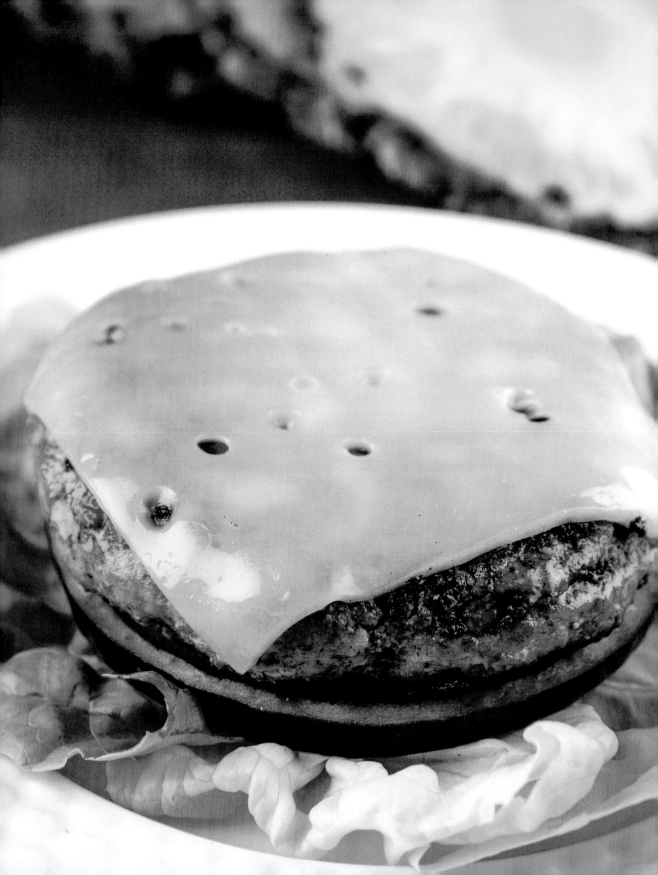

Hawaiian Hula Turkey Burgers

269 cal

🕐30m GF I can't decide what I love more about these—the fruity tropical flavor or awesome meatloaf-like texture!

¾ **cup chopped sweet onion**

½ **cup canned crushed pineapple packed in juice, thoroughly drained**

2½ **tablespoons Clean & Hungry Teriyaki Sauce (recipe and store-bought alternatives on page 342)**

1 **pound raw lean ground turkey (7% fat or less)**

¼ **cup egg whites (about 2 large eggs' worth)**

½ **teaspoon garlic powder**

½ **teaspoon onion powder**

½ **teaspoon each salt and black pepper**

4 **slices reduced-fat Swiss cheese**

¼th of recipe (1 patty): 269 calories, 11.5g total fat (5g sat fat), 542mg sodium, 9g carbs, 1g fiber, 5.5g sugars, 32g protein

You'll Need: skillet, nonstick spray, small blender or food processor, fine-mesh strainer, large bowl, grill pan (or large skillet) with a lid

Prep: 10 minutes • **Cook:** 20 minutes

1. Bring a skillet sprayed with nonstick spray to medium-high heat. Cook and stir onion until softened and lightly browned, about 4 minutes.

2. Transfer onion to a small blender or food processor. Add drained pineapple, and puree until smooth.

3. Transfer puree to a fine-mesh strainer, and thoroughly drain excess liquid.

4. Place drained puree in a large bowl. Mix in teriyaki sauce. Add all remaining ingredients *except* cheese. Mix thoroughly.

5. Bring a grill pan (or large skillet) sprayed with nonstick spray to medium-high heat. Firmly form mixture into 4 mounds in the pan, evenly spaced. Flatten into patties, each about ¾ inch thick.

6. Cook until golden brown and cooked through, about 6 minutes per side, flipping carefully.

7. Reduce heat to low. Top patties with cheese. Cover and cook until melted, about 1 minute.

MAKES 4 SERVINGS

Chew on This...

Although Hawaiians are said to consume the most SPAM in the United States, these Hawaiian burgers are purely turkey based.

Gobble 'Em Up Fajita Burgers

184 cal

   These patties are EXPLODING with tasty Mexican flavors!

½ cup finely chopped onion

½ cup finely chopped red bell pepper

1 pound raw lean ground turkey (7% fat or less)

¼ cup egg whites (about 2 large eggs' worth)

¾ teaspoon chili powder

½ teaspoon salt

¼ teaspoon ground cumin

¼th of recipe (1 patty): 184 calories, 7.5g total fat (3g sat fat), 413mg sodium, 3.5g carbs, 1g fiber, 1.5g sugars, 24.5g protein

You'll Need: skillet, nonstick spray, large bowl, grill pan (or large skillet)

Prep: 15 minutes • **Cook:** 15 minutes

1. Bring a skillet sprayed with nonstick spray to medium-high heat. Add onion and pepper. Cook and stir until softened and lightly browned, about 4 minutes.

2. Transfer to a large bowl. Add remaining ingredients, and mix thoroughly.

3. Evenly form into 4 patties, each about ½ inch thick.

4. Bring a grill pan (or large skillet) sprayed with nonstick spray to medium-high heat. Cook patties until golden brown and cooked through, about 5 minutes per side.

MAKES 4 SERVINGS

Chew on This...

Rumor has it, the average American eats a burger three times a week! Good thing this book has many burger options to zazzle up your routine.

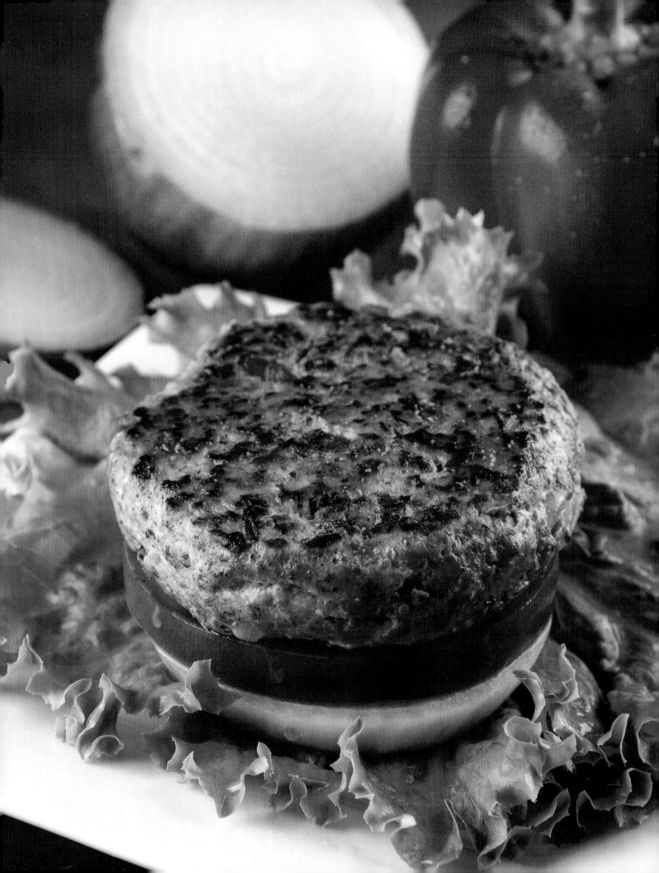

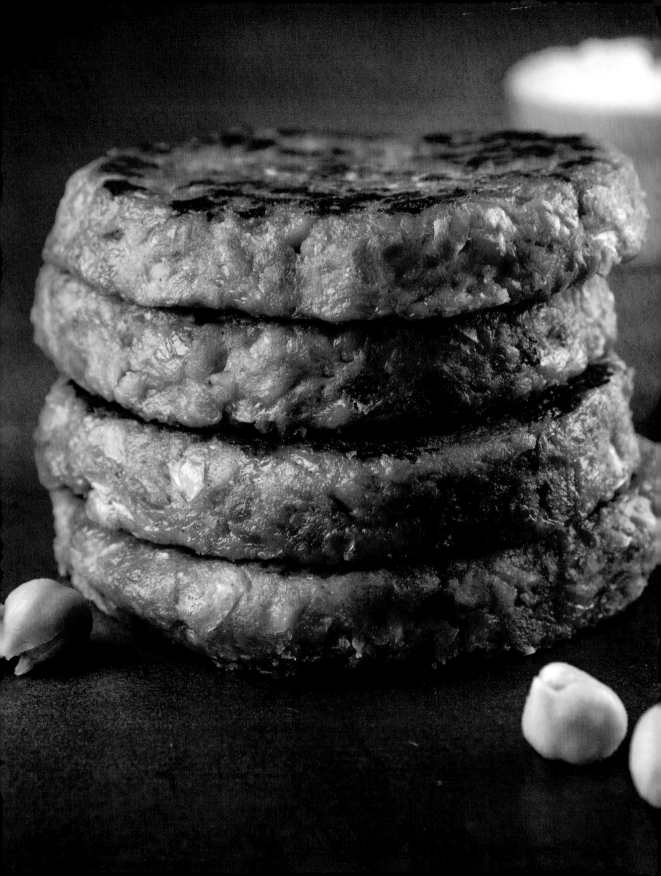

Caramelized Onion Chickpea Burgers

220 cal

(V) I can almost guarantee you've NEVER had a meatless burger quite like one of these. If they were sold in stores, my freezer would be CRAMMED with boxes of 'em.

2 cups finely chopped sweet onions

1 tablespoon chopped garlic

1 tablespoon whipped butter

One 15-ounce can chickpeas (garbanzo beans), drained and rinsed

½ cup shredded reduced-fat cheddar cheese

¼ cup whole-wheat flour

¼ cup egg whites (about 2 large eggs' worth)

½ teaspoon salt

¼ teaspoon onion powder

¼ teaspoon paprika

⅛ teaspoon black pepper

Optional topping: Clean & Hungry Ranch Dressing (recipe on page 339)

¼th of recipe (1 patty): 220 calories, 6g total fat (2.5g sat fat), 592mg sodium, 30.5g carbs, 7g fiber, 4.5g sugars, 12.5g protein

You'll Need: skillet, nonstick spray, large bowl, potato masher, grill pan (or large skillet)

Prep: 15 minutes • **Cook:** 30 minutes

1. Bring a skillet sprayed with nonstick spray to medium-low heat. Add onions, garlic, and butter. Stirring often, cook until onions have caramelized, about 18 minutes.

2. Place chickpeas in a large bowl, and thoroughly mash with a potato masher. Add caramelized onions and remaining ingredients. Mix thoroughly.

3. Firmly form into 4 patties, each about ½ inch thick.

4. Bring a grill pan (or large skillet) sprayed with nonstick spray to medium heat. Cook patties until golden brown and cooked through, about 5 minutes per side.

MAKES 4 SERVINGS

Freeze It: Burger Edition

To Freeze: Tightly wrap each cooled patty in foil or plastic wrap. (Reserve any cheese for later.) Place individually wrapped patties in a sealable container or bag, seal, and store in the freezer.

To Thaw: Bring a grill pan (or skillet) with a lid sprayed with nonstick spray to medium heat. Cook unwrapped patties until hot and slightly softened, 4 to 6 minutes per side. Or place a single unwrapped patty on a microwave-safe plate. Microwave on high for about 45 seconds per side. Top with cheese (if applicable), and cook until melted.

Garlic & Onion Butternut Turnip Fries

(196 cal)

(5i) (V) (GF)   These fries are so amazing that I would marry them. (But then I'd eat them and be widowed.) Heads up: This is a fork 'n knife recipe, for sure! If you use your hands, prepare to get messy . . . And butternut-squash-fry fans: Also check out the Squashed & Sweet Potatoed Home Fries on page 33.

12 ounces (about ½ medium) butternut squash

12 ounces (about 1 medium) turnip

¼ teaspoon salt

2 teaspoons whipped butter

2 cups sliced sweet onions

1 tablespoon chopped garlic

½ of recipe (about 1 cup): 196 calories, 2.5g total fat (1.5g sat fat), 433mg sodium, 43g carbs, 8.5g fiber, 15g sugars, 4.5g protein

You'll Need: 2 baking sheets, nonstick spray, skillet, large bowl

Prep: 15 minutes • **Cook:** 35 minutes

1. Preheat oven to 425 degrees. Spray 2 baking sheets with nonstick spray.

2. Peel squash and turnip, and cut into French-fry-shaped spears. Thoroughly pat dry. Lay spears on the sheets, evenly spaced.

3. Sprinkle with ⅛ teaspoon salt. Bake for 20 minutes.

4. Flip spears and bake until mostly tender on the inside and crispy on the outside, about 15 minutes.

5. Meanwhile, melt butter in a skillet over medium-high heat. Add onions, garlic, and remaining ⅛ teaspoon salt. Cook and stir until softened and lightly browned, about 6 minutes. Transfer to a large bowl, and cover to keep warm.

6. Add baked spears to the large bowl, and toss to mix.

MAKES 2 SERVINGS

Chew on This . . .

Sources say Americans eat potatoes more than any other vegetable, and mostly in the form of French fries!

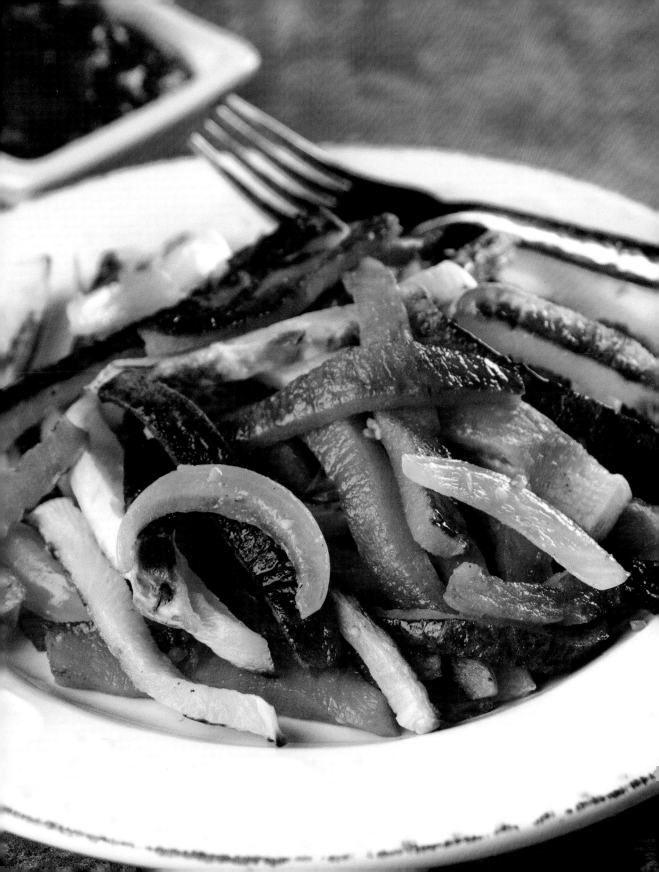

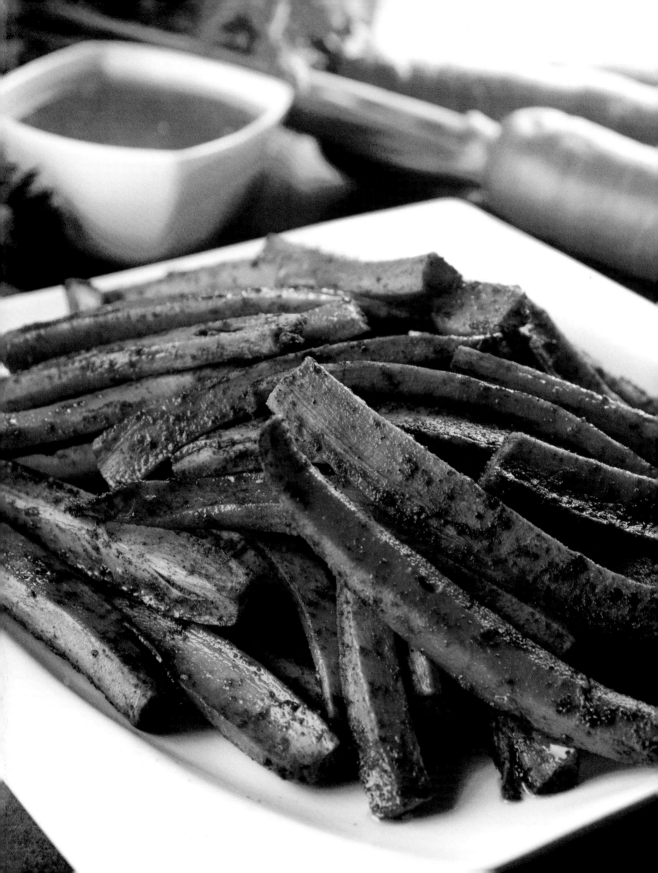

Cinnamon Spice Skinny Carrot Fries

131 cal

   With the honey and cinnamon, these fries almost taste like dessert . . .

1 pound (about 8 large) carrots

1 tablespoon honey

2 teaspoons cinnamon

¼ teaspoon salt

½ of recipe: 131 calories, 0.5g total fat (0g sat fat), 447mg sodium, 32g carbs, 7.5g fiber, 19g sugars, 2g protein

You'll Need: baking sheet, nonstick spray, large bowl
Prep: 20 minutes • **Cook:** 30 minutes

1. Preheat oven to 425 degrees. Spray a baking sheet with nonstick spray.
2. Peel carrots, and cut into French-fry-shaped spears. Place in a large bowl.
3. Drizzle with honey, and toss to coat. Sprinkle with cinnamon and salt, and again toss to coat.
4. Lay spears on the baking sheet in a single layer, evenly spaced. Bake for 15 minutes.
5. Flip spears. Bake for 10 minutes.
6. Set oven to broil. Broil until fries are tender on the inside and slightly crispy on the outside, about 2 minutes.

MAKES 2 SERVINGS

Chew on This . . .

Ancient Greeks called the carrot a philtron, which means "love charm." Maybe that's why I'm nose-over-toes IN LOVE with these carrot fries!

HG Fry FYIs

- If consuming HG fries the day after they're made, reheat them in a toaster oven for crispiest and best results.

- Some of these recipes feature a crispy coating made with whole-wheat panko breadcrumbs. You can find these crumbs at select supermarkets, most natural-food stores, and online. If you can't get your hands on the whole-wheat ones, standard panko breadcrumbs are your next best bet.

Turnip the Yum Poutine

217 cal

(GF) French fries topped with gravy and cheese?! Yes, please! P.S. Grab a fork and knife for this one . . .

1½ pounds (about 2 medium) turnips

¼ teaspoon black pepper

1 cup reduced-sodium beef broth

1½ tablespoons arrowroot powder

1 teaspoon reduced-sodium/lite soy sauce

½ teaspoon onion powder

⅛ teaspoon ground thyme

1 tablespoon whipped butter

2 sticks light string cheese, sliced into bite-sized pieces

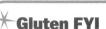

Gluten FYI

Some soy sauce contains gluten. If you avoid gluten, read labels carefully. Or grab a product labeled gluten-free.

½ of recipe: 217 calories, 6.5g total fat (3g sat fat), 752mg sodium, 29.5g carbs, 6.5g fiber, 13.5g sugars, 11.5g protein

You'll Need: 2 baking sheets, nonstick spray, medium bowl, small pot with a lid, plate

Prep: 15 minutes • **Cook:** 35 minutes

1. Preheat oven to 425 degrees. Spray 2 baking sheets with nonstick spray.

2. Peel turnips, and cut into French-fry-shaped spears.

3. Evenly lay spears on the baking sheets, and sprinkle with pepper. Bake for 15 minutes.

4. Flip spears. Bake until tender on the inside and crispy on the outside, about 15 more minutes.

5. Meanwhile, make the gravy. In a medium bowl, combine broth with arrowroot powder. Stir to dissolve. Add soy sauce, onion powder, and thyme. Mix well.

6. Melt butter in a small pot over medium heat. Carefully add broth mixture. Cook and stir until thickened to the consistency of gravy, about 2 minutes. Cover to keep warm.

7. Arrange spears on the centers of the baking sheets. Top with string cheese pieces.

8. Bake until cheese has softened, about 2 minutes.

9. Plate fries, and top with gravy.

MAKES 2 SERVINGS

Chew on This . . .

Our neighbors to the north swear by poutine, but Jones Soda may have gone too far when it released a limited-edition poutine-flavored pop in Canada.

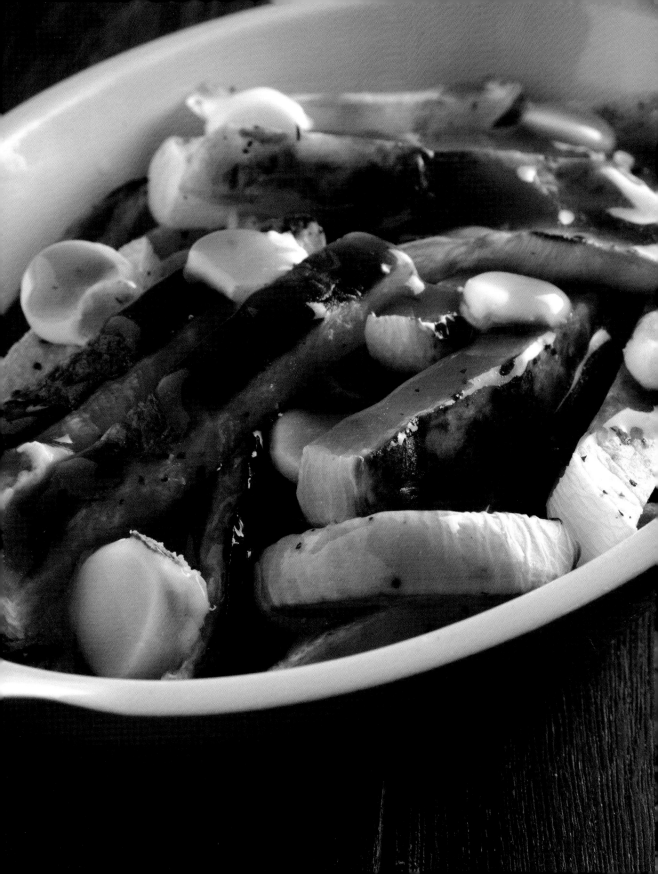

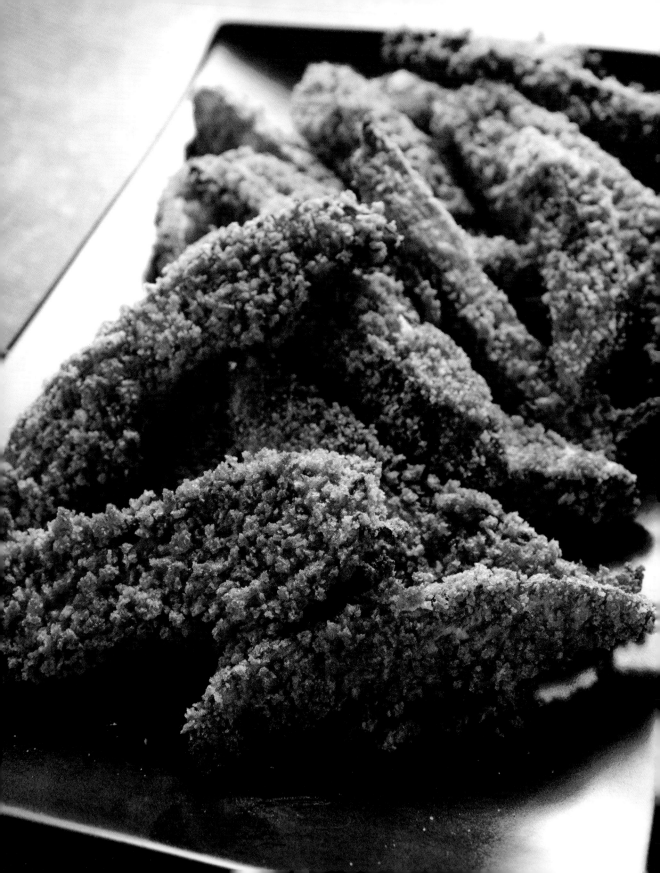

Hella Good Bella Fries

123 cal

  V Bet you've never turned mushrooms into French fries! The game's about to change . . .

2 large portabella mushroom caps (stems removed)

¼ cup egg whites (about 2 large eggs' worth)

½ cup whole-wheat panko breadcrumbs

1 teaspoon garlic powder

1 teaspoon onion powder

¼ teaspoon salt

⅛ teaspoon black pepper

Optional dip: Clean & Hungry Ketchup (recipe and store-bought alternatives on page 343)

½ of recipe (about 10 fries): 123 calories, 0.5g total fat (0g sat fat), 378mg sodium, 21.5g carbs, 4g fiber, 4g sugars, 9g protein

You'll Need: large baking sheet, nonstick spray, large bowl, medium-large bowl

Prep: 15 minutes • **Cook:** 15 minutes

1. Preheat oven to 425 degrees. Spray a large baking sheet with nonstick spray.

2. Slice mushroom caps into French-fry-shaped spears.

3. Place in a large bowl. Top with egg whites, and flip to coat.

4. In a medium-large bowl, mix breadcrumbs with seasonings.

5. One at a time, shake spears to remove excess egg, and coat with seasoned crumbs.

6. Evenly lay on the baking sheet, and top with any remaining seasoned crumbs. Bake for 6 minutes.

7. Carefully flip spears. Bake until lightly browned and crispy, about 6 more minutes.

MAKES 2 SERVINGS

Chew on This . . .

Mushrooms are everywhere . . . literally! They're found on every continent in the world and in all types of cuisine.

Crunch a Bunch Zucchini Fries

114 cal

  A fried zucchini swap with under 150 calories per serving?! It has arrived . . .

1 pound (about 2 medium) zucchini

¼ cup egg whites (about 2 large eggs' worth)

½ cup whole-wheat panko breadcrumbs

¾ teaspoon garlic powder

¾ teaspoon onion powder

½ teaspoon Italian seasoning

¼ teaspoon salt

⅛ teaspoon black pepper

Optional seasonings: additional salt and black pepper

Optional dip: Clean & Hungry Ketchup (recipe and store-bought alternatives on page 343)

½ of recipe (about 20 fries): 114 calories, 1g total fat (0g sat fat), 359mg sodium, 21.5g carbs, 4g fiber, 6.5g sugars, 6.5g protein

You'll Need: large baking sheet, nonstick spray, large bowl, medium-large bowl

Prep: 15 minutes • **Cook:** 20 minutes

1. Preheat oven to 400 degrees. Spray a large baking sheet with nonstick spray.

2. Slice off and discard zucchini ends. Cut zucchini into French-fry-shaped spears.

3. Place in a large bowl. Top with egg whites, and flip to coat.

4. In a medium-large bowl, mix breadcrumbs with seasonings.

5. One at a time, shake zucchini spears to remove excess egg, and lightly coat with seasoned crumbs.

6. Evenly lay spears on the baking sheet, and top with any remaining seasoned crumbs. Bake for 10 minutes.

7. Carefully flip spears. Bake until lightly browned and crispy, about 10 more minutes.

MAKES 2 SERVINGS

Chew on This . . .

The world's heaviest recorded zucchini weighed nearly 65 pounds. That thing would've made a lot of zucchini fries!

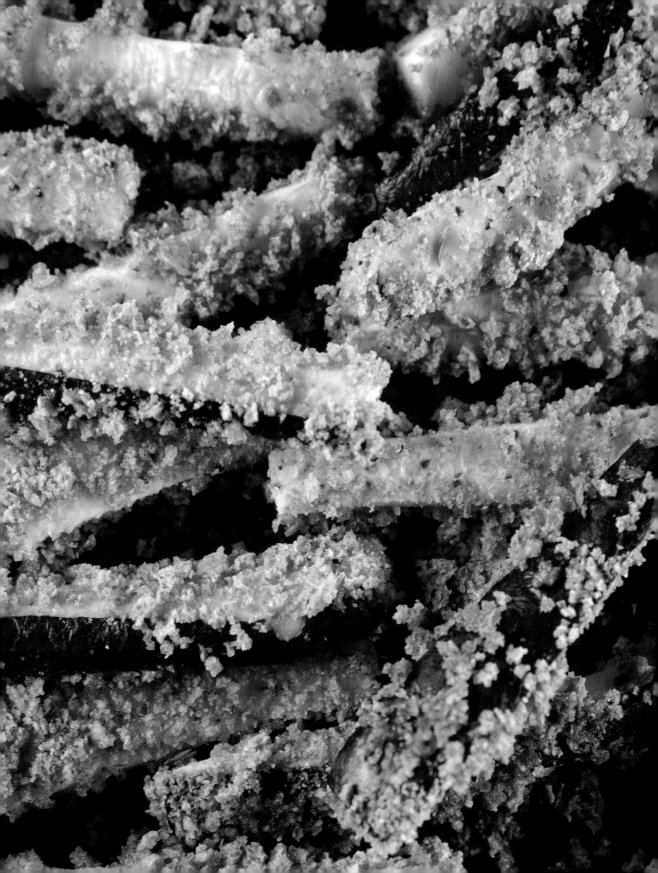

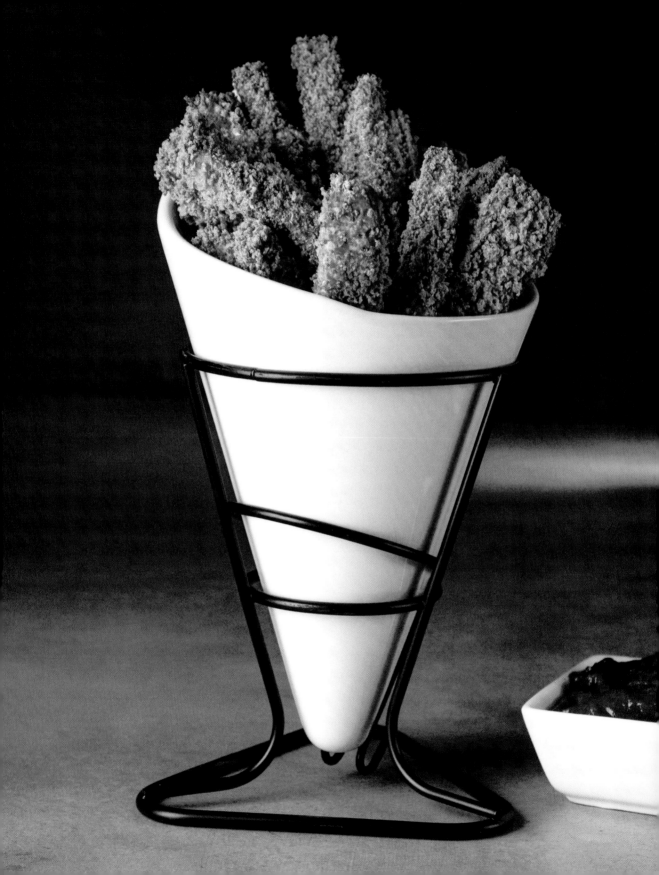

First-Prize Eggplant Fries

80 cal

5i **V**   Yup: I made French fries out of eggplant! Crunchy outside, soft inside . . . It doesn't get any better than this!

12 ounces (about 1 medium) eggplant

½ cup egg whites (about 4 large eggs' worth)

¾ cup whole-wheat panko breadcrumbs

½ teaspoon garlic powder

½ teaspoon onion powder

½ teaspoon Italian seasoning

½ teaspoon salt

¼ teaspoon black pepper

Optional dip: Clean & Hungry Ketchup (recipe and store-bought alternatives on page 343)

¼th of recipe (about 12 fries): 80 calories, 0.5g total fat (0g sat fat), 340mg sodium, 15.5g carbs, 4g fiber, 3.5g sugars, 4g protein

You'll Need: 2 large baking sheets, nonstick spray, large bowl, medium-large bowl

Prep: 15 minutes • **Cook:** 25 minutes

1. Preheat oven to 400 degrees. Spray 2 large baking sheets with nonstick spray.

2. Peel eggplant. Slice off and discard ends. Cut eggplant into French-fry-shaped spears.

3. Place in a large bowl. Top with egg whites, and flip to coat.

4. In a medium-large bowl, mix breadcrumbs with seasonings.

5. One at a time, shake spears to remove excess egg, and lightly coat with seasoned crumbs.

6. Evenly lay spears on the baking sheets, and top with any remaining seasoned crumbs. Bake for 12 minutes.

7. Remove baking sheets, and return them to the oven on the opposite racks. Bake until lightly browned and crispy, about 12 more minutes.

MAKES 4 SERVINGS

Chew on This . . .

Rumor has it the eggplant originated in India, where it's been called the King of Vegetables. Does that make these adorable li'l veggie fries princes and princesses?!

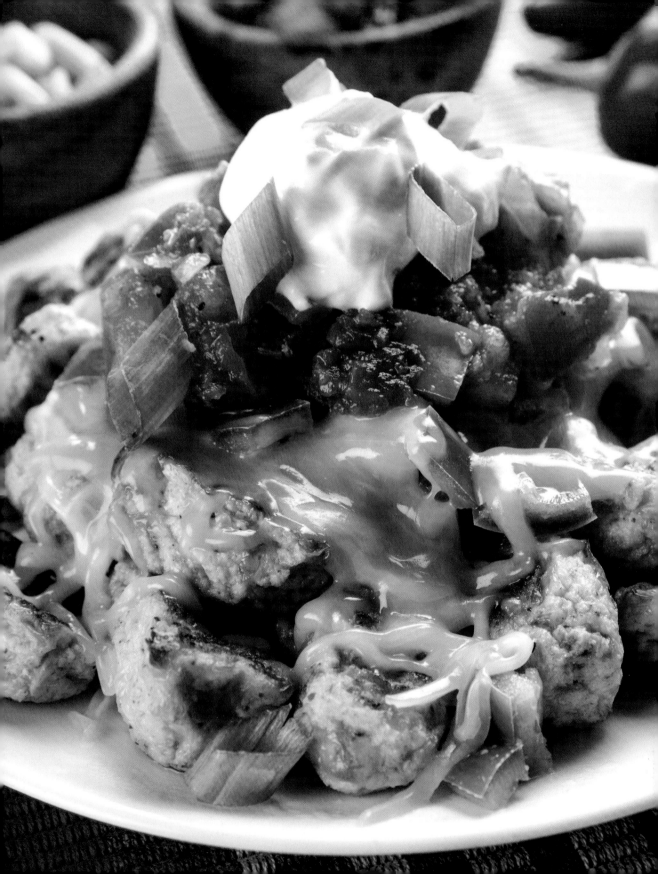

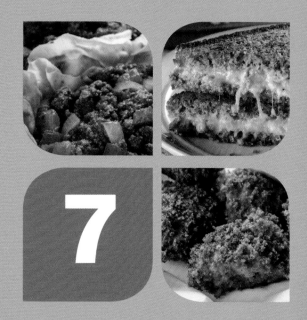

I Kid You Not!

Gooey grilled cheese, saucy sloppy joes, tuna melts, crispy chicken nuggets, tater tots . . . Are you sensing a theme here? Our childhood cravings are all centered around CARBS. Why? Research shows that kids are biologically drawn to starchy carbs because these foods help their brains and bodies grow. Now that we're all grown up, we still want to enjoy these kid favorites without all the extra calories and carbs. This chapter will let you do just that!

White Pizza-fied Grilled Cheese

327 cal

  This sandwich is the perfect mashup of two beloved foods. Hooray for that!

¼ cup shredded part-skim mozzarella cheese

2 tablespoons light/low-fat ricotta cheese

2 tablespoons bagged sun-dried tomatoes (not packed in oil), chopped

2 tablespoons chopped fresh basil

⅛ teaspoon garlic powder

Dash each salt and black pepper

2 slices whole-grain bread with 60 to 80 calories per slice

2 teaspoons whipped butter

Entire recipe: 327 calories, 12.5g total fat (6.5g sat fat), 653mg sodium, 37.5g carbs, 7.5g fiber, 9.5g sugars, 17.5g protein

You'll Need: small bowl, skillet, nonstick spray

Prep: 10 minutes • **Cook:** 5 minutes

1. In a small bowl, mix all ingredients *except* bread and butter. Mix well.

2. Evenly top one bread slice with mixture. Top with remaining bread slice.

3. Spread the top of the sandwich with 1 teaspoon butter.

4. Bring a skillet sprayed with nonstick spray to medium heat. Place sandwich in the skillet, buttered side down.

5. Spread the top with remaining 1 teaspoon butter. Cook until bread is golden brown and cheese has melted, about 2 minutes per side, flipping carefully.

MAKES 1 SERVING

Chew on This...

April is National Grilled Cheese Sandwich Month. October is National Pizza Month. I encourage you to eat this sandwich in April, October, or any other month of the year!

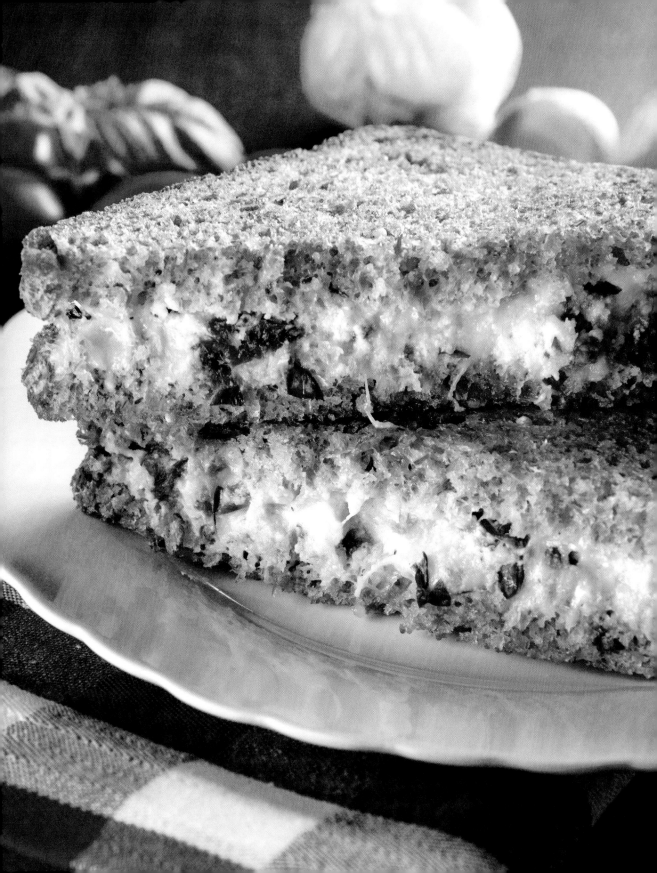

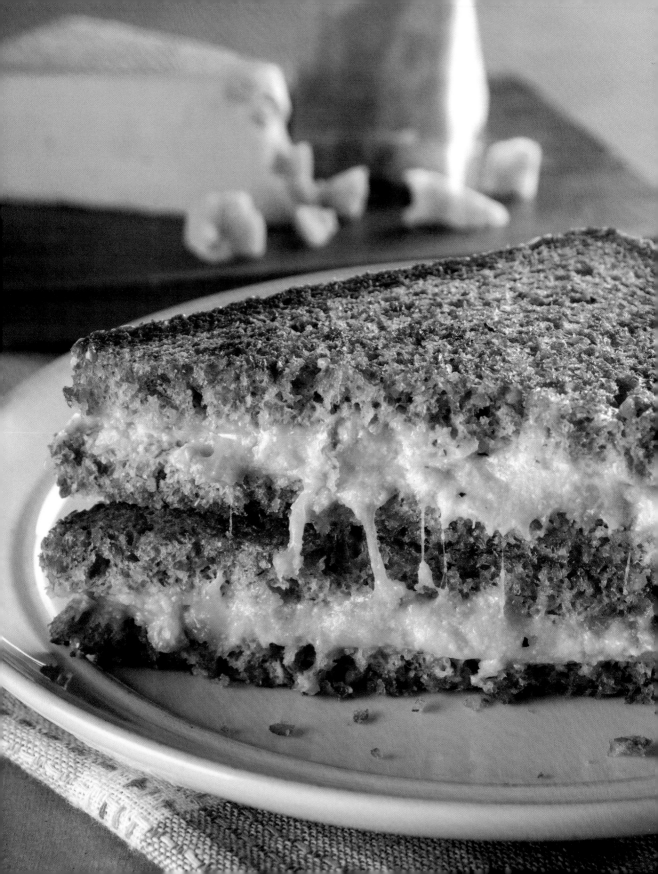

Easy-Peasy Grilled Cheesy

331 cal

  4 fantastic cheeses + 2 slices of toasty bread = a recipe for happiness!

2 tablespoons light/low-fat ricotta cheese

2 tablespoons shredded part-skim mozzarella cheese

2 tablespoons shredded reduced-fat cheddar cheese

2 tablespoons shredded reduced-fat Monterey or Colby Jack cheese

⅛ teaspoon garlic powder

Dash each salt and black pepper

2 slices whole-grain bread with 60 to 80 calories per slice

2 teaspoons whipped butter

Entire recipe: 331 calories, 15.5g total fat (8.5g sat fat), 735mg sodium, 30.5g carbs, 5.5g fiber, 5g sugars, 20g protein

You'll Need: small bowl, skillet, nonstick spray

Prep: 5 minutes • **Cook:** 5 minutes

1. In a small bowl, mix all ingredients *except* bread and butter.

2. Evenly top one bread slice with mixture. Top with remaining bread slice.

3. Spread the top of the sandwich with 1 teaspoon butter.

4. Bring a skillet sprayed with nonstick spray to medium heat. Place sandwich in the skillet, buttered side down.

5. Spread the top with remaining 1 teaspoon butter. Cook until bread is golden brown and cheese has melted, about 2 minutes per side, flipping carefully.

MAKES 1 SERVING

Chew on This . . .

A competitive eater in Texas once ate 13 grilled cheese sandwiches in just 60 seconds. That is completely unnecessary!

Sloppy Jane Lettuce Cups

192 cal

GF Who needs an oversized carby bun? Enjoy sloppy joe goodness served in crispy lettuce leaves!

1¼ cups canned crushed tomatoes

2 tablespoons tomato paste

1 tablespoon honey

1 tablespoon red wine vinegar

2 teaspoons molasses

1 pound raw extra-lean ground beef (4% fat or less)

¼ teaspoon each salt and black pepper

1 cup chopped onion

1 cup chopped red bell pepper

1 tablespoon apple cider vinegar

10 large iceberg or butter lettuce leaves

⅕th of recipe (2 lettuce cups): 192 calories, 4g total fat (1.5g sat fat), 309mg sodium, 17g carbs, 3g fiber, 11g sugars, 21g protein

You'll Need: medium bowl, large skillet, nonstick spray
Prep: 15 minutes • **Cook:** 20 minutes

1. In a medium bowl, combine crushed tomatoes, tomato paste, honey, red wine vinegar, and molasses. Mix until uniform.

2. Bring a large skillet sprayed with nonstick spray to medium-high heat. Add beef, and sprinkle with salt and black pepper. Cook and crumble for about 5 minutes, until mostly cooked.

3. Reduce heat to medium. Add onion, bell pepper, and apple cider vinegar. Cook, stir, and crumble for about 6 minutes, until beef is fully cooked and veggies have softened.

4. Reduce heat to low. Add tomato mixture. Cook and stir until hot, about 5 minutes.

5. Let cool slightly. Evenly distribute mixture among lettuce leaves, about ⅓ cup each.

MAKES 5 SERVINGS

Chew on This . . .

Sloppy joes have also been called slush burgers and yip yips. (I briefly considered calling this recipe Yip Yip Slush Cups, but I went with Sloppy Jane Lettuce Cups instead!)

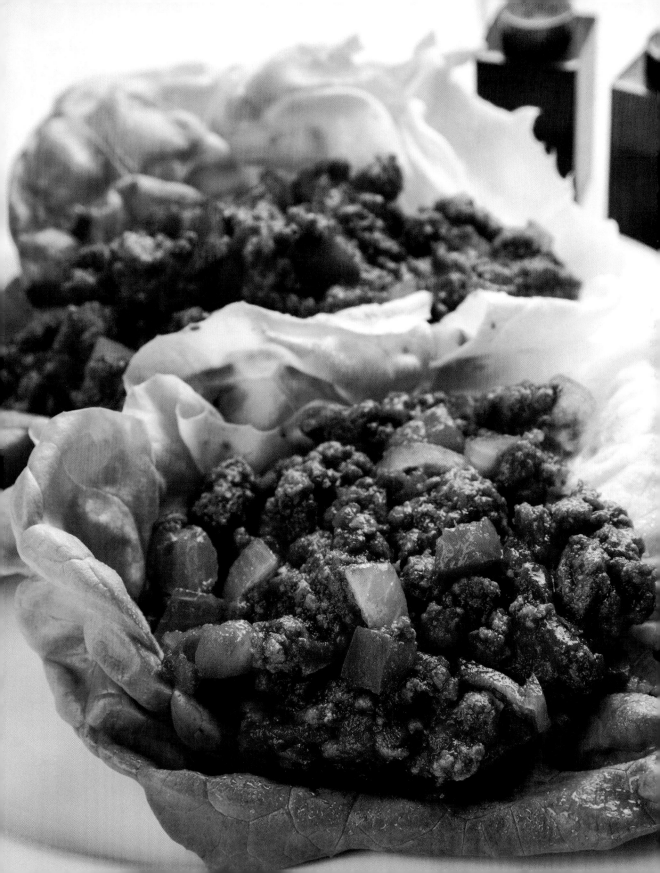

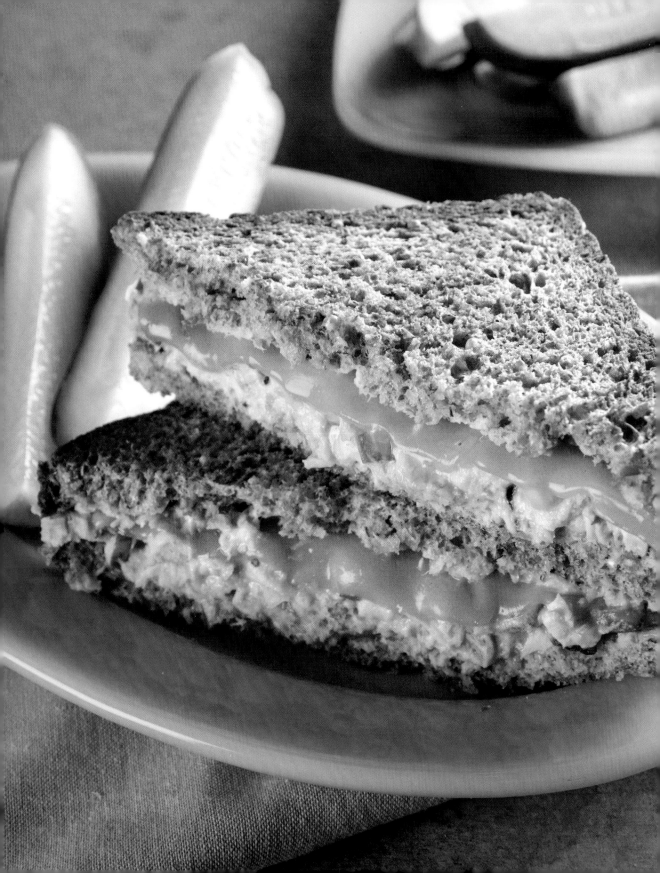

Looney Tuna Mega Melt

335 cal

15m This toasty HG makeover has all the flavor but less than half the calories of the original. Success!

2 slices whole-grain bread with 60 to 80 calories per slice

One 2.6-ounce pouch albacore tuna in water, thoroughly drained and flaked

2 tablespoons finely chopped cucumber

1 tablespoon finely chopped onion

1 tablespoon light mayonnaise

1 teaspoon Dijon mustard

⅛ teaspoon garlic powder

⅛ teaspoon onion powder

Dash black pepper

1 slice reduced-fat cheddar cheese

Entire recipe: 335 calories, 11.5g total fat (3.5g sat fat), 749mg sodium, 31.5g carbs, 5.5g fiber, 5.5g sugars, 28.5g protein

You'll Need: baking sheet, medium bowl

Prep: 5 minutes • **Cook:** 10 minutes

1. Preheat oven to 450 degrees.

2. Lightly toast bread, and lay on a baking sheet.

3. In a medium bowl, mix all remaining ingredients *except* cheese.

4. Evenly top one bread slice with the tuna mixture. Top with cheese and the other bread slice.

5. Bake until bread is fully toasted and cheese has melted, about 5 minutes.

MAKES 1 SERVING

Chew on This . . .

Tuna is one of the most consumed types of fish in America, and the classic tuna melt is super popular. But the average tuna melt clocks in at approximately 800 calories!

So Money Honey Mustard Chicken Nuggets

219 cal

 5i **30m** These sweet 'n savory bites are not only delicious, but also healthy. Clucky you!

¼ cup whole-wheat panko breadcrumbs

½ teaspoon onion powder

½ teaspoon garlic powder

⅛ teaspoon each salt and black pepper

2 tablespoons Dijon mustard

1 tablespoon honey

8 ounces raw boneless skinless chicken breast, cut into 10 nuggets

½ of recipe (5 nuggets): 219 calories, 3g total fat (0.5g sat fat), 517mg sodium, 16.5g carbs, 1g fiber, 9.5g sugars, 26.5g protein

You'll Need: baking sheet, nonstick spray, 2 wide bowls
Prep: 10 minutes • **Cook:** 20 minutes

1. Preheat oven to 375 degrees. Spray a baking sheet with nonstick spray.

2. In a wide bowl, mix breadcrumbs with seasonings.

3. In another wide bowl, thoroughly mix mustard with honey.

4. Add chicken to mustard mixture, and toss to coat.

5. One at a time, shake chicken nuggets to remove excess mustard mixture, and coat with seasoned crumbs.

6. Evenly place nuggets on the baking sheet, and top with any remaining seasoned crumbs. Bake for 8 minutes.

7. Flip chicken. Bake until lightly browned and crispy, 8 to 10 minutes.

MAKES 2 SERVINGS

HG Tip

Mix up some extra honey mustard (1 part honey to 2 parts mustard) to use as dipping sauce!

Chew on This . . .

Chicken nuggets have been enjoyed in America since the '50s, but many varieties contain lots of oil and questionable ingredients. (Not these!)

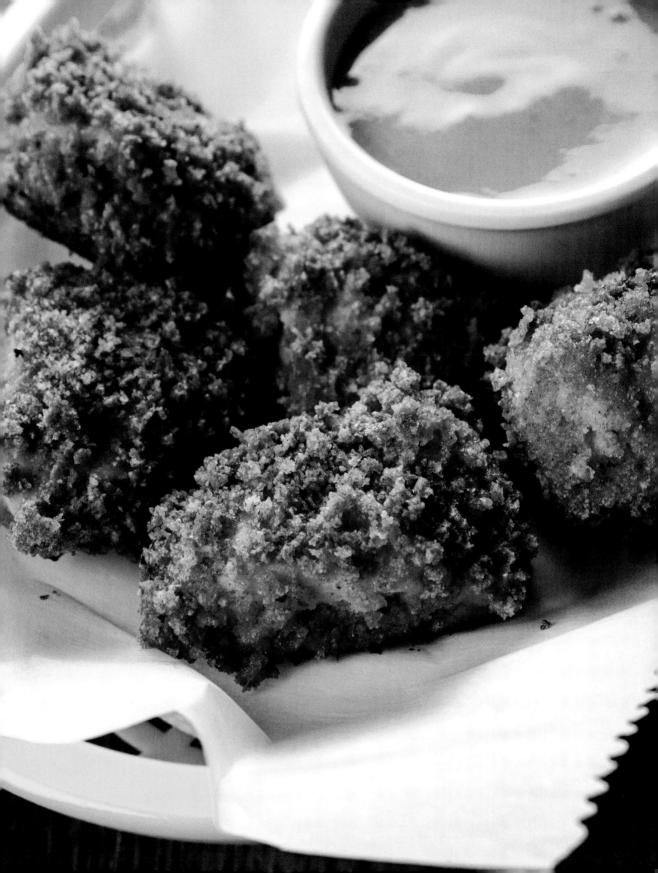

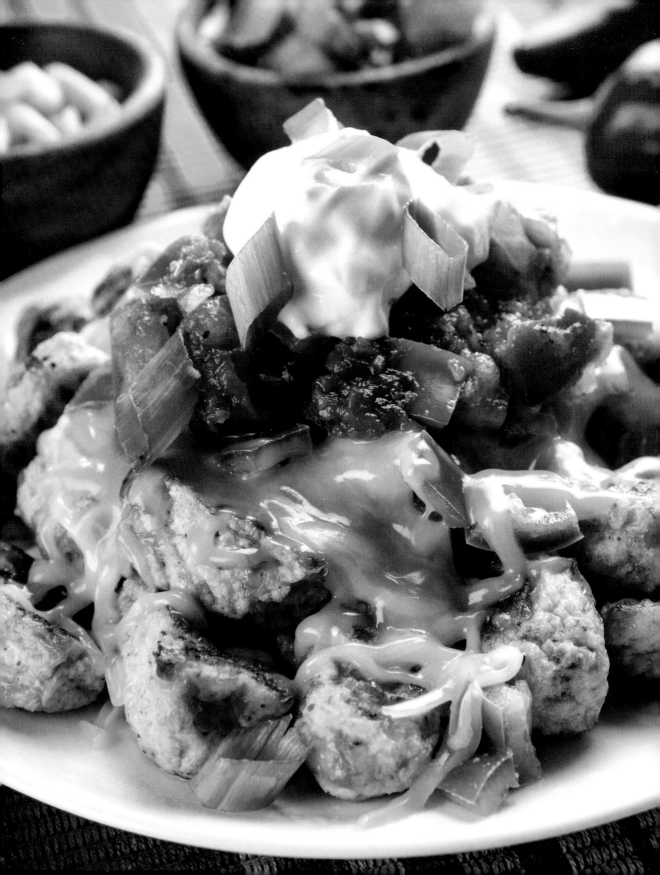

Tater Tot-chos

210 cal

V Traditional tots are made with potatoes; nachos are typically made with corn chips. My Tater Tot-chos are made with CAULIFLOWER! And don't miss the Reconstructed Nachos on page 262!

2 cups roughly chopped cauliflower

¼ cup egg whites (about 2 large eggs' worth)

¼ cup whole-wheat panko breadcrumbs

1 tablespoon grated Parmesan cheese

¼ teaspoon garlic powder

¼ teaspoon onion powder

¼ teaspoon ground cumin

¼ teaspoon salt

⅛ teaspoon black pepper

⅛ teaspoon chili powder

½ cup shredded reduced-fat Mexican-blend cheese

2 tablespoons seeded and chopped jalapeño peppers

¼ cup Clean & Hungry Salsa (recipe and store-bought alternatives on page 334)

2 tablespoons light sour cream

2 tablespoons chopped scallions

½ of recipe (14 tots): 210 calories, 9g total fat (5g sat fat), 768mg sodium, 17.5g carbs, 4g fiber, 6g sugars, 16.5g protein

You'll Need: baking sheet, parchment paper, food processor, large microwave-safe bowl, fine-mesh strainer, clean dish towel (or paper towels)

Prep: 20 minutes • **Cook:** 30 minutes • **Cool:** 10 minutes

1. Preheat oven to 400 degrees. Line a baking sheet with parchment paper.

2. Pulse cauliflower in a food processor until reduced to the consistency of coarse breadcrumbs.

3. Place cauliflower crumbs in a large microwave-safe bowl; cover and microwave for 2 minutes.

4. Uncover and stir. Re-cover and microwave for another 2 minutes, or until hot and soft.

5. Transfer to a fine-mesh strainer to drain. Let cool for 10 minutes, or until cool enough to handle.

6. Using a clean dish towel (or paper towels), firmly press out as much liquid as possible—there will be a lot.

7. Return cauliflower crumbs to the large bowl. Add egg whites, breadcrumbs, Parm, and seasonings. Add 2 tablespoons Mexican-blend cheese, and mix thoroughly.

8. Firmly and evenly form mixture into 28 tots, each about 1 inch long, ½ inch wide, and ½ inch thick.

9. Evenly lay tots on the baking sheet. Bake for 10 minutes.

10. Carefully flip. Bake until golden brown and crispy, 10 to 12 minutes.

11. Arrange tots on the center of the sheet, so they are touching. Sprinkle with remaining 6 tablespoons Mexican-blend cheese, and top with jalapeño peppers.

12. Bake until cheese has melted, about 3 minutes.

13. Serve topped with salsa, sour cream, and scallions.

MAKES 2 SERVINGS

Fully Loaded Tater Tots

185 cal

V These Fully Loaded Tater Tots are loaded up on the inside as opposed to being topped or smothered . . . Neatness counts!

2 cups roughly chopped cauliflower

½ cup shredded reduced-fat cheddar cheese

¼ cup finely chopped scallions

¼ cup egg whites (about 2 large eggs' worth)

¼ cup whole-wheat panko breadcrumbs

2 tablespoons light sour cream

¼ teaspoon garlic powder

¼ teaspoon onion powder

¼ teaspoon salt

⅛ teaspoon black pepper

Optional dip: additional light sour cream

½ of recipe (14 tots): 185 calories, 7.5g total fat (4.5g sat fat), 612mg sodium, 15.5g carbs, 3.5g fiber, 4.5g sugars, 14.5g protein

You'll Need: baking sheet, parchment paper, food processor, large microwave-safe bowl, fine-mesh strainer, clean dish towel (or paper towels)
Prep: 25 minutes • **Cook:** 30 minutes • **Cool:** 10 minutes

1. Preheat oven to 400 degrees. Line a baking sheet with parchment paper.

2. Pulse cauliflower in a food processor until reduced to the consistency of coarse breadcrumbs.

3. Place cauliflower crumbs in a large microwave-safe bowl; cover and microwave for 2 minutes.

4. Uncover and stir. Re-cover and microwave for another 2 minutes, or until hot and soft.

5. Transfer to a fine-mesh strainer to drain. Let cool for 10 minutes, or until cool enough to handle.

6. Using a clean dish towel (or paper towels), firmly press out as much liquid as possible—there will be a lot.

7. Return cauliflower crumbs to the large bowl. Add remaining ingredients. Mix thoroughly.

8. Firmly and evenly form mixture into 28 tots, each about 1 inch long, ½ inch wide, and ½ inch thick.

9. Place tots on the baking sheet, evenly spaced. Bake for 10 minutes.

10. Carefully flip. Bake until golden brown and crispy, 10 to 12 minutes.

MAKES 2 SERVINGS

Chew on This . . .

The frozen food company known for tater tots, Ore-Ida, originally set out to add French fries to its corn business. Rather than discard the leftover scraps of potato, the brand turned 'em into tots! I, for one, am incredibly grateful.

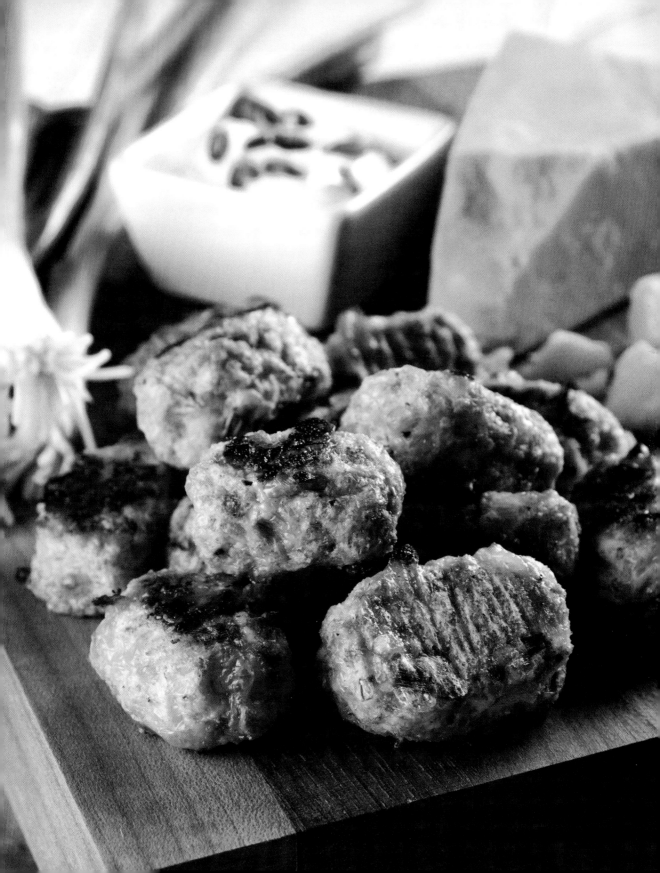

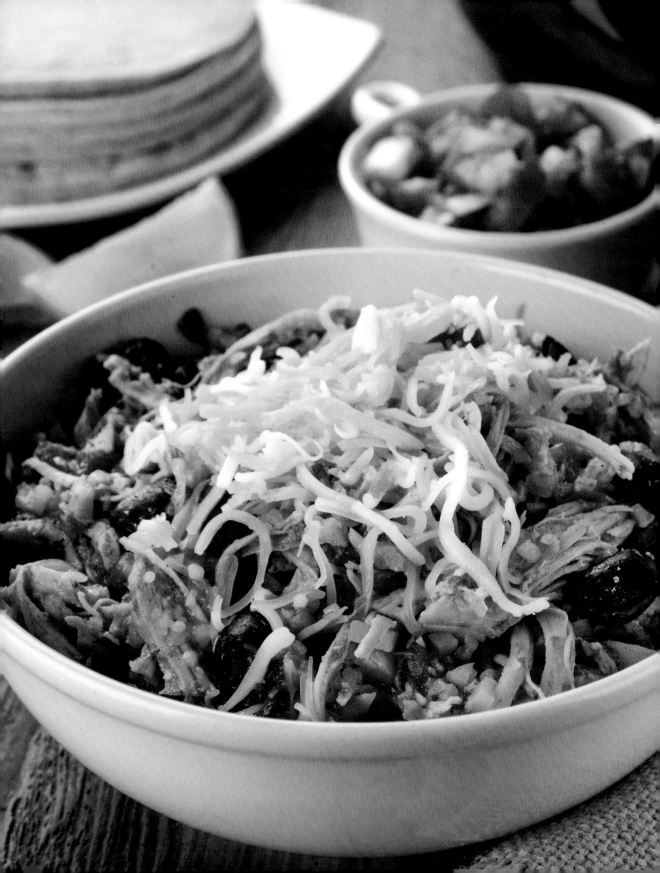

8

Mmmmm, Mexican!

I've read that a whopping 74 percent of Americans reach for Mexican food monthly. In fact, recent fast-food analysis shows that Mexican food has actually been making the biggest gains over other food types! The bummer is that a meal at a Mexican restaurant can easily exceed 1,000 calories. This chapter offers ten spectacular options under 375 calories a pop . . .

Tiki Time
BBQ Chicken Tacos

GF Skip the fried shells and fatty beef, and enjoy these fruity 'n saucy soft chicken tacos! (For an a.m. taco fix, check out the Rise & Shine Breakfast Tacos on page 29.)

¾ **cup finely chopped pineapple**

8 ounces raw boneless skinless chicken breast

⅛ **teaspoon each salt and black pepper**

½ **cup chopped red onion**

¼ **cup chopped fresh cilantro**

1 tablespoon seeded and finely chopped jalapeño pepper

1½ **teaspoons plain rice vinegar**

2 tablespoons Clean & Hungry BBQ Sauce (recipe and store-bought alternatives on page 335)

½ **teaspoon chili powder**

Four 6-inch corn tortillas

½ **of recipe (2 tacos):** 302 calories, 4.5g total fat (0.5g sat fat), 293mg sodium, 36g carbs, 4.5g fiber, 11g sugars, 28.5g protein

You'll Need: heavy-duty foil, baking sheet, nonstick spray, meat mallet, medium bowl, medium-large bowl, microwave-safe plate

Prep: 15 minutes • **Cook:** 30 minutes

1. Preheat oven to 375 degrees. Lay a large piece of heavy-duty foil on a baking sheet, and spray with nonstick spray.

2. Place pineapple on the center of the foil.

3. Pound chicken to ½-inch thickness. Sprinkle with salt and black pepper, and place over pineapple.

4. Cover with another large piece of foil. Fold together and seal all four edges of the foil pieces, forming a well-sealed packet.

5. Bake for 25 minutes, or until chicken is cooked through.

6. Meanwhile, in a medium bowl, mix onion, cilantro, jalapeño pepper, and vinegar.

7. Cut packet to release hot steam before opening entirely.

8. Transfer chicken to a medium-large bowl. Shred with two forks.

9. Add cooked pineapple, BBQ sauce, and chili powder to the chicken. Mix well.

10. On a microwave-safe plate, microwave tortillas for 30 seconds, or until warm.

11. Evenly distribute chicken mixture among the tortillas, and top with onion mixture.

MAKES 2 SERVINGS

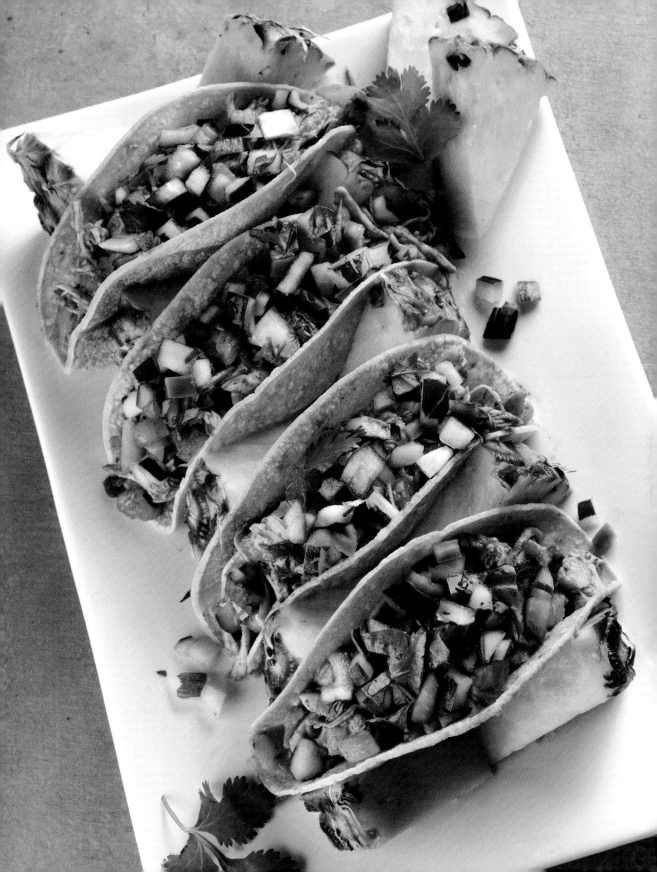

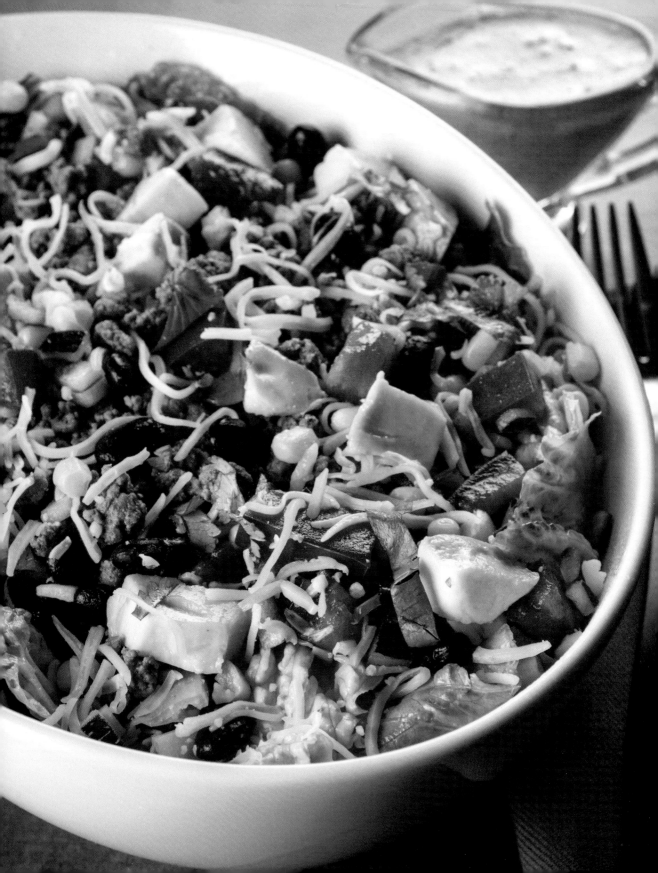

Mexicali Madness Chopped Salad

370 cal

30m **GF** Obsession confession: I am completely obsessed with chopped salads! This one is a total calorie bargain and extremely filling. And the dressing is incredible!

DRESSING

3 tablespoons fat-free plain Greek yogurt

1 tablespoon fat-free milk

1 tablespoon chopped fresh cilantro

1½ teaspoons plain rice vinegar

1 teaspoon honey

⅛ teaspoon ground cumin

⅛ teaspoon chili powder

Dash salt

SALAD

3 cups chopped romaine lettuce

4 ounces raw extra-lean ground beef (4% fat or less)

⅛ teaspoon ground cumin

⅛ teaspoon chili powder

⅛ teaspoon each salt and black pepper

2 tablespoons canned black beans, drained and rinsed

¼ cup chopped tomato

2 tablespoons finely chopped red onion

2 tablespoons frozen sweet corn kernels, thawed

2 tablespoons shredded reduced-fat Mexican-blend cheese

1 ounce (about 2 tablespoons) chopped avocado

1 tablespoon chopped fresh cilantro

Entire recipe: 370 calories, 12.5g total fat (4.5g sat fat), 749mg sodium, 29g carbs, 8g fiber, 13g sugars, 37g protein

You'll Need: small bowl, large plate or large bowl, skillet, nonstick spray
Prep: 20 minutes • **Cook:** 5 minutes

1. In a small bowl, mix dressing ingredients.

2. Place lettuce on a large plate or in a large bowl.

3. Bring a skillet sprayed with nonstick spray to medium-high heat. Add beef, and sprinkle with seasonings. Cook and crumble for about 3 minutes, until fully cooked.

4. Reduce heat to low. Add beans, and cook and stir until hot and well mixed, about 1 minute.

5. Add beef mixture to the large bowl. Top with remaining ingredients.

6. Drizzle with dressing, or serve it on the side.

MAKES 1 SERVING

Chew on This...

Think it's smart to order salad at a Mexican restaurant? Think about this: A taco salad usually has at least 900 calories! (The beef, the cheese, the dressing, that shell?! It adds up!)

Slow-Cooker Chicken Burrito Bonanza

GF The great thing about this dish is that there are so many ways to enjoy it. On a salad, in a tortilla (HG recipe on page 196), in lettuce cups . . . even stuffed inside an egg-white omelette for breakfast!

1½ pounds raw boneless skinless chicken breast

¼ teaspoon black pepper

½ teaspoon salt

1 cup chopped onion

One 15-ounce can black beans, drained and rinsed

One 14.5-ounce can diced tomatoes, drained

One 4-ounce can diced green chiles, drained

1½ cups reduced-sodium chicken broth

1 tablespoon chili powder

1 tablespoon ground cumin

½ teaspoon onion powder

½ teaspoon garlic powder

½ teaspoon paprika

4 cups cauliflower rice/crumbles

½ cup shredded reduced-fat Mexican-blend cheese

Optional seasonings: additional salt and black pepper

⅛th of recipe (about 1 cup): 214 calories, 4.5g total fat (1.5g sat fat), 640mg sodium, 18g carbs, 5.5g fiber, 4.5g sugars, 26g protein

You'll Need: slow cooker, large bowl, slotted spoon

Prep: 15 minutes

Cook: 3 to 4 hours or 7 to 8 hours, plus 55 minutes

1. Place chicken in a slow cooker, and season with pepper and ¼ teaspoon salt. Top with onion, beans, tomatoes, and chiles.

2. Add broth and seasonings, including remaining ¼ teaspoon salt. Gently stir.

3. Cover and cook on high for 3 to 4 hours or on low for 7 to 8 hours, until chicken is fully cooked.

4. Transfer chicken to a large bowl. Shred with two forks.

5. Return shredded chicken to the slow cooker, and mix well.

6. Add cauliflower rice/crumbles, and stir to mix.

7. If cooking on low heat, increase heat to high. Cover and cook for 55 minutes, or until cauliflower is tender.

8. Serve with a slotted spoon, draining the liquid. Top each serving with 1 tablespoon cheese.

MAKES 8 SERVINGS

Need-to-Know Info

Use store-bought cauliflower crumbles/rice, or DIY! See page 346 for the 411.

Chew on This . . .

"Burrito" is Spanish for "little donkey." That's adorable, but Slow-Cooker Chicken Little Donkey Bonanza would be a weird and confusing name for this recipe!

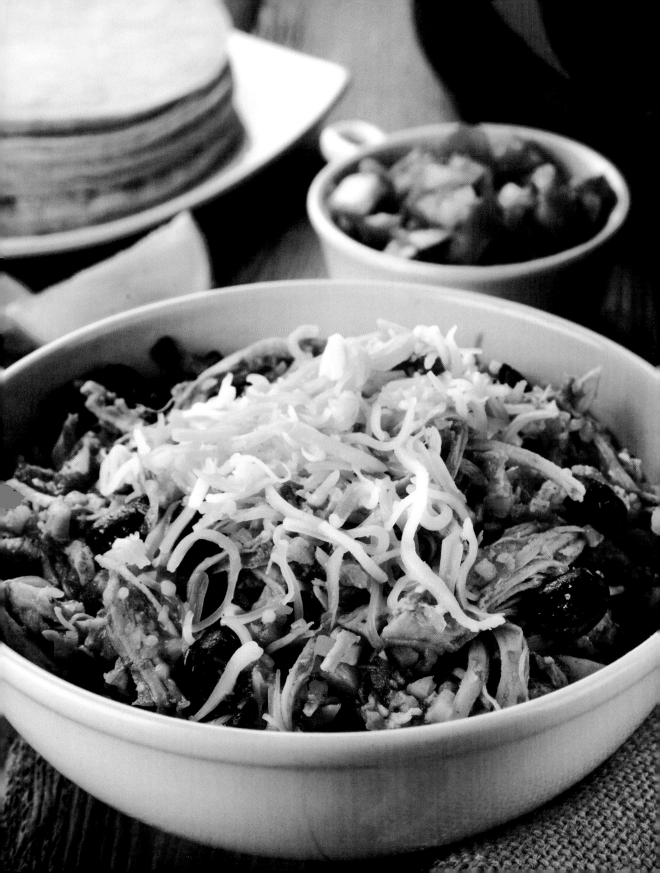

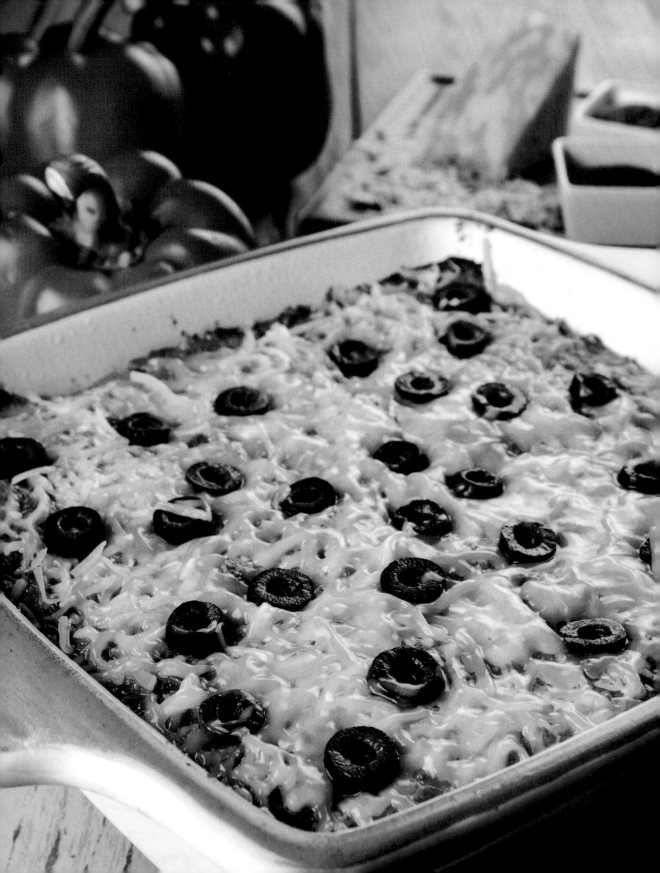

Mexilicious Spaghetti Squash Casserole

330 cal

GF Americans love Mexican food. Americans love casseroles. So it stands to reason that Americans will have major love for this Mexilicious casserole! I sure do. So much flavor, and the portion size is HUGE. Pssst . . . More spaghetti-squash recipes await on page 363!

5 cups cooked spaghetti squash, drained of excess moisture

1 pound raw extra-lean ground beef (4% fat or less)

2½ teaspoons chili powder

2 teaspoons ground cumin

¼ teaspoon onion powder

¼ teaspoon garlic powder

¼ teaspoon paprika

¼ teaspoon each salt and black pepper

½ cup chopped bell pepper

½ cup chopped onion

2 cups canned crushed tomatoes

½ cup egg whites (about 4 large eggs' worth)

½ cup shredded reduced-fat Mexican-blend cheese

¼ cup sliced black olives

¼th of casserole: 330 calories, 9.5g total fat (4g sat fat), 738mg sodium, 26.5g carbs, 6.5g fiber, 10.5g sugars, 34g protein

You'll need: 8-inch by 8-inch baking pan, nonstick spray, large bowl, large skillet

Prep: 15 minutes • **Cook:** 45 minutes • **Cool:** 10 minutes

Plus prep and cook times for spaghetti squash (page 350) if not made in advance.

1. Preheat oven to 400 degrees. Spray an 8-inch by 8-inch baking pan with nonstick spray.

2. Place spaghetti squash in a large bowl.

3. Bring a large skillet sprayed with nonstick spray to medium-high heat. Add beef, and sprinkle with 1 teaspoon chili powder, 1 teaspoon cumin, and ⅛ teaspoon each of the remaining seasonings. Cook and crumble for about 5 minutes, until mostly cooked.

4. Add bell pepper and onion to the skillet. Cook and stir for about 4 minutes, until beef is fully cooked and veggies have softened. Transfer to the large bowl.

5. Add canned crushed tomatoes, egg whites, and remaining 1½ teaspoons chili powder, 1 teaspoon cumin, and ⅛ teaspoon each of the remaining seasonings. Mix thoroughly.

6. Transfer mixture to the baking pan, and smooth out the top. Bake until slightly firm, about 25 minutes.

7. Sprinkle with cheese and olives. Bake until cheese has melted and lightly browned, about 10 minutes.

8. Let stand for 10 minutes before slicing.

MAKES 4 SERVINGS

Chew on This . . .

In other parts of the world, squash is often made into candy. Guess they love squash even more than we do!

Clean & Hungry Whole-Wheat Tortillas

78 cal

5i 30m V   It's SO easy to make your own tortillas . . . Try it and see! Then use 'em to make lean 'n clean burritos, wraps, and quesadillas (like the recipe on the next page!). These are also essential for page 218's moo shu.

¾ cup egg whites (about 6 large eggs' worth)

½ cup whole-wheat flour

½ teaspoon baking powder

¼ teaspoon each salt and black pepper

Store-Bought Alternatives

I've got to be honest: It's hard to find clean tortillas that are low in calories. My top pick? La Tortilla Factory Whole Wheat Organic Tortillas, with 100 calories each.

¼th of recipe (1 tortilla): 78 calories, 0.5g total fat (0g sat fat), 280mg sodium, 12g carbs, 2g fiber, 0.5g sugars, 7g protein

You'll Need: blender or food processor, large skillet, nonstick spray, offset spatula or flexible rubber spatula

Prep: 10 minutes • **Cook:** 15 minutes

1. Place all ingredients in a blender or food processor. Add ½ cup water, and blend until uniform.

2. Bring a large skillet sprayed with nonstick spray to medium heat. Pour ¼th of the batter (about ½ cup) into the skillet, quickly tilting the skillet in all directions to evenly distribute.

3. Cook until edges are firm and bottom is lightly browned, about 2 minutes.

4. Carefully flip with an offset spatula or flexible rubber spatula.

5. Cook until lightly browned on the other side, about 1 minute.

6. Repeat three times to make three more tortillas. If needed, remove skillet from heat and re-spray after making each tortilla.

7. Let cool. Cover and refrigerate until ready to use.

MAKES 4 SERVINGS

Freeze It: Tortilla Edition

To Freeze: Stack them with a layer of wax paper in between each tortilla. Place them in a freezer bag, seal, and lay flat in the freezer.

To Thaw: Place one tortilla between 2 damp paper towels on a microwave-safe plate. Microwave for 30 seconds, or until thawed.

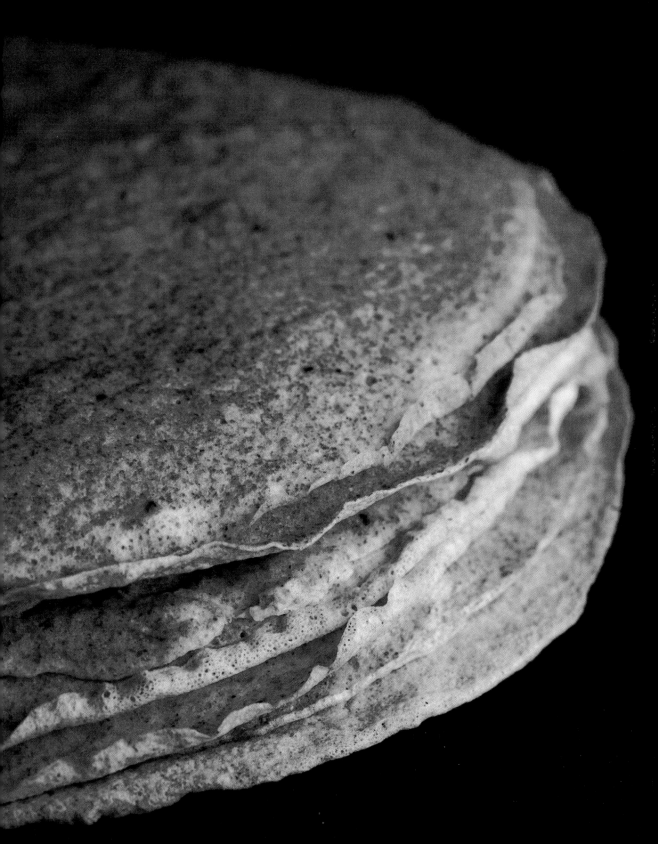

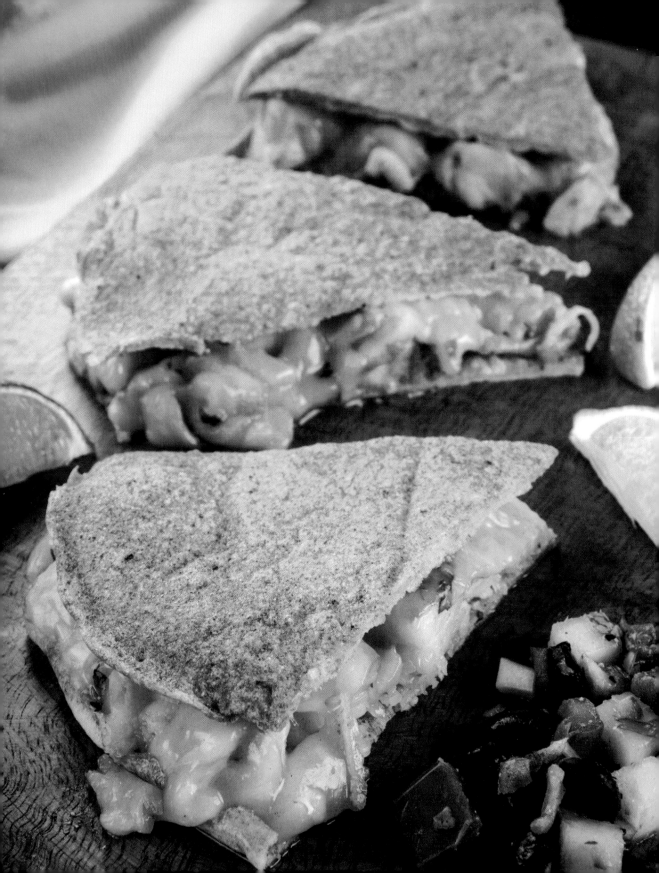

Blackened Better-Than-Ever Shrimp Quesadillas

239 cal

5i **30m** Ah, the quesadilla. Mexico's grilled cheese! While many quesadilla recipes have come out of the Hungryland kitchen over the years, this may actually be the BEST one ever. Wanna go all out? Top it off with some Best in the Southwest Guac Dip (page 269). Insanity!

¼ teaspoon garlic powder

¼ teaspoon onion powder

⅛ teaspoon paprika

Dash cayenne pepper

Dash ground cumin

Dash each salt and black pepper

6 ounces (about 12) raw large shrimp, peeled, tails removed, deveined

2 Clean & Hungry Whole-Wheat Tortillas (recipe and store-bought alternatives on page 196)

½ cup shredded reduced-fat Mexican blend cheese

1 tablespoon chopped fresh cilantro

Optional toppings: Clean & Hungry Salsa or Trop 'Til You Drop Island Salsa (recipes and store-bought alternatives on page 334 and 207), light sour cream

½ of recipe (3 wedges): 239 calories, 7g total fat (3.5g sat fat), 832mg sodium, 14g carbs, 2g fiber, 0.5g sugars, 29.5g protein

You'll Need: medium bowl, large skillet, nonstick spray
Prep: 10 minutes • **Cook:** 10 minutes

1. Mix seasonings in a medium bowl. Add shrimp, and toss to coat.

2. Bring a large skillet sprayed with nonstick spray to medium heat. Cook shrimp for 2 minutes.

3. Flip shrimp. Cook for about 2 more minutes, until cooked through and blackened.

4. Roughly chop shrimp.

5. Clean skillet. Re-spray, and return to medium heat. Lay a tortilla in the skillet, and sprinkle with ¼ cup cheese.

6. Top tortilla with chopped shrimp and cilantro. Sprinkle with remaining ¼ cup cheese, and top with remaining tortilla.

7. Cook until cheese has melted and tortillas have browned, 1 to 2 minutes per side, flipping carefully and pressing lightly to seal.

8. Cut into 6 wedges.

MAKES 2 SERVINGS

Outside-In Chicken Enchiladas

270 cal

GF   Who needs tortillas? These unique high-protein enchiladas deliver an explosion of enchilada flavor into your face!

SAUCE

1 cup canned crushed tomatoes

2 tablespoons chopped fresh cilantro

1 teaspoon chili powder

½ teaspoon garlic powder

½ teaspoon onion powder

¼ teaspoon ground cumin

⅛ teaspoon salt

ENCHILADAS

½ cup refried beans

¼ teaspoon chili powder

½ teaspoon ground cumin

¼ teaspoon salt

½ cup shredded reduced-fat Mexican blend cheese

Four 5-ounce raw boneless skinless chicken breast cutlets

⅛ teaspoon black pepper

¼ cup chopped scallions

Optional toppings: sliced black olives, fresh cilantro

¼th of recipe (1 enchilada): 270 calories, 7g total fat (2.5g sat fat), 645mg sodium, 11g carbs, 3g fiber, 2.5g sugars, 38.5g protein

You'll Need: 8-inch by 8-inch baking pan, nonstick spray, 2 medium bowls, meat mallet, toothpicks, foil

Prep: 20 minutes • **Cook:** 25 minutes

1. Preheat oven to 400 degrees. Spray an 8-inch by 8-inch baking pan with nonstick spray.

2. In a medium bowl, mix sauce ingredients.

3. Place beans in another medium bowl. Add chili powder, ¼ teaspoon cumin, and ⅛ teaspoon salt. Mix well. Stir in ¼ cup cheese.

4. Pound chicken to ½-inch thickness. Season with pepper, remaining ¼ teaspoon cumin, and remaining ⅛ teaspoon salt.

5. Evenly distribute bean mixture among the chicken cutlets. Carefully roll up each chicken cutlet over the mixture. Secure with toothpicks.

6. Place cutlets in the baking pan. Top with sauce and remaining ¼ cup cheese.

7. Cover pan with foil. Bake for 25 minutes, or until chicken is cooked through and cheese has melted.

8. Top with scallions.

MAKES 4 SERVINGS

Chew on This...

Enchiladas first appeared in print wayyyy back in 1831, where they were featured in the first Mexican cookbook.

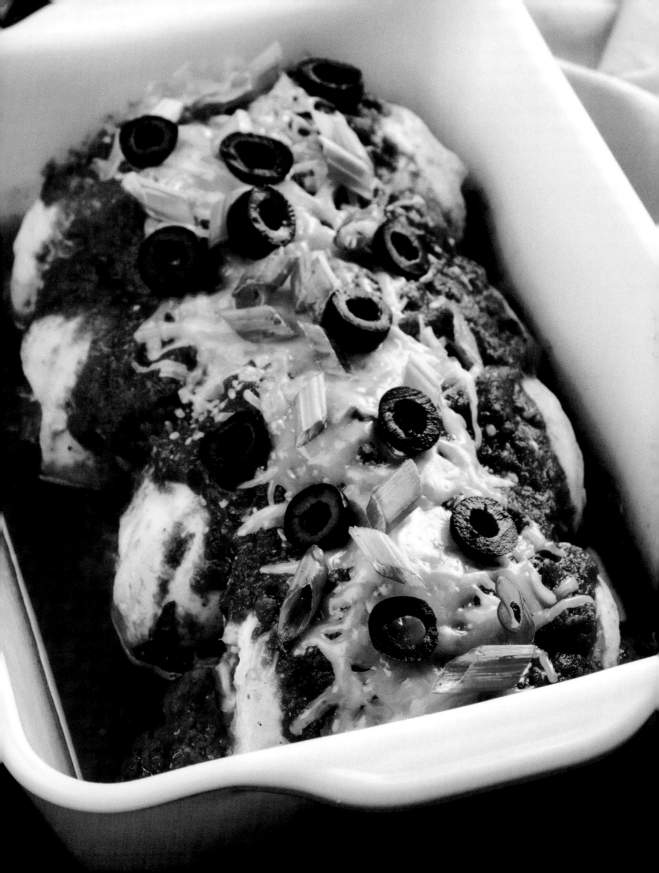

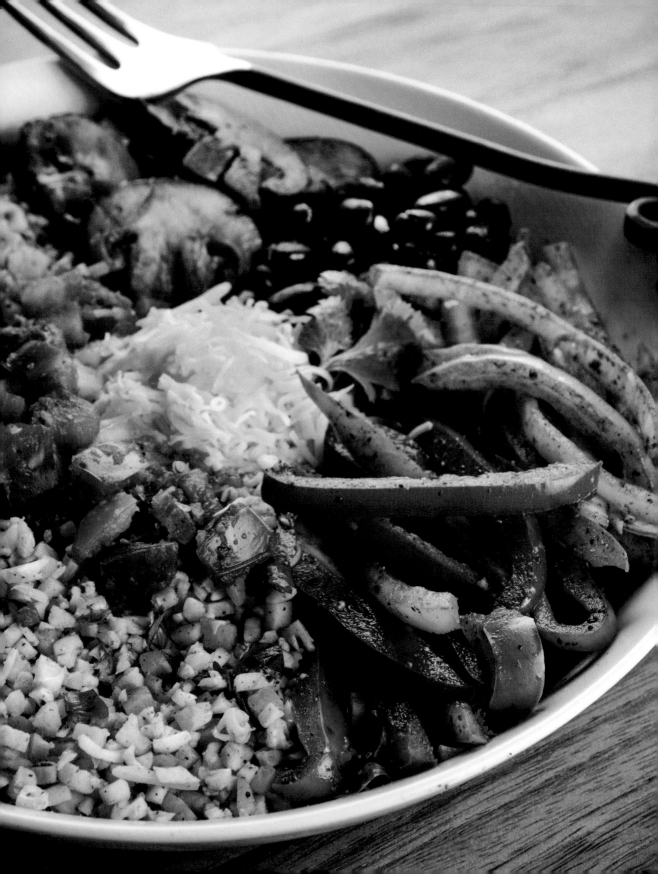

Need a Fajita Veggie Rice Bowl

269 cal

🕐 30m Ⓥ GF Obsession confession: The only time I eat real rice is with sushi—and in limited quantities. Why waste all those carby calories when you can have cauliflower rice!? For more cauliflower-rice creations, flip to page 362.

2 cups cauliflower rice/crumbles

1 teaspoon chopped garlic

⅛ teaspoon each salt and black pepper

¾ teaspoon chili powder

½ teaspoon ground cumin

¼ teaspoon paprika

2 tablespoons chopped fresh cilantro

½ cup sliced onion

½ cup sliced mushrooms

¼ cup sliced red bell pepper

¼ cup sliced green bell pepper

⅓ cup canned black beans, drained and rinsed

3 tablespoons shredded reduced-fat Mexican-blend cheese

2 tablespoons Clean & Hungry Salsa (recipe and store-bought alternatives on page 334)

Optional topping: light sour cream

Entire recipe: 269 calories, 6g total fat (3g sat fat), 863mg sodium, 41.5g carbs, 13.5g fiber, 12g sugars, 18g protein

You'll Need: skillet, nonstick spray, medium-large bowl

Prep: 10 minutes • **Cook:** 15 minutes

1. Bring a skillet sprayed with nonstick spray to medium-high heat. Add cauliflower rice/crumbles, chopped garlic, salt, black pepper, ½ teaspoon chili powder, ¼ teaspoon cumin, and ⅛ teaspoon paprika. Cook and stir until softened, about 5 minutes.

2. Transfer to a medium-large bowl. Stir in cilantro, and cover to keep warm.

3. Remove skillet from heat; clean, if needed. Re-spray, and return to medium-high heat. Add remaining veggies and remaining ¼ teaspoon chili powder, ¼ teaspoon cumin, and ⅛ teaspoon paprika. Cook and stir until mostly softened, about 4 minutes.

4. Reduce heat to low. Add beans, and cook and stir until hot, about 1 minute.

5. Transfer to the medium-large bowl, and top with cheese and salsa.

MAKES 1 SERVING

Chew on This . . .

The first fajitas were made from meat trimmings and given to Mexican cowboys as a form of payment. Talk about a hearty paycheck!

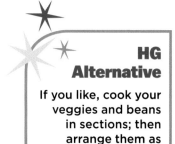

HG Alternative

If you like, cook your veggies and beans in sections; then arrange them as pictured!

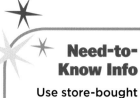

Need-to-Know Info

Use store-bought cauliflower crumbles/rice, or DIY! See page 346 for the 411.

Mexican Street Corn Obsession

188 cal

30m · **V** · **GF**   This dish seriously gave me the chills the first time I ate it—creamy, cheesy perfection! Bookmark this one . . . You'll want to make it again and again and again!

½ cup light mayonnaise

2 tablespoons fat-free plain Greek yogurt

1½ teaspoons honey

½ teaspoon ground cumin

½ teaspoon chili powder

¼ teaspoon salt

2 tablespoons chopped fresh cilantro

½ cup crumbled feta cheese

½ cup chopped red onion

4 cups frozen sweet corn kernels

Optional topping: additional fresh cilantro

Optional garnish: lime wedges

⅙th of recipe (about ⅔ cup): 188 calories, 8g total fat (2g sat fat), 382mg sodium, 25g carbs, 1.5g fiber, 7.5g sugars, 5g protein

You'll Need: medium bowl, large skillet with a lid, nonstick spray, large bowl

Prep: 15 minutes • **Cook:** 10 minutes

1. In a medium bowl, combine mayo, yogurt, honey, and seasonings. Mix until uniform.

2. Stir in cilantro and ¼ cup feta cheese.

3. Bring a large skillet sprayed with nonstick spray to medium-high heat. Cook onion until slightly softened, about 3 minutes.

4. Add corn and 2 tablespoons water to the skillet. Cover and cook for 2 minutes, or until corn has thawed and water has evaporated.

5. Uncover, and cook and stir until onion is soft and corn has blackened, about 6 minutes.

6. Transfer to a large bowl. Add mayo mixture, and stir to coat.

7. Top with remaining ¼ cup feta cheese.

MAKES 6 SERVINGS

Chew on This . . .

A cob of corn almost always has an even number of rows. Weird but true!

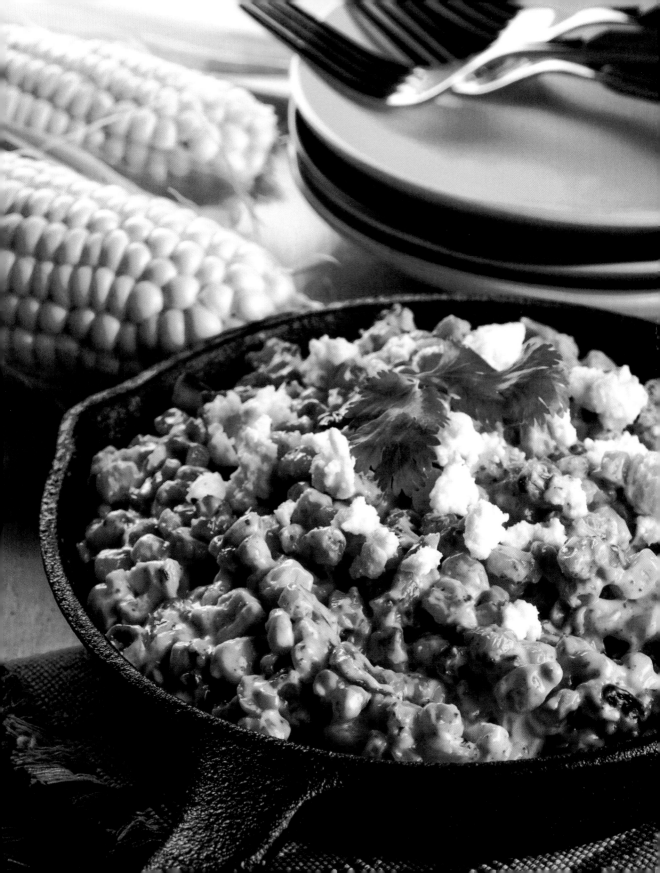

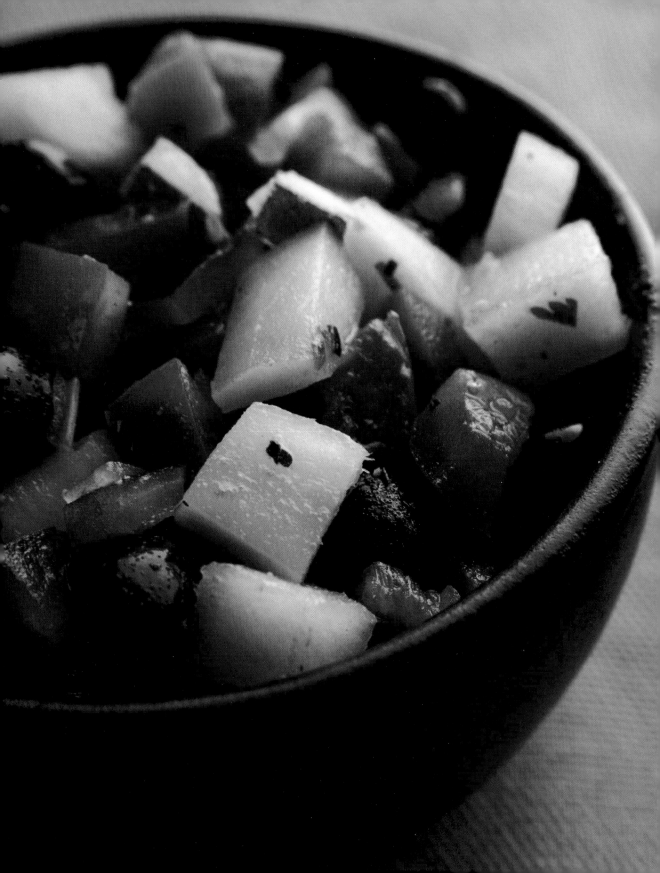

Trop 'Til You Drop Island Salsa

25 cal

15m **V** **GF**   This stuff is excellent over grilled chicken, on salad, with my Crispy Crunchy Tortilla Chips (page 265) . . . I'd even eat it straight from a spoon! P.S. Don't miss the Let's Get Tropical Guacamole on page 270!

½ cup chopped mango

½ cup canned black beans, drained and rinsed

⅓ cup seeded and chopped tomatoes

¼ cup finely chopped red onion

¼ cup finely chopped red bell pepper

1 tablespoon seeded and chopped jalapeño pepper

1 tablespoon chopped fresh cilantro

2 teaspoons lime juice

¼ teaspoon salt

⅛ teaspoon black pepper

⅛ teaspoon ground cumin

⅛th of recipe (about ¼ cup): 25 calories, 0g total fat (0g sat fat), 108mg sodium, 5.5g carbs, 1g fiber, 2g sugars, 1g protein

You'll Need: medium-large sealable container
Prep: 15 minutes

1. In a medium-large sealable container, combine all ingredients. Mix until uniform.
2. Seal, and refrigerate until ready to use.

MAKES 8 SERVINGS

Chew on This . . .

In the early '90s, salsa surpassed ketchup as America's most popular condiment. It's since lost its standing, but it's number one in my book!

Hungry for More Mexican Munchies?

Uno Huevo Ranchero (page 21) • That's Good Stuffed Breakfast Peppers (page 26)

Rise & Shine Breakfast Tacos (page 29) • Fully Loaded Dan-Good Chili (page 95)

Overflowing with Chili Acorn Squash (page 96) • Messy Mexican Skillet Pizza (page 122)

Gobble 'Em Up Fajita Burgers (page 154) • Tater Tot-chos (page 183)

Whoop, Whoop Tortilla Soup (page 242) • Reconstructed Nachos (page 262)

Crispy Crunchy Tortilla Chips (page 265) • Ultimate Ate-Layer Dip (page 266)

Best in the Southwest Guac Dip (page 269) • Let's Get Tropical Guacamole (page 270)

Clean & Hungry Salsa (page 334)

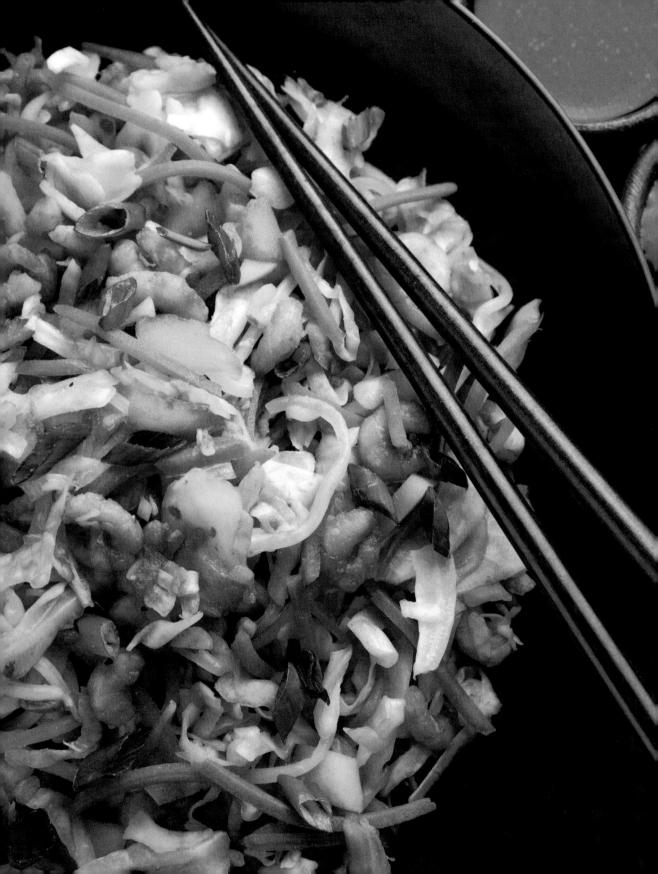

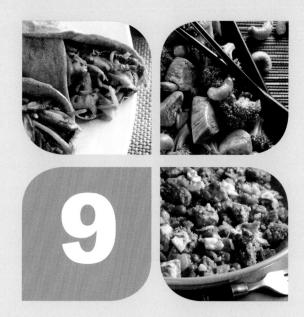

9

Chinese, Please!

Chinese food is super popular here in the States. Sources say more than three-quarters of us eat it at least once a month, and we have more Chinese restaurants here than McDonald's, Burger King, and KFC locations combined! But there's no need to spend extra calories (and a lot of money) on Chinese food, as it's often laden with too much oil and obscene amounts of carbs. Just whip up the incredible recipes on the pages that follow. They're super easy . . . I promise!

Saucy Sweet & Sour Chicken

 I absolutely love this dish. The pineapple juice and honey make it perfectly sweet & tangy!

One 16-ounce can pineapple chunks packed in juice (not drained)

2 tablespoons arrowroot powder

3 tablespoons plain rice vinegar

1 tablespoon honey

1 tablespoon reduced-sodium/lite soy sauce

1½ teaspoons tomato paste

½ teaspoon chopped garlic

⅛ teaspoon crushed red pepper

⅛ teaspoon ground ginger

1½ cups broccoli florets

1 cup chopped red bell pepper

1 cup chopped onion

1 pound raw boneless skinless chicken breast, cut into bite-sized pieces

¼ teaspoon each salt and black pepper

2 cups bean sprouts

¼th of recipe (about 1½ cups): 284 calories, 3g total fat (0.5g sat fat), 359mg sodium, 33.5g carbs, 4.5g fiber, 23.5g sugars, 29g protein

You'll Need: small bowl, extra-large skillet with a lid, nonstick spray, large bowl

Prep: 15 minutes • **Cook:** 20 minutes

1. To make the sauce, drain the juice from the pineapple into a small bowl. Add arrowroot powder, and stir to dissolve. Add vinegar, honey, soy sauce, tomato paste, garlic, crushed red pepper, and ginger. Mix until uniform.

2. Bring an extra-large skillet sprayed with nonstick spray to medium-high heat. Add broccoli, bell pepper, onion, and ¼ cup water. Cover and cook for 6 minutes, or until veggies are tender and water has evaporated. Transfer to a large bowl.

3. Remove skillet from heat. Re-spray, and return to medium-high heat. Add chicken, and sprinkle with salt and black pepper. Cook and stir for about 5 minutes, until cooked through.

4. Add bean sprouts, pineapple, cooked veggies, and sauce to the skillet. Cook and stir until sprouts have softened, sauce has thickened, and entire dish is hot and well mixed, about 4 minutes.

MAKES 4 SERVINGS

Gluten Alert

My Chinese food recipes call for soy sauce. Some soy sauce contains gluten. If you avoid gluten, check the ingredient lists. Or grab a product marked gluten-free.

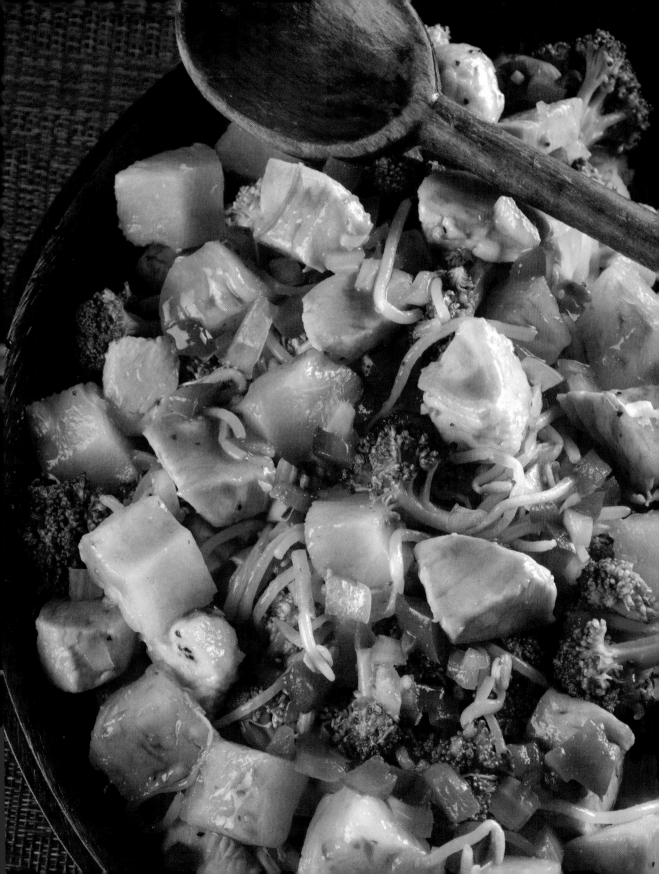

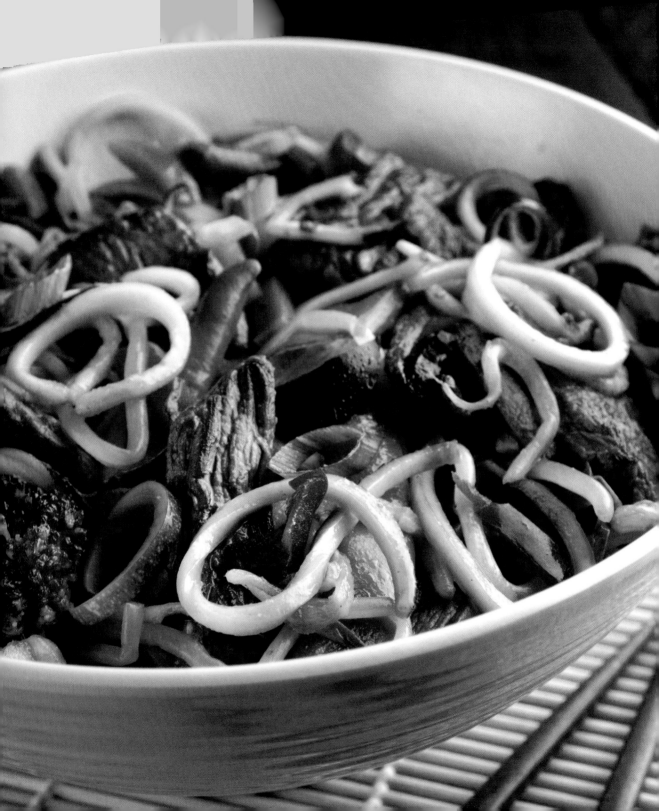

Beef Zucchini So Low Mein

302 cal

30m GF Using zucchini noodles to make lo mein is one of the smartest swaps to ever emerge from the HG kitchen! Beef fans will flip over this Chinese-food makeover.

2 tablespoons reduced-sodium/lite soy sauce

2 teaspoons honey

1 teaspoon sesame oil

½ teaspoon crushed garlic

½ teaspoon onion powder

1 cup frozen Asian-style stir-fry vegetables

1 cup bean sprouts

1 cup quartered mushrooms

1 pound spiralized zucchini (about 2 medium zucchini)

8 ounces thinly sliced raw flank steak

¼ teaspoon garlic powder

¼ cup chopped scallions

Need-to-Know Info

It's super easy to spiralize zucchini. Get the 411 on page 349!

HG Tip

Freeze your beef slightly before cutting it. This will make it easier to thinly slice.

½ of recipe (about 2 cups): 302 calories, 9.5g total fat (3g sat fat), 641mg sodium, 24g carbs, 5g fiber, 17g sugars, 32g protein

You'll Need: small bowl, extra-large skillet, nonstick spray, strainer

Prep: 15 minutes • **Cook:** 15 minutes

1. To make the sauce, in a small bowl, combine soy sauce, honey, oil, crushed garlic, and ¼ teaspoon onion powder. Mix until uniform.

2. Bring an extra-large skillet sprayed with nonstick spray to medium-high heat. Add frozen veggies, bean sprouts, and mushrooms. Cook and stir until frozen veggies are hot and fresh veggies have mostly softened, about 4 minutes.

3. Add zucchini to the skillet. Cook and stir until hot and slightly softened, about 3 minutes.

4. Transfer to a strainer, and thoroughly drain excess liquid.

5. Remove skillet from heat, re-spray, and return to medium-high heat. Add beef, and sprinkle with garlic powder and remaining ¼ teaspoon onion powder. Cook and stir for about 3 minutes, until mostly cooked.

6. Return drained veggies to the skillet, add scallions, and top with sauce. Cook and stir until sauce is evenly distributed and mostly absorbed and entire dish is hot and well mixed, about 2 minutes.

MAKES 2 SERVINGS

Chew on This...

An order of restaurant beef lo mein: 700+ calories. A heaping serving of HG beef lo mein: 302 calories. I win! (You win too, since you now have this recipe.)

Nuts About Cashew Chicken

30m **GF**   Cashews and chicken are one of the best couples of all time! This dish is amazing.

1 teaspoon arrowroot powder

2½ tablespoons reduced-sodium/lite soy sauce

1 teaspoon sesame oil

1 packet natural no-calorie sweetener

½ teaspoon chopped garlic

½ teaspoon chopped ginger

½ teaspoon onion powder

5 cups broccoli florets

8 ounces raw boneless skinless chicken breast, cut into bite-sized pieces

¼ teaspoon garlic powder

⅓ cup chopped scallions

1 ounce (about ¼ cup) cashews

½ of recipe (about 1¾ cups): 344 calories, 12.5g total fat (2g sat fat), 807mg sodium, 25.5g carbs, 7g fiber, 6.5g sugars, 36.5g protein

You'll Need: small bowl, large skillet with a lid, large bowl, nonstick spray

Prep: 10 minutes • **Cook:** 15 minutes

1. To make the sauce, in a small bowl, combine arrowroot powder with 1 tablespoon water. Stir to dissolve. Add soy sauce, oil, sweetener, garlic, ginger, and ¼ teaspoon onion powder. Mix well.

2. Bring a large skillet to medium heat. Add broccoli and ½ cup water. Cover and cook for 6 minutes, or until broccoli is tender and water has evaporated. Transfer to a large bowl.

3. Remove skillet from heat. Spray with nonstick spray, and return to medium heat. Add chicken, and sprinkle with garlic powder and remaining ¼ teaspoon onion powder. Cook and stir for about 5 minutes, until cooked through.

4. Reduce heat to medium low. Add cooked broccoli, scallions, cashews, and sauce. Cook and stir until sauce has slightly thickened and entire dish is hot and well mixed, about 2 minutes.

MAKES 2 SERVINGS

Chew on This . . .

Cashews grow in apple-like fruits and their shells are actually poisonous. I'll stick to shelled cashews from the grocery store, thankyouverymuch.

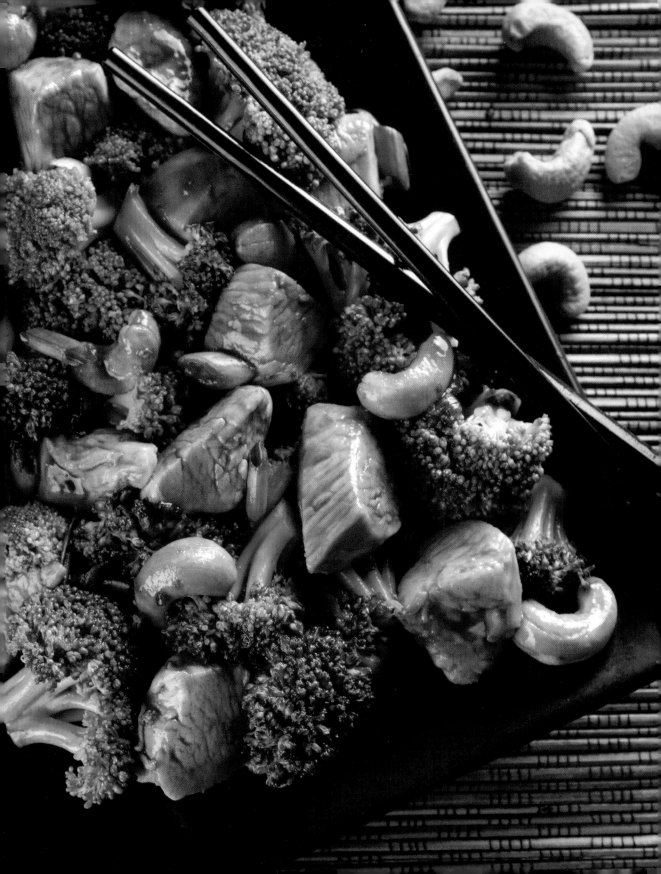

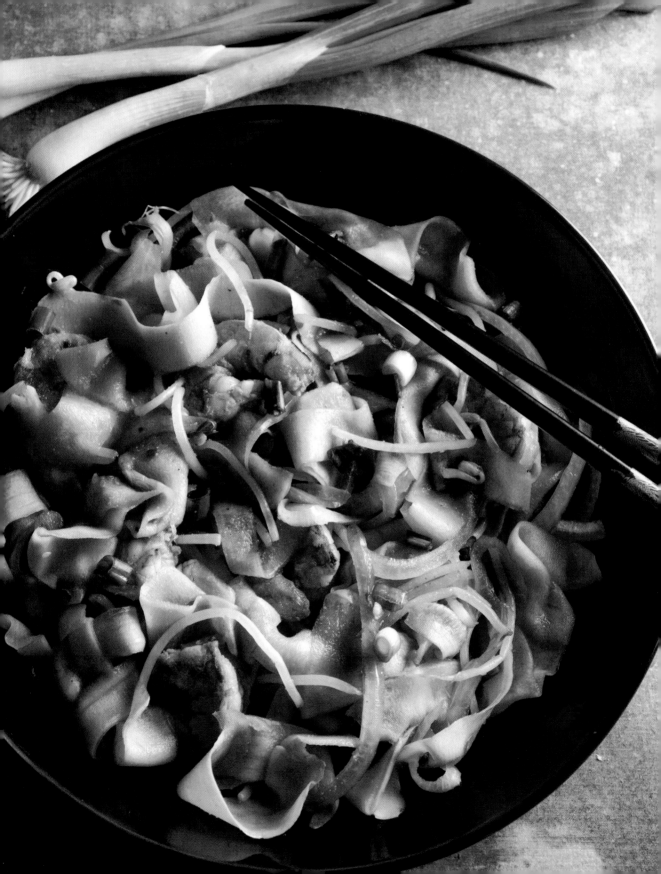

So Much Shrimp Chow Fun

254 cal

GF Saucy shrimp + DIY squash noodles = crazy delicious! For more veggie-noodle goodness, flip to page 362.

1½ tablespoons reduced-sodium/lite soy sauce

1 teaspoon sesame oil

1 packet natural no-calorie sweetener

¾ teaspoon chopped garlic

½ teaspoon onion powder

1 pound (about 2 medium) yellow squash

2 cups bean sprouts

1 cup thinly sliced onion

8 ounces (about 16) raw large shrimp, peeled, tails removed, deveined

¼ teaspoon garlic powder

1 cup chopped scallions

HG FYI

This recipe calls for a standard veggie peeler (as opposed to a veggie spiralizer). The standard peeler gives you wider noodles, perfect for chow fun.

½ of recipe (about 2 cups): 254 calories, 4.5g total fat (1g sat fat), 764mg sodium, 27.5g carbs, 6.5g fiber, 15.5g sugars, 29g protein

You'll Need: small bowl, veggie peeler, large skillet, nonstick spray, strainer
Prep: 20 minutes • **Cook:** 15 minutes

1. To make the sauce, in a small bowl, combine soy sauce, oil, sweetener, chopped garlic, and ¼ teaspoon onion powder. Mix well.

2. Slice off and discard squash ends. Using a veggie peeler, slice squash into wide strips, rotating the squash after each slice.

3. Bring a large skillet sprayed with nonstick spray to medium-high heat. Add squash and bean sprouts. Cook and stir until slightly softened, about 4 minutes.

4. Transfer to a strainer, and thoroughly drain excess liquid.

5. Remove skillet from heat. Re-spray, and return to medium-high heat. Cook and stir onion until mostly softened, about 3 minutes.

6. Add shrimp, and season with garlic powder and remaining ¼ teaspoon onion powder. Cook and stir for about 3 minutes, until onion has fully softened and shrimp are fully cooked.

7. Reduce heat to medium low. Add scallions and drained veggies, and drizzle with sauce. Cook and stir until hot and well mixed, about 2 minutes.

MAKES 2 SERVINGS

Chew on This...

Chow-fun noodles are extra wide . . . but YOU won't be if this recipe finds its way into your regular rotation.

Veggie Moo Shu Madness

262 cal

  I could eat this one all day long! And I just might . . .

2 teaspoons reduced-sodium/lite soy sauce

2 teaspoons sesame oil

2 teaspoons plain rice vinegar

1 packet natural no-calorie sweetener

½ teaspoon chopped garlic

½ teaspoon ground ginger

2 cups bagged broccoli cole slaw

1 cup bean sprouts

1 cup thinly sliced shiitake mushrooms

½ cup canned bamboo shoots, drained

¼ cup thinly sliced scallions

4 Clean & Hungry Whole-Wheat Tortillas (recipe and store-bought alternatives on page 196)

Optional: Clean & Hungry Teriyaki Sauce (recipe and store-bought alternatives on page 342)

½ of recipe (2 wraps): 262 calories, 5.5g total fat (0.5g sat fat), 778mg sodium, 37g carbs, 8g fiber, 6g sugars, 19g protein

You'll Need: medium bowl, extra-large skillet with a lid, nonstick spray, microwave-safe plate

Prep: 10 minutes • **Cook:** 10 minutes

1. To make the sauce, in a medium bowl, combine soy sauce, oil, vinegar, sweetener, garlic, and ginger. Mix well.

2. Bring an extra-large skillet sprayed with nonstick spray to medium-high heat. Add broccoli cole slaw, bean sprouts, mushrooms, and ¼ cup water. Cover and cook for 4 minutes, or until veggies have mostly softened and water has evaporated.

3. Add bamboo shoots, scallions, and sauce. Cook and stir until hot and well mixed, about 2 minutes.

4. On a microwave-safe plate, microwave tortillas for 10 seconds, or until warm.

5. If you like, spread teriyaki sauce on tortillas.

6. Distribute veggie mixture among the bottom halves of the tortillas (about ¾ cup each), and roll up tortillas.

MAKES 2 SERVINGS

Chew on This . . .

American-style Chinese moo shu is typically wrapped in tortillas. That is so like us—stuffing food inside more food! Luckily, this recipe features my famous low-calorie tortillas.

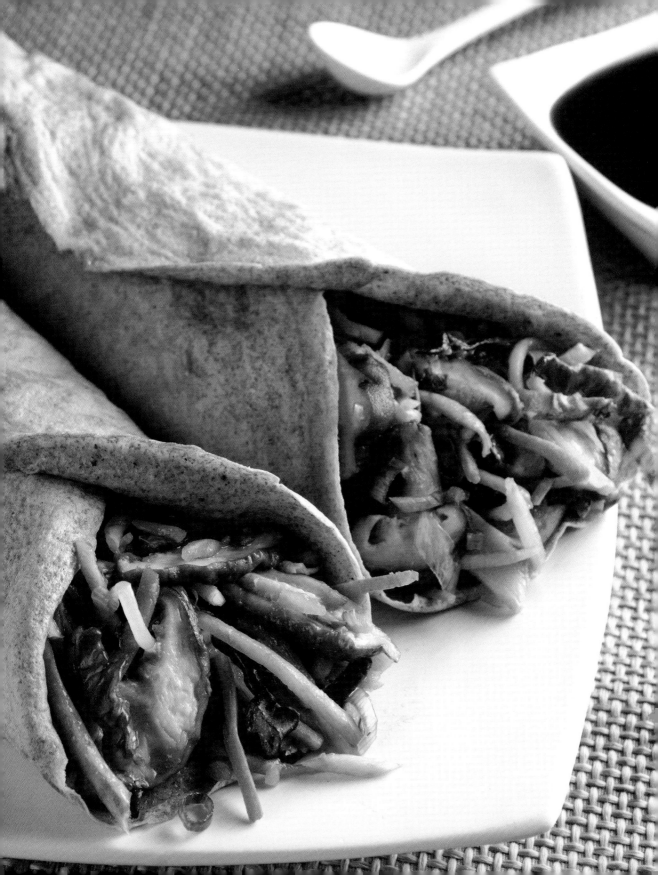

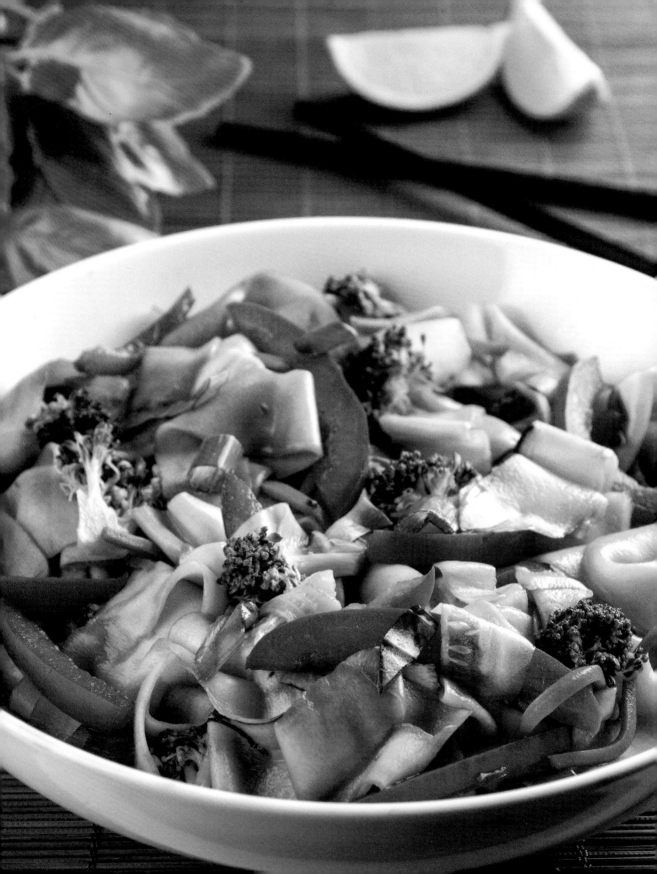

Let's Get Drunken Noodles

132 cal

(V) (30m) (GF)   Obsession confession: This recipe was inspired by some crazy delicious drunken noodles I once ate in Las Vegas. You'll want to eat these every day. Find more veggie-noodle recipes on page 362!

2 tablespoons reduced-sodium/lite soy sauce

2 teaspoons molasses

1½ teaspoons lime juice

1 packet natural no-calorie sweetener

1 teaspoon chopped garlic

⅛ teaspoon red pepper flakes

1 pound (about 2 medium) zucchini

⅛ teaspoon salt

1 cup sliced red bell pepper

1 cup shredded carrots

1 cup small broccoli florets

¼ cup chopped scallions

2 tablespoons chopped fresh basil

½ of recipe (about 2 cups): 132 calories, 1g total fat (<0.5g sat fat), 765mg sodium, 27.5g carbs, 6.5g fiber, 17g sugars, 6.5g protein

You'll Need: small bowl, veggie peeler, extra-large skillet with a lid, nonstick spray, strainer

Prep: 15 minutes • **Cook:** 15 minutes

1. To make the sauce, in a small bowl, combine soy sauce, molasses, lime juice, sweetener, garlic, and pepper flakes. Mix until uniform.

2. Slice off and discard zucchini ends. Using a veggie peeler, slice zucchini into wide strips, rotating the zucchini after each slice.

3. Bring an extra-large skillet sprayed with nonstick spray to medium-high heat. Add zucchini, and sprinkle with salt. Cook and stir until hot and slightly softened, about 4 minutes.

4. Transfer zucchini to a strainer, and thoroughly drain excess liquid.

5. Remove skillet from heat. Re-spray, and bring to medium heat. Add bell pepper, carrots, broccoli, and ¼ cup water. Cover and cook for 4 minutes, until veggies have softened and water has evaporated.

6. Return drained zucchini to the skillet. Add scallions, basil, and sauce. Cook and stir until sauce is evenly distributed and mostly absorbed and entire dish is hot, about 2 minutes.

MAKES 2 SERVINGS

HG FYI

You won't need a veggie spiralizer for this dish; a traditional veggie peeler is perfect for getting nice wide noodles.

Chew on This . . .

Some people believe that "drunken noodles" originated when an intoxicated man threw together the dish in a drunken haze. Jury's still out, but these noodles are definitely IN.

Egg Roll in a Bowl

269 cal

 GF This recipe is one of my absolute favorites! You'll NEVER miss that greasy shell.

1 tablespoon reduced-sodium/lite soy sauce

1 teaspoon sesame oil

½ teaspoon crushed garlic

½ teaspoon ground ginger

Dash black pepper

4 cups bagged coleslaw mix

1 cup bean sprouts

3 ounces ready-to-eat bay (small) shrimp

⅓ cup chopped scallions

¼ cup canned sliced water chestnuts, drained and chopped

Entire recipe: 269 calories, 6g total fat (0.5g sat fat), 807mg sodium, 27g carbs, 8g fiber, 14g sugars, 28g protein

You'll Need: small bowl, large skillet with a lid, nonstick spray

Prep: 10 minutes • **Cook:** 15 minutes

1. To make the sauce, in a small bowl, combine soy sauce, oil, garlic, ginger, and pepper. Mix until uniform.

2. Bring a large skillet sprayed with nonstick spray to medium-high heat. Add coleslaw, bean sprouts, and ½ cup water. Cover and cook for 8 minutes, or until fully softened.

3. Uncover and, if needed, cook and stir until water has evaporated, 2 to 3 minutes.

4. Add sauce and remaining ingredients. Cook and stir until hot and well mixed, about 2 minutes.

MAKES 1 SERVING

Chew on This...

And the bronze medal goes to . . . egg rolls! The fried favorites are the third most popular Chinese dish in America.

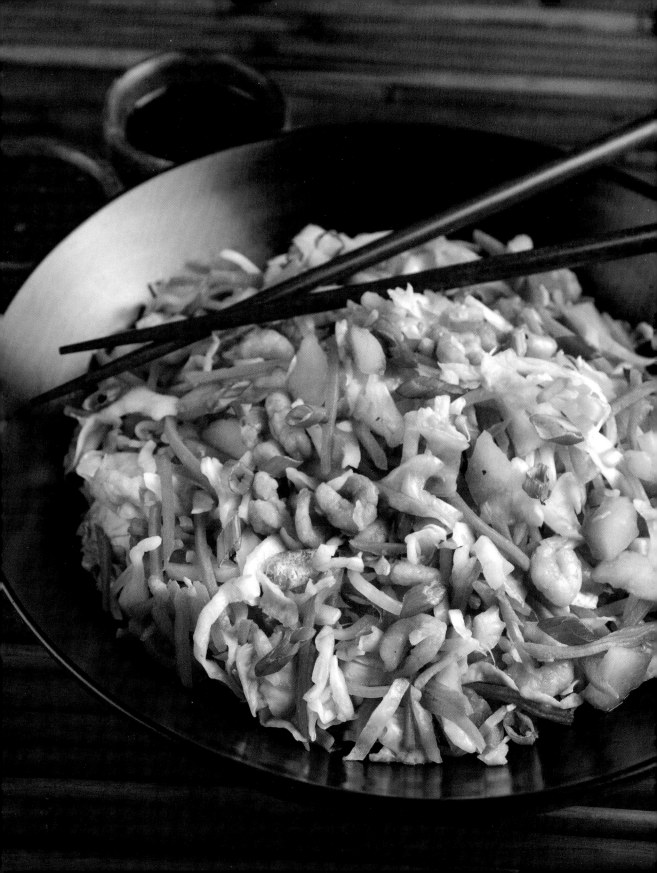

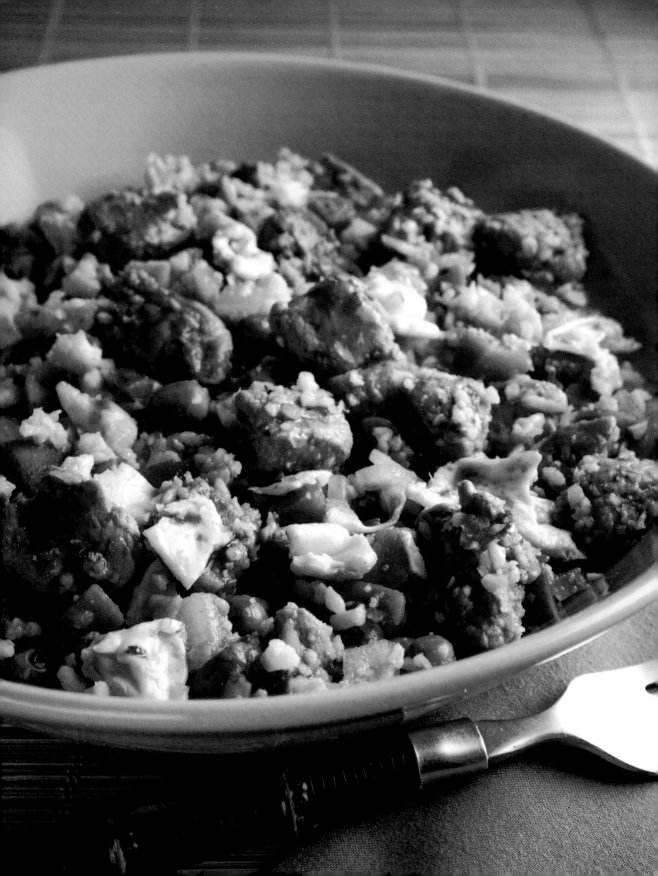

Grab-a-Fork Pork Fried Rice

197 cal

30m **GF** Obsession confession: This one is neither fried nor rice. It's cooked in a skillet with barely any oil, and the rice is made of cauliflower! For more fun with cauliflower, flip to page 362.

⅓ cup egg whites (about 3 large eggs' worth)

8 ounces raw pork tenderloin, trimmed of excess fat, chopped

⅛ teaspoon garlic powder

⅛ teaspoon ground ginger

⅛ teaspoon each salt and black pepper

4 cups cauliflower rice/ crumbles

2 cups frozen peas and carrots

1 cup chopped onion

1 tablespoon sesame oil

2 teaspoons chopped garlic

¼ cup Clean & Hungry Teriyaki Sauce (recipe and store-bought alternatives on page 342)

Optional seasoning: additional salt

¼th of recipe (about 1¾ cups): 197 calories, 5g total fat (1g sat fat), 325mg sodium, 19.5g carbs, 6g fiber, 7.5g sugars, 19g protein

You'll Need: extra-large skillet, nonstick spray, medium bowl

Prep: 15 minutes • **Cook:** 15 minutes

1. Bring an extra-large skillet sprayed with nonstick spray to medium heat. Scramble egg whites until fully cooked, about 3 minutes, using a spatula to break them into bite-sized pieces. Transfer to a medium bowl.

2. Remove skillet from heat; clean, if needed. Re-spray, and bring to medium-high heat. Add pork, and sprinkle with seasonings. Cook and stir until browned on all sides, about 2 minutes.

3. Add cauliflower rice/crumbles, frozen veggies, onion, oil, and garlic. Cook and stir until pork is fully cooked and veggies are soft, 6 to 8 minutes.

4. Reduce heat to medium low. Add scrambled egg whites and teriyaki sauce. Cook and stir until hot and well mixed, about 2 minutes.

MAKES 4 SERVINGS

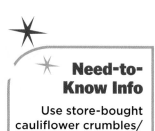

Need-to-Know Info

Use store-bought cauliflower crumbles/ rice, or DIY! See page 346 for the 411.

Aloha Chicken Fried Rice

282 cal

GF People are TOO obsessed with fried rice for me to stop after just one recipe . . . so here's another! This one has juicy pineapple and tender chicken. And remember to check out all the cauliflower rice recipes on page 362.

½ cup egg whites (about 4 large eggs' worth)

1 pound raw boneless skinless chicken breast, cut into bite-sized pieces

¼ teaspoon each salt and black pepper

2 cups frozen Asian-style stir-fry vegetables

4 cups cauliflower rice/crumbles

1 cup bean sprouts

¾ cup chopped onion

1 tablespoon sesame oil

1 teaspoon chopped garlic

½ cup chopped pineapple

½ cup canned water chestnuts, drained and chopped

¼ cup Clean & Hungry Teriyaki Sauce (recipe and store-bought alternatives on page 342)

¼ cup chopped scallions

Optional seasonings: additional salt and black pepper

¼th of recipe (about 2 cups): 282 calories, 7g total fat (1g sat fat), 400mg sodium, 21g carbs, 6g fiber, 9g sugars, 34g protein

You'll Need: extra-large skillet, nonstick spray, medium bowl
Prep: 20 minutes • **Cook:** 25 minutes

1. Bring an extra-large skillet sprayed with nonstick spray to medium heat. Scramble egg whites until fully cooked, 3 to 4 minutes, breaking them up into bite-sized pieces. Transfer to a medium bowl.

2. Remove skillet from heat; clean, if needed. Re-spray, and bring to medium-high heat. Add chicken, and season with salt and pepper. Cook and stir until browned on all sides, about 3 minutes.

3. Add frozen veggies. Cook and stir until veggies have thawed and excess water has evaporated, about 4 minutes.

4. Add cauliflower rice/crumbles, bean sprouts, onion, oil, and garlic. Cook and stir until veggies have mostly softened and any excess water has evaporated, 6 to 8 minutes.

5. Add scrambled egg whites, pineapple, water chestnuts, and teriyaki sauce. Cook and stir until hot and well mixed, about 2 minutes.

6. Top with scallions.

MAKES 4 SERVINGS

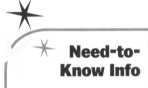

Need-to-Know Info

Use store-bought cauliflower crumbles/rice, or DIY! See page 346 for the 411.

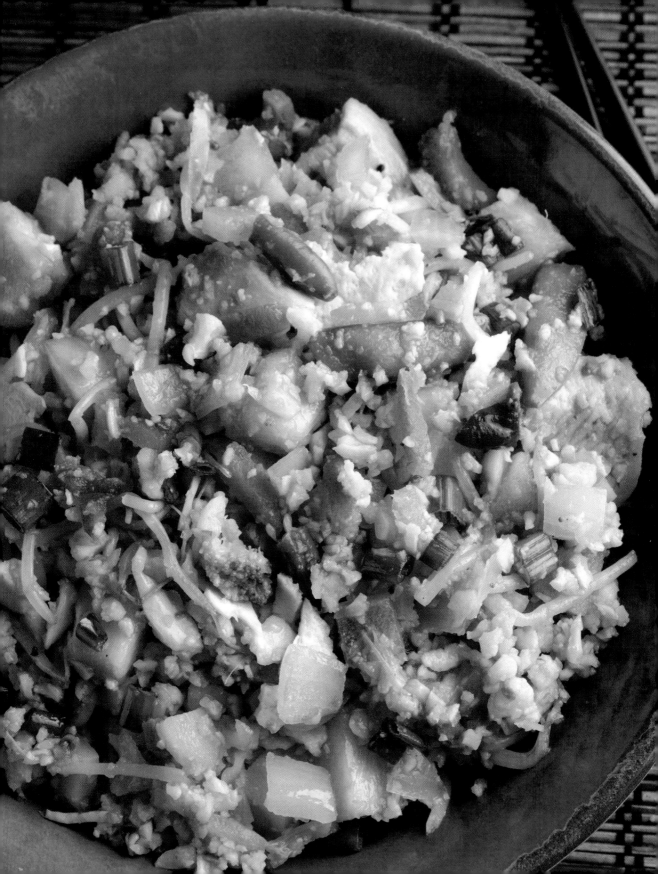

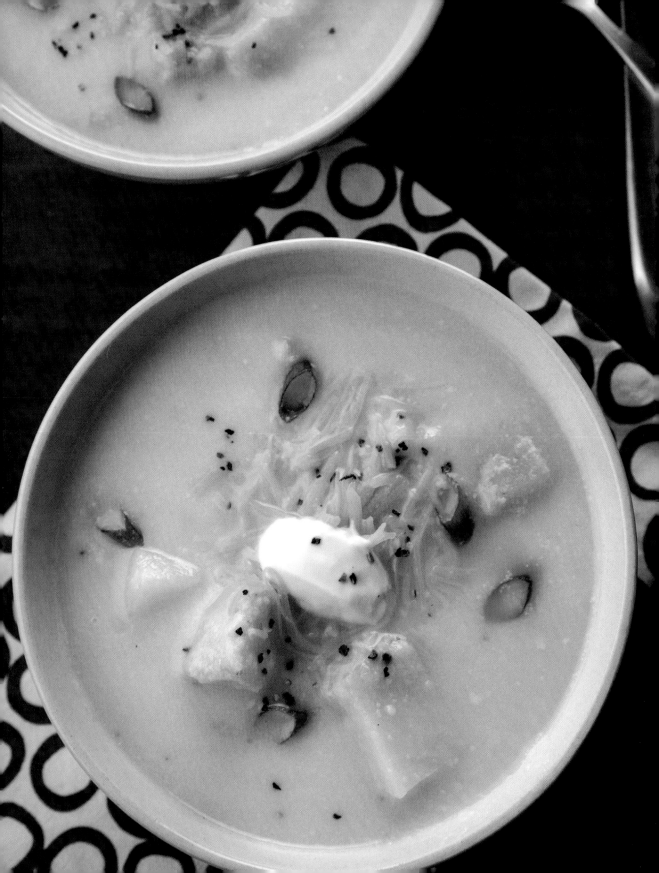

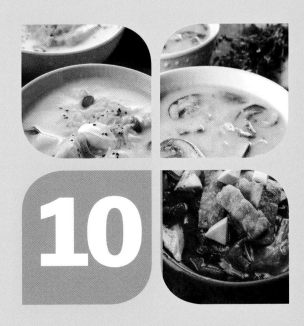

Souped Up!

Americans reportedly eat more than 10 billion bowls of soup each year. (That's actually only about 30 bowls per person . . . and I think I might be responsible for more than my share!) Artist Andy Warhol even turned soup cans into a pop-culture phenomenon; he painted them after eating the stuff daily for two straight decades! But since there's nothing like hot, comforting, homemade soup, I'm serving up nine new recipes you'll wanna stick your spoon in as soon as humanly possible.

I Dream of Cream of Mushroom Soup

GF This may be my BEST soup recipe ever! Pureed cauliflower makes it feel super rich and creamy while keeping the calorie count low . . .

4 cups roughly chopped cauliflower

2 cups fat-free milk

2 tablespoons whipped butter

4 cups thinly sliced brown mushrooms

1 cup chopped onion

1 cup chicken broth

1 tablespoon chopped garlic

1 teaspoon salt

¼ teaspoon black pepper

⅙th of recipe (about 1 cup): 93 calories, 2.5g total fat (1g sat fat), 604mg sodium, 13g carbs, 2g fiber, 7.5g sugars, 5.5g protein

You'll Need: large pot, strainer, blender or food processor
Prep: 15 minutes • **Cook:** 40 minutes

1. Bring a large pot of water to a boil. Cook cauliflower until very tender, about 15 minutes.

2. Transfer cauliflower to a strainer to drain.

3. Place drained cauliflower in a blender or food processor. Add milk, and puree until smooth.

4. Melt butter in the (empty) pot over medium-high heat. Add mushrooms and onion. Cook and stir until mostly softened and browned, about 8 minutes.

5. Add cauliflower puree and remaining ingredients. Cook and stir until hot and well mixed, about 2 minutes.

MAKES 6 SERVINGS

Hey, Vegetarians!

The recipes in this chapter call for chicken broth, which provides maximum flavor. For a vegetarian spin, feel free to use veggie broth in the I Dream of Cream of Mushroom Soup, Best-Ever Cream of Broccoli Soup, Oh Wow Corn Chowder, and Locked & Loaded Baked Potato Soup.

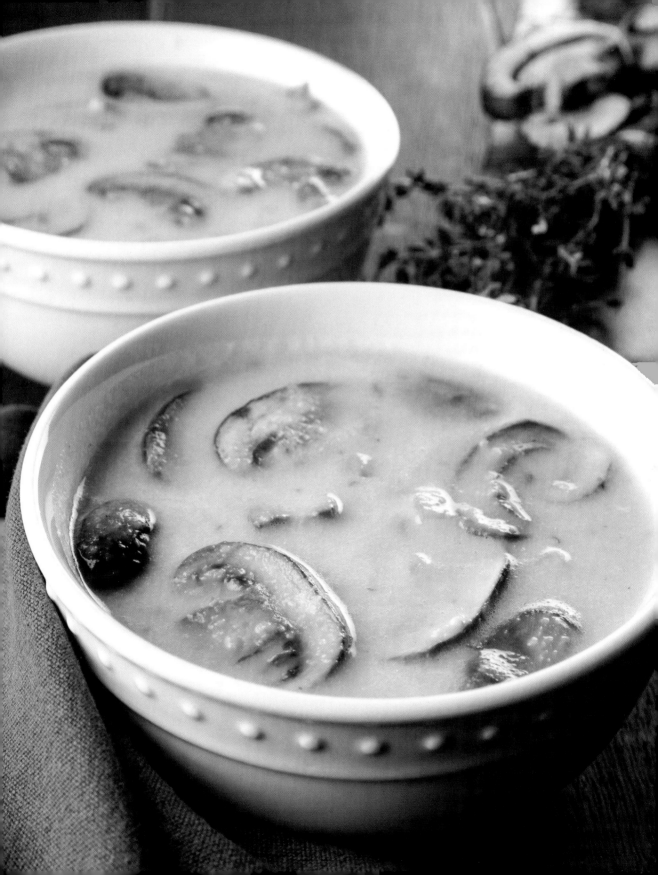

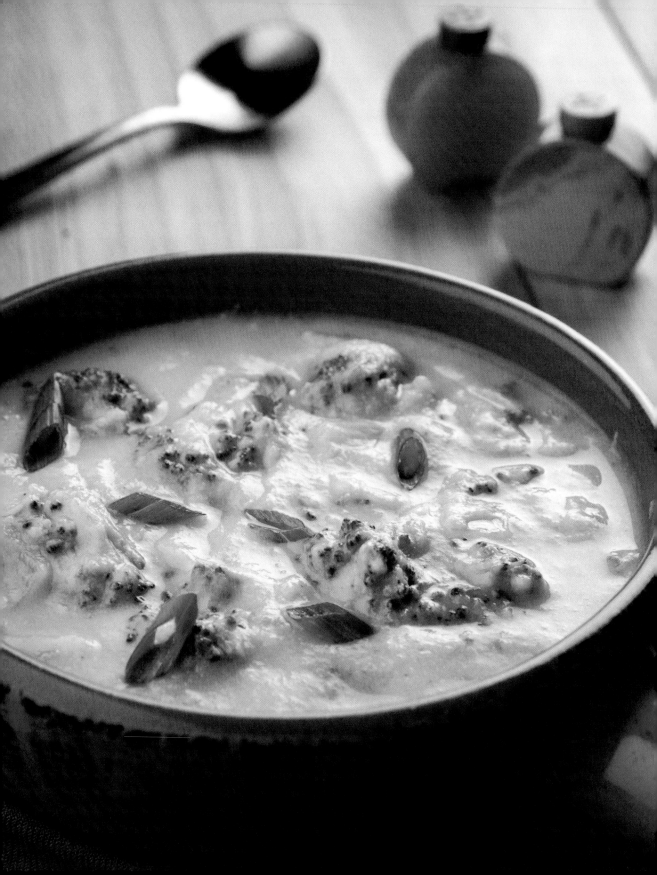

Best-Ever Cream of Broccoli Soup

124 cal

 I am IN LOVE with this soup. Someone get us a room.

3 cups chopped cauliflower

3 cups chopped broccoli

2 cups fat-free milk

½ cup shredded reduced-fat cheddar cheese

1 cup chopped onion

1 cup chicken broth

1½ tablespoons chopped garlic

½ teaspoon salt

¼ teaspoon black pepper

Optional topping: chopped scallions

Optional seasonings: salt and additional black pepper

⅕th of recipe (about 1 cup): 124 calories, 3g total fat (1.5g sat fat), 563mg sodium, 16.5g carbs, 3.5g fiber, 8.5g sugars, 9.5g protein

You'll Need: large pot with a lid, strainer, blender or food processor, nonstick spray

Prep: 15 minutes • **Cook:** 45 minutes

1. Bring a large pot of water to a boil. Add cauliflower and 1 cup broccoli. Cook until very tender, about 15 minutes.

2. Transfer veggies to a strainer to drain.

3. Place drained veggies in a blender or food processor. Add milk and cheese, and puree until mostly smooth and uniform.

4. Spray the (empty) pot with nonstick spray, and bring to medium-high heat. Cook and stir onion until mostly softened, about 4 minutes.

5. Add veggie puree, remaining 2 cups broccoli, and remaining ingredients. Bring to a boil.

6. Reduce to a simmer. Cover and cook for 15 minutes, or until broccoli is tender.

MAKES 5 SERVINGS

Chew on This...

While it may seem strange to us North Americans, soup is eaten for breakfast in countries all over the world!

Wham, Bam, Thank You Clam Chowder

107 cal

 Pureed cauliflower does it again! The creaminess here is unimaginably good.

4 cups roughly chopped cauliflower

2 cups fat-free milk

1 cup chopped onion

1 cup chopped celery

10 ounces (about 2 small) white potatoes cut into ½-inch pieces

1 cup chicken broth

1½ tablespoons chopped garlic

¼ teaspoon black pepper

Two 10-ounce cans baby clams (not drained)

Optional seasonings: salt, additional black pepper

⅛th of recipe (about 1 cup): 107 calories, <0.5g total fat (0g sat fat), 530mg sodium, 16.5g carbs, 2.5g fiber, 5.5g sugars, 11g protein

You'll Need: large pot with a lid, strainer, blender or food processor, nonstick spray

Prep: 25 minutes • **Cook:** 1 hour

1. Bring a large pot of water to a boil. Cook cauliflower until very tender, about 15 minutes.

2. Transfer cauliflower to a strainer to drain.

3. Transfer drained cauliflower to a blender or food processor. Add milk, and puree until smooth.

4. Spray the (empty) pot with nonstick spray, and bring to medium-high heat. Add onion and celery. Cook and stir until slightly softened, about 4 minutes.

5. Add cauliflower puree, potatoes, broth, garlic, and pepper. Bring to a boil.

6. Reduce to a simmer. Cover and cook for 20 minutes, or until potatoes are tender.

7. Add clams and the liquid from the cans. Cook and stir until hot and well mixed, about 2 minutes.

MAKES 8 SERVINGS

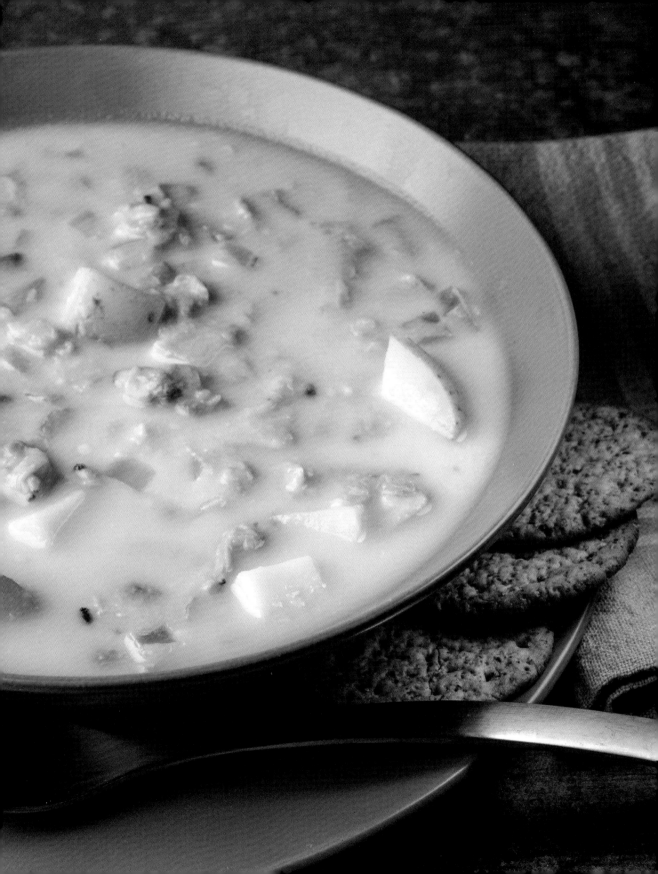

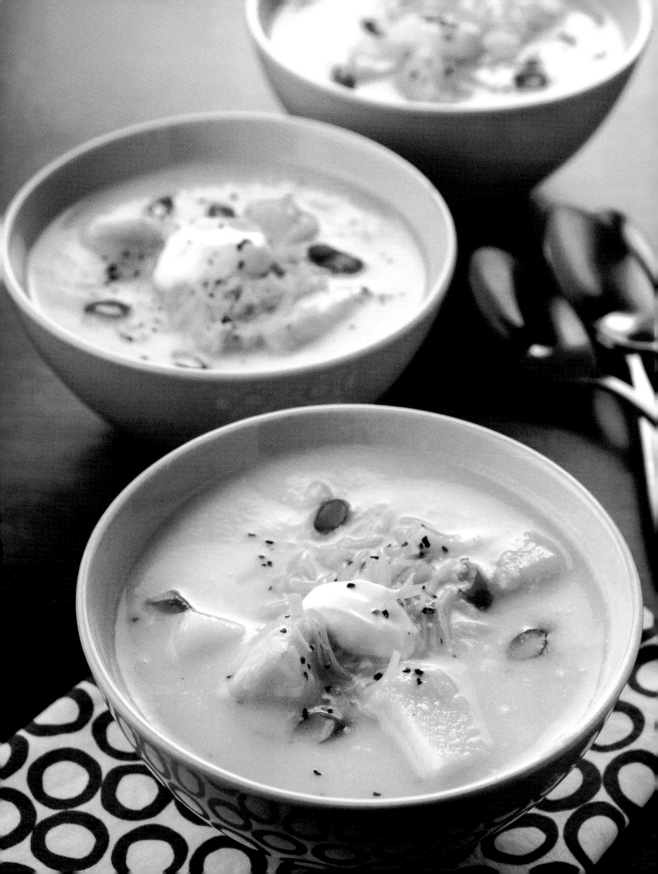

Locked & Loaded
Baked Potato Soup

177 cal

 This soup tastes exactly like a steamy baked potato with all the fixins . . .

4 cups roughly chopped cauliflower

2 cups fat-free milk

⅓ cup plus 5 tablespoons shredded reduced-fat cheddar cheese

⅓ cup plus 5 tablespoons chopped scallions

12 ounces (about 2 small) white potatoes cut into ½-inch pieces

1 cup chicken broth

1½ tablespoons chopped garlic

¼ teaspoon each salt and black pepper

5 tablespoons light sour cream

Optional seasonings: additional salt and black pepper

⅕th of recipe (about 1 cup): 177 calories, 4.5g total fat (2.5g sat fat), 480mg sodium, 23.5g carbs, 4g fiber, 9.5g sugars, 11g protein

You'll Need: large pot with a lid, strainer, blender or food processor

Prep: 15 minutes • **Cook:** 55 minutes

1. Bring a large pot of water to a boil. Cook cauliflower until very tender, about 15 minutes.

2. Transfer cauliflower to a strainer to drain.

3. Place drained cauliflower in a blender or food processor. Add milk and ⅓ cup cheese, and puree until mostly smooth and uniform.

4. Place cauliflower puree and ⅓ cup scallions in the (empty) pot. Add potatoes, broth, garlic, salt, and pepper. Bring to a boil.

5. Reduce to a simmer. Cover and cook for 20 minutes, or until potatoes are tender.

6. Top each serving with 1 tablespoon each cheese, scallions, and sour cream.

MAKES 5 SERVINGS

Chew on This . . .

Americans can't get enough potatoes! Spuds are said to be the leading veggie crop in the US, with 50 percent of those potatoes going on to become processed foods.

Oh Wow Corn Chowder

GF Yum, yum, yum! This chowder tastes so incredibly decadent, you might have trouble believing it's clean and low-calorie . . . but it totally is!

3 cups roughly chopped cauliflower

2 cups fat-free milk

3 cups frozen sweet corn kernels, thawed

1 cup chopped sweet onion

10 ounces (about 2 small) white potatoes cut into ½-inch pieces

1 cup chicken broth

2 teaspoons chopped garlic

2 packets natural no-calorie sweetener

½ teaspoon salt

¼ teaspoon black pepper

½ cup chopped scallions

Optional topping: additional chopped scallions

⅙th of recipe (about 1 cup): 161 calories, 1g total fat (0g sat fat), 407mg sodium, 33g carbs, 4g fiber, 11g sugars, 7g protein

You'll Need: large pot with a lid, strainer, blender or food processor, nonstick spray

Prep: 15 minutes • **Cook:** 55 minutes

1. Bring a large pot of water to a boil. Cook cauliflower until very tender, about 15 minutes.

2. Transfer cauliflower to a strainer to drain.

3. Place drained cauliflower in a blender or food processor. Add milk and 1½ cups corn. Puree until smooth.

4. Spray the (empty) pot with nonstick spray, and bring to medium-high heat. Add cauliflower puree, remaining 1½ cups corn, and all remaining ingredients *except* scallions. Bring to a boil.

5. Reduce to a simmer. Cover and cook for 20 minutes, or until potatoes are tender.

6. Add scallions. Cook and stir until softened, about 2 minutes.

MAKES 6 SERVINGS

Chew on This . . .

North American settlers used corn for currency. I'd bet this corn chowder would have earned top value!

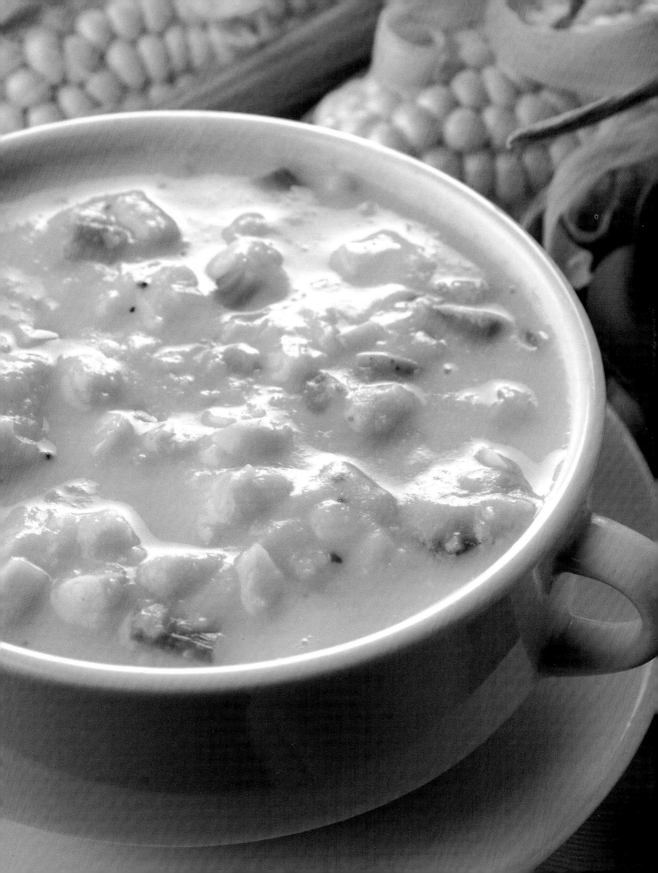

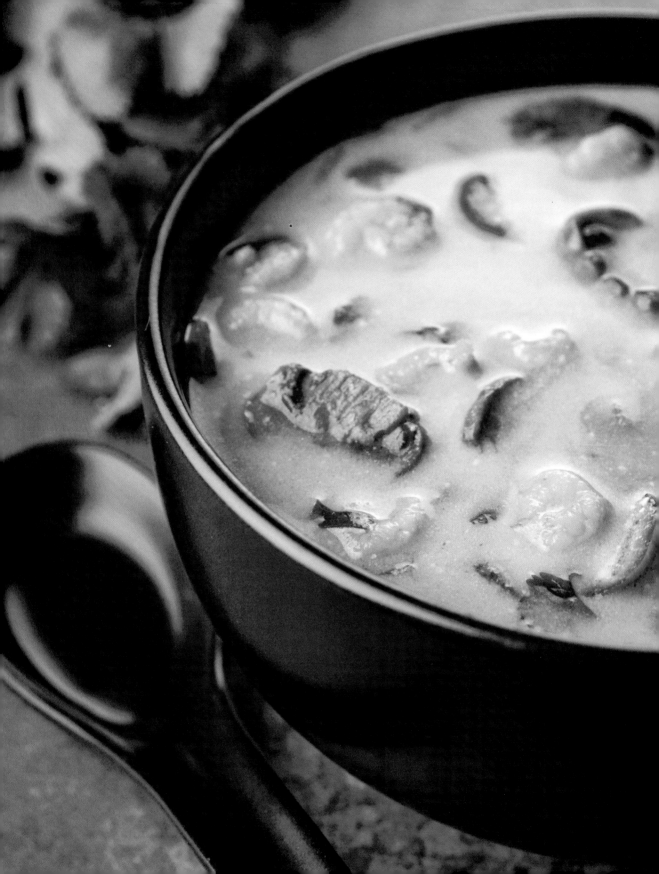

Thai Oh My
Coconut Shrimp Soup

101 cal

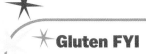 The calorie count here is crazy low, and this soup is really filling! Give it a Thai (ha!) . . .

2 cups thinly sliced mushrooms

1 cup chopped onion

1 tablespoon crushed ginger

1 tablespoon lime zest

1½ teaspoons chopped garlic

½ teaspoon cayenne pepper

4 cups reduced-sodium chicken broth

1 cup canned lite coconut milk

2 tablespoons lime juice

1 tablespoon reduced-sodium/lite soy sauce

8 ounces ready-to-eat bay (small) shrimp

½ cup chopped fresh cilantro

Optional: thinly sliced jalapeño pepper

⅙th of recipe (about 1 cup): 101 calories, 3.5g total fat (2g sat fat), 558mg sodium, 6g carbs, 1g fiber, 3g sugars, 11g protein

You'll Need: large pot, nonstick spray

Prep: 20 minutes • **Cook:** 30 minutes

1. Bring a large pot sprayed with nonstick spray to medium-high heat. Add mushrooms, onion, ginger, lime zest, garlic, and cayenne pepper. Cook and stir until veggies have softened and lightly browned, about 4 minutes.

2. Add all remaining ingredients *except* shrimp and cilantro. Mix well, and bring to a boil.

3. Reduce to a simmer. Cook for 15 minutes.

4. Add shrimp and cilantro. Cook and stir until hot and well mixed, about 2 minutes.

MAKES 6 SERVINGS

Gluten FYI

Some soy sauce contains gluten. If you avoid gluten, check the ingredient lists. Or grab a product marked gluten-free.

Chew on This . . .

Thai food is traditionally eaten with the spoon in the right hand while seated on the floor. I can personally attest to the fact that this soup tastes just as good via a left hand at a kitchen table.

Whoop, Whoop Tortilla Soup

153 cal

GF Please enjoy this tasty soup, complete with crispy baked-not-fried tortilla strips! And for more slow-cooker creations, flip to page 366.

SOUP

1 pound raw boneless skinless chicken breast

¼ teaspoon salt

⅛ teaspoon black pepper

1½ teaspoons ground cumin

1½ teaspoons chili powder

½ teaspoon garlic powder

½ teaspoon onion powder

4 cups chicken broth

One 14.5-ounce can fire-roasted diced tomatoes (not drained)

1½ cups chopped onion

1 cup chopped bell pepper

2 tablespoons seeded and finely chopped jalapeño pepper

1 tablespoon lime juice

TORTILLA STRIPS

Four 6-inch corn tortillas

¼ teaspoon ground cumin

¼ teaspoon chili powder

TOPPING

4 ounces chopped avocado (about ½ cup or 1 medium avocado)

⅛th of recipe (about 1 cup plus toppings): 153 calories, 4g total fat (0.5g sat fat), 611mg sodium, 13.5g carbs, 3g fiber, 4g sugars, 15g protein

You'll Need: slow cooker, baking sheet, nonstick spray, large bowl

Prep: 20 minutes • **Cook:** 3 to 4 hours or 7 to 8 hours

1. Place chicken in a slow cooker. Sprinkle with salt, black pepper, and ¼ teaspoon of each of the remaining seasonings.

2. Add chicken broth and all remaining soup ingredients, including remaining 1¼ teaspoons cumin, 1¼ teaspoons chili powder, ¼ teaspoon garlic powder, and ¼ teaspoon onion powder. Stir to mix.

3. Cover and cook on high for 3 to 4 hours or on low for 7 to 8 hours, until chicken is fully cooked.

4. Meanwhile, prepare tortilla strips. Preheat oven to 400 degrees. Spray a baking sheet with nonstick spray.

5. Cut tortillas into thin 2-inch-long strips, and lay on the baking sheet. Lightly spray with nonstick spray, and sprinkle with seasonings.

6. Bake for 4 minutes.

7. Flip tortilla strips. Bake until crispy, about 4 more minutes.

8. Transfer chicken to a large bowl. Shred with two forks.

9. Return chicken to the slow cooker, and mix well.

10. Top each serving with ⅛th of the tortilla strips (about 8 pieces) and ½ ounce (about 1 tablespoon) avocado.

MAKES 8 SERVINGS

Chew on This . . .

Traditional Mexican tortilla soup sometimes includes epazote, a Mexican herb that can be poisonous in very large quantities. No worries. This recipe doesn't contain any of it at all!

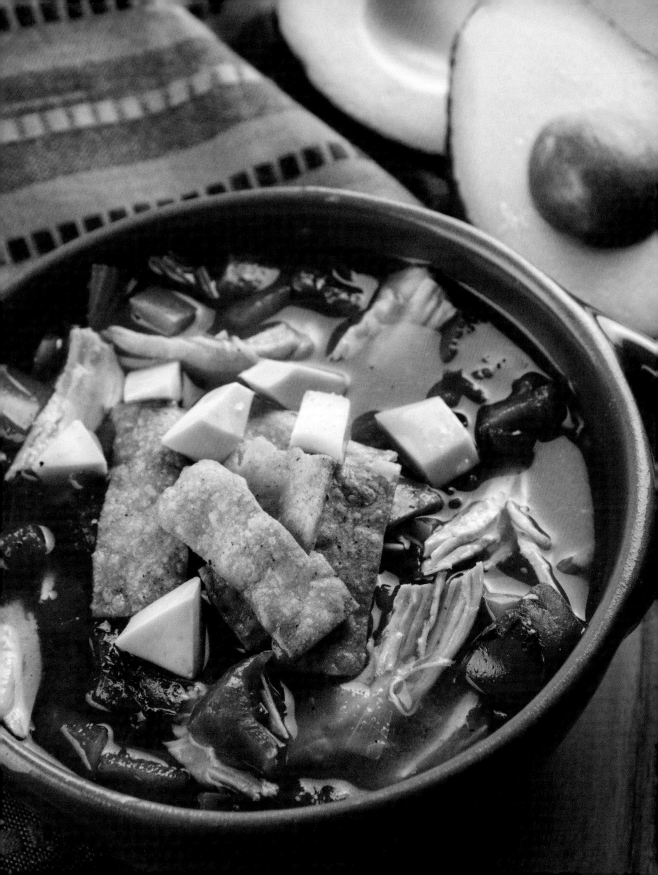

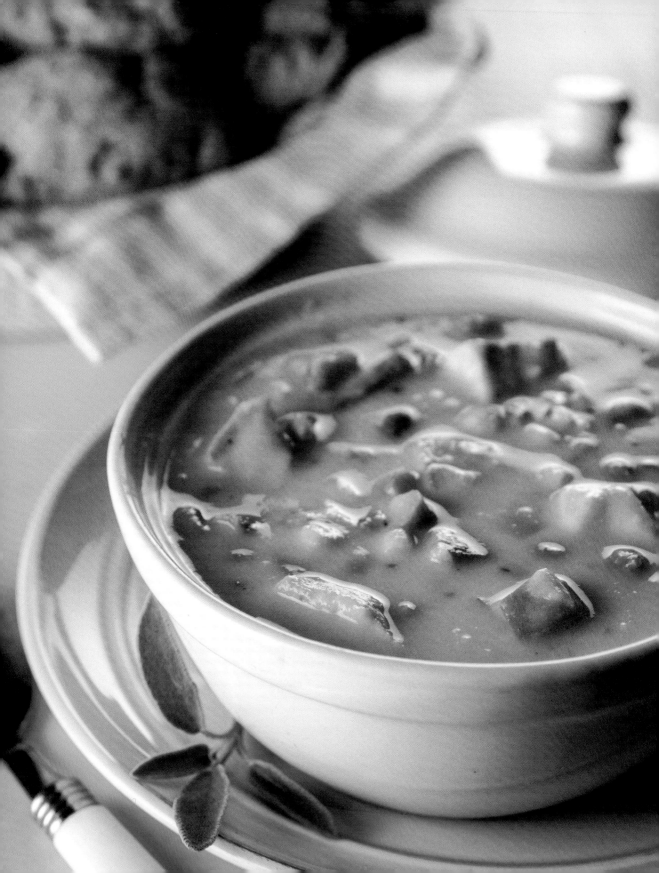

Chicken Pot Pie Soup

172 cal

GF This soup is SO creamy, which is quite a coup, given its lean & clean ingredients! And it's amazing with my Cauliflower Power Biscuit Bakes (page 34).

4 cups roughly chopped cauliflower

10 ounces raw boneless skinless chicken breast

¾ teaspoon salt

½ teaspoon black pepper

2 cups fat-free milk

½ cup shredded reduced-fat cheddar cheese

1 cup chopped onion

2 cups frozen petite mixed vegetables

1 cup chicken broth

1½ tablespoons chopped garlic

⅛ teaspoon ground thyme

Dash ground sage

Optional seasonings: additional salt and black pepper

⅙th of recipe (about 1 cup): 172 calories, 3.5g total fat (1.5g sat fat), 597mg sodium, 16g carbs, 3g fiber, 8.5g sugars, 18.5g protein

You'll Need: large pot, meat mallet, large skillet, nonstick spray, strainer, blender or food processor
Prep: 10 minutes • **Cook:** 35 minutes

1. Bring a large pot of water to a boil. Cook cauliflower until very tender, about 15 minutes.

2. Meanwhile, pound chicken to a ½-inch thickness. Season with ¼ teaspoon each salt and pepper. Bring a large skillet sprayed with nonstick spray to medium heat. Cook chicken for about 4 minutes per side, until cooked through.

3. Transfer cauliflower to a strainer to drain.

4. Chop chicken into bite-sized pieces.

5. Place drained cauliflower in a blender or food processor. Add milk and cheese, and puree until mostly smooth and uniform.

6. Spray the (empty) pot with nonstick spray, and bring to medium-high heat. Cook and stir onion until mostly softened, about 4 minutes.

7. Add cauliflower puree, chopped chicken, and remaining ingredients, including the remaining ½ teaspoon salt and ¼ teaspoon pepper. Cook and stir until frozen veggies have thawed and soup is hot and well mixed, about 5 minutes.

MAKES 6 SERVINGS

Chew on This . . .

Back in the days of the Roman Empire, chicken pot pies were sometimes served with LIVE birds under the shell that would burst out when served. Talk about a show!

Chicken Veggie-Noodle Soup

GF This soup combines three of my personal obsessions: chicken, spiralized veggie noodles, and a slow cooker! Does it get any better? Flip to page 362 for more veggie noodles and page 366 for more slow-cooker creations.

1 pound raw boneless skinless chicken breasts, halved

¼ teaspoon each salt and black pepper

6 cups reduced-sodium chicken broth

½ cup chopped carrots

½ cup chopped celery

½ cup chopped onion

2 teaspoons chopped garlic

2 teaspoons Italian seasoning

½ teaspoon onion powder

¼ teaspoon ground thyme

2 bay leaves

1 pound spiralized zucchini (about 2 medium zucchini)

Optional seasonings: additional salt and black pepper

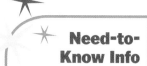

Need-to-Know Info

It's super easy to spiralize zucchini. Get the 411 on page 349!

⅛th of recipe (about 1 cup): 99 calories, 2g total fat (0.5g sat fat), 528mg sodium, 5g carbs, 1g fiber, 3g sugars, 14.5g protein

You'll Need: slow cooker, large bowl

Prep: 15 minutes

Cook: 3 to 4 hours or 7 to 8 hours, plus 10 minutes

1. Place chicken in a slow cooker, and season with salt and pepper. Add all remaining ingredients *except* zucchini. Mix well.

2. Cover and cook on high for 3 to 4 hours or on low for 7 to 8 hours, until chicken is fully cooked and veggies have softened.

3. If cooking at high heat, decrease heat to low. Remove and discard bay leaves.

4. Transfer chicken to a large bowl. Shred chicken with two forks.

5. Return shredded chicken to the slow cooker. Stir in zucchini, re-cover, and cook for 10 minutes, or until zucchini has slightly softened.

MAKES 8 SERVINGS

Freeze It: Soup Edition

To Freeze: Distribute single servings into sealable microwave-safe containers with a little room at the top. (Reserve any toppings.) Let cool completely, seal, and freeze.

To Thaw: Vent the lid, and microwave until hot, stopping occasionally to stir. Add any toppings just before serving.

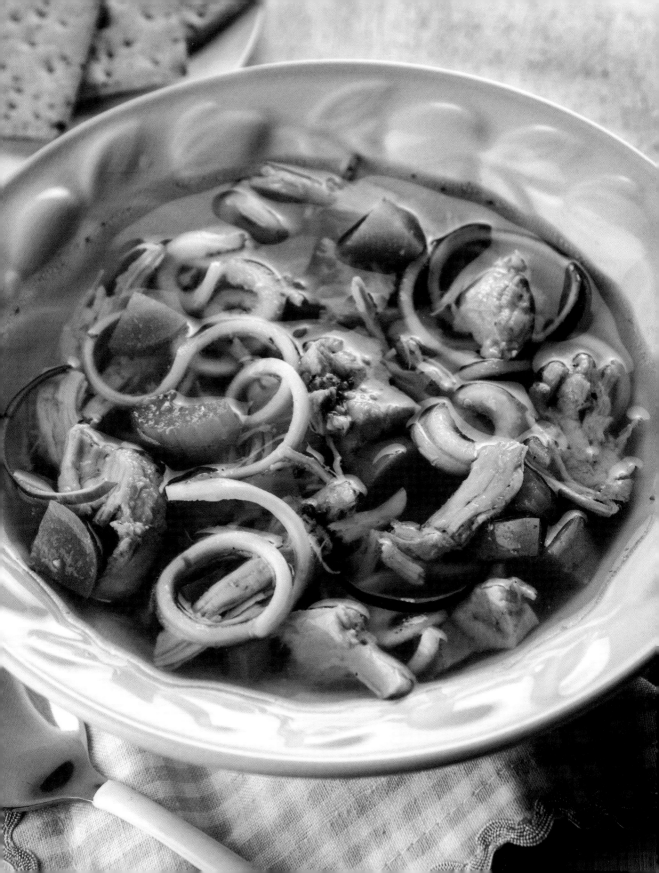

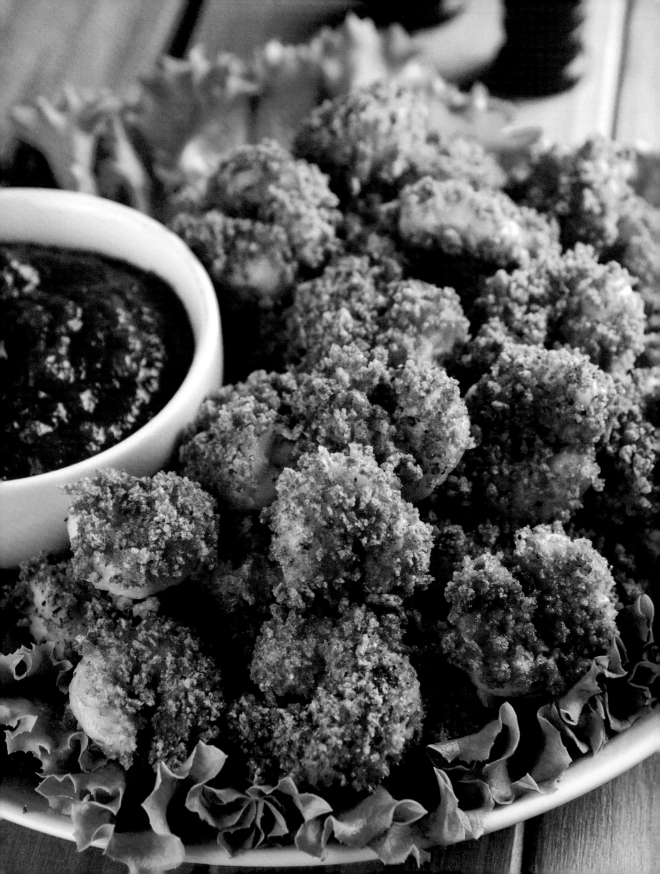

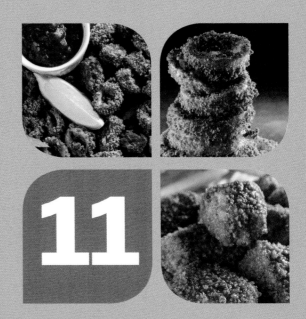

Raising the Bar!

Jalapeño poppers, Buffalo wings, onion rings . . . Nothing says OBSESSED like these typically greasy bar-food favorites! Like the chapter name implies, I'm raising the bar when it comes to the classic finger foods. Gone are the excess calories; here to stay are the iconic flavors and decadence!

Make You Holler Jalapeño Poppers

111 cal

🟢5i 🟣V These truly delicious apps taste EXACTLY like restaurant poppers, but they have a tiny fraction of the calories!

½ cup whole-wheat panko breadcrumbs

⅛ teaspoon each salt and black pepper

½ teaspoon garlic powder

½ teaspoon onion powder

⅓ cup light/reduced-fat cream cheese, room temperature

¼ cup shredded reduced-fat cheddar cheese

6 jalapeño peppers

¼ cup egg whites (about 2 large eggs' worth)

¼th of recipe (3 poppers): 111 calories, 5.5g total fat (3.5g sat fat), 241mg sodium, 10g carbs, 1.5g fiber, 2.5g sugars, 5.5g protein

You'll Need: baking sheet, nonstick spray, 2 wide bowls, small bowl

Prep: 25 minutes • **Cook:** 30 minutes

1. Preheat oven to 375 degrees. Spray a baking sheet with nonstick spray.

2. In a wide bowl, combine breadcrumbs, salt, black pepper, and ¼ teaspoon each garlic powder and onion powder. Mix well.

3. In a small bowl, combine cream cheese, cheddar, and remaining ¼ teaspoon each garlic powder and onion powder. Mix thoroughly.

4. Halve jalapeño peppers lengthwise, and remove seeds and stems.

5. Evenly spoon and spread cheese mixture into the pepper halves.

6. Place egg whites in a second wide bowl. One at a time, coat pepper halves with egg whites, shake to remove excess, and coat with seasoned crumbs.

7. Evenly place on the baking sheet, stuffed sides up. Top with any remaining seasoned crumbs.

8. Bake until outsides are crispy and peppers have softened, 25 to 30 minutes.

MAKES 4 SERVINGS

HG Tips
Use a spoon to seed your jalapeños. When handling jalapeños, don't touch your eyes—that pepper juice can STING. And wash your hands well immediately afterward.

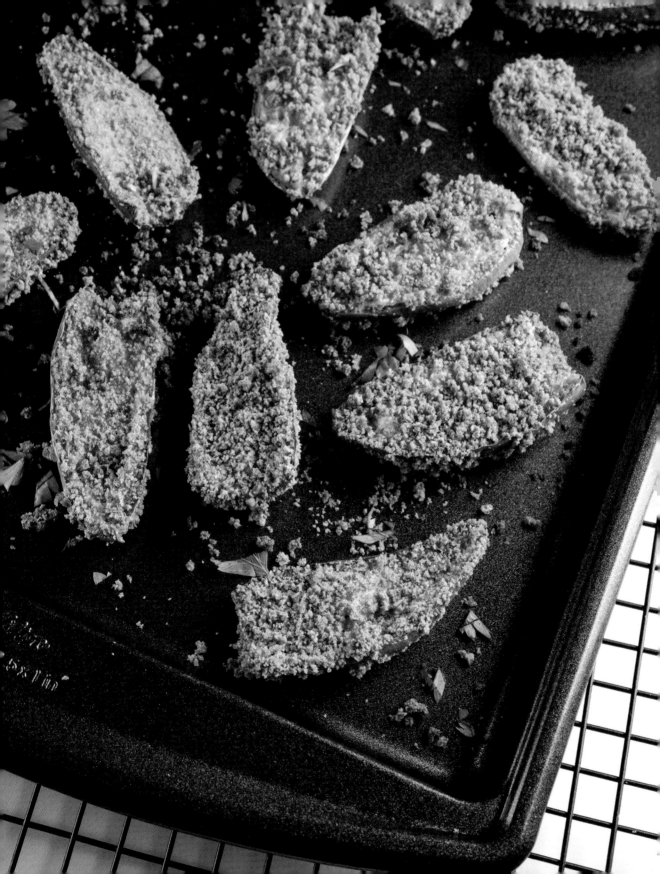

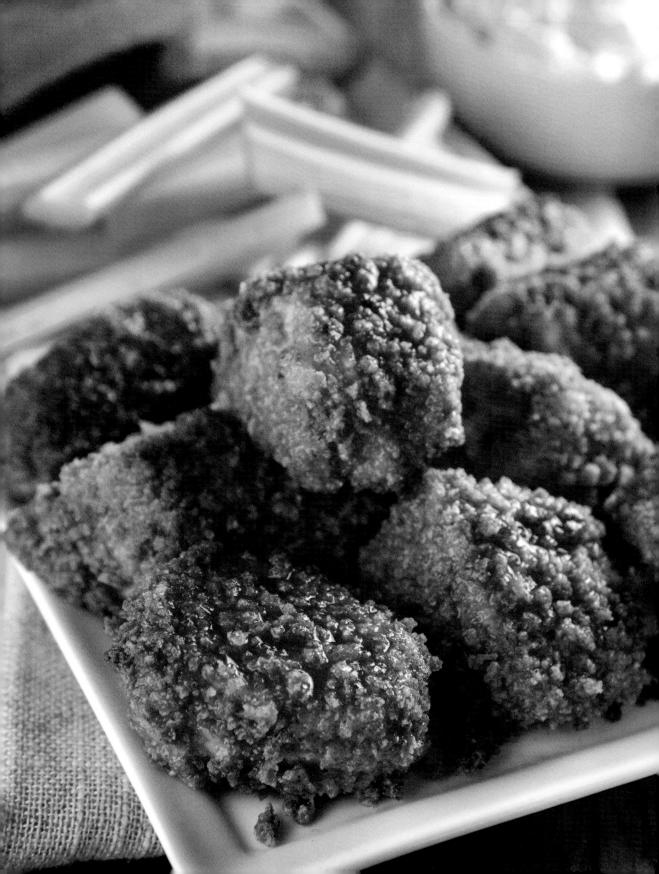

Bangin' Boneless Buffalo Wings

174 cal

5i **30m**   I love, love, love these boneless hot wings! Make a couple of batches for your next get-together . . .

¼ **cup whole-wheat panko breadcrumbs**

⅛ **teaspoon onion powder**

⅛ **teaspoon garlic powder**

Dash cayenne pepper

8 ounces raw boneless skinless chicken breast, cut into 10 nuggets

2 tablespoons egg whites (about 1 large egg's worth)

2 tablespoons Frank's RedHot Original Cayenne Pepper Sauce

Optional dip: Clean & Hungry Chunky Blue Cheese Dressing or Clean & Hungry Ranch Dressing (recipes on pages 338 and 339)

½ of recipe (5 wings): 174 calories, 3g total fat (0.5g sat fat), 648mg sodium, 7g carbs, 1g fiber, 0.5g sugars, 27.5g protein

You'll Need: baking sheet, nonstick spray, 2 wide bowls, small bowl, medium-large bowl

Prep: 10 minutes • **Cook:** 20 minutes

1. Preheat oven to 375 degrees. Spray a baking sheet with nonstick spray.

2. In a wide bowl, mix breadcrumbs with seasonings.

3. Place chicken in another wide bowl. Top with egg whites, and flip to coat.

4. One at a time, shake chicken nuggets to remove excess egg, and lightly coat with seasoned crumbs.

5. Evenly lay nuggets on the baking sheet. Bake for 8 minutes.

6. Flip chicken. Bake until light golden brown and crispy, 8 to 10 minutes.

7. Meanwhile, in a small bowl, combine hot sauce with 2 teaspoons water. Mix well.

8. Transfer chicken to a medium-large bowl. Drizzle with sauce, and gently toss to coat.

MAKES 2 SERVINGS

Chew on This . . .

Only 50 years ago, the wings were the cheapest part of the chicken. Today, they're the most desirable and the most expensive. Luckily, my Buffalo wings are made from more-affordable chicken breast. I'm saving you cash and calories!

Oh Yes We Did Onion Rings

169 cal

5i **30m** **V** Even virtuous veggies become calorie clogged when you batter and deep-fry them! This baked recipe makeover will save you oodles of calories and fat grams. Bonus: No scary deep fryer required!

1 large (about 14 ounces) onion

¼ cup egg whites (about 2 large eggs' worth)

⅔ cup whole-wheat panko breadcrumbs

1 teaspoon garlic powder

1 teaspoon onion powder

¼ teaspoon salt

⅛ teaspoon black pepper

2 tablespoons whole-wheat flour

Optional dip: Clean & Hungry Ketchup (recipe and store-bought alternatives on page 343)

½ of recipe (about 12 rings): 169 calories, 0.5g total fat (0g sat fat), 368mg sodium, 34g carbs, 4.5g fiber, 7g sugars, 7.5g protein

You'll Need: 2 large baking sheets, nonstick spray, wide bowl, medium-large bowl, large sealable plastic bag

Prep: 15 minutes • **Cook:** 15 minutes

1. Preheat oven to 450 degrees. Spray 2 large baking sheets with nonstick spray.

2. Slice off onion ends and remove outer layer. Cut into ½-inch-wide slices, and separate into rings.

3. Place egg whites in a wide bowl.

4. In a medium-large bowl, mix breadcrumbs with seasonings.

5. Add onion rings to a large sealable plastic bag. Sprinkle with flour. Seal bag, and shake to mix.

6. Coat rings with the egg whites by dipping them into the bowl, two at a time. Shake rings to remove excess egg. Lightly coat with seasoned crumbs.

7. Evenly place on the baking sheets, and top with any remaining seasoned crumbs.

8. Bake for 6 minutes, with one baking sheet on the top rack and one on the bottom.

9. Carefully remove baking sheets, and return them to the oven on the opposite racks.

10. Bake until golden brown, about 6 more minutes.

MAKES 2 SERVINGS

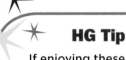

HG Tip

If enjoying these the day after they're made, heat them in a toaster oven for crispiest results!

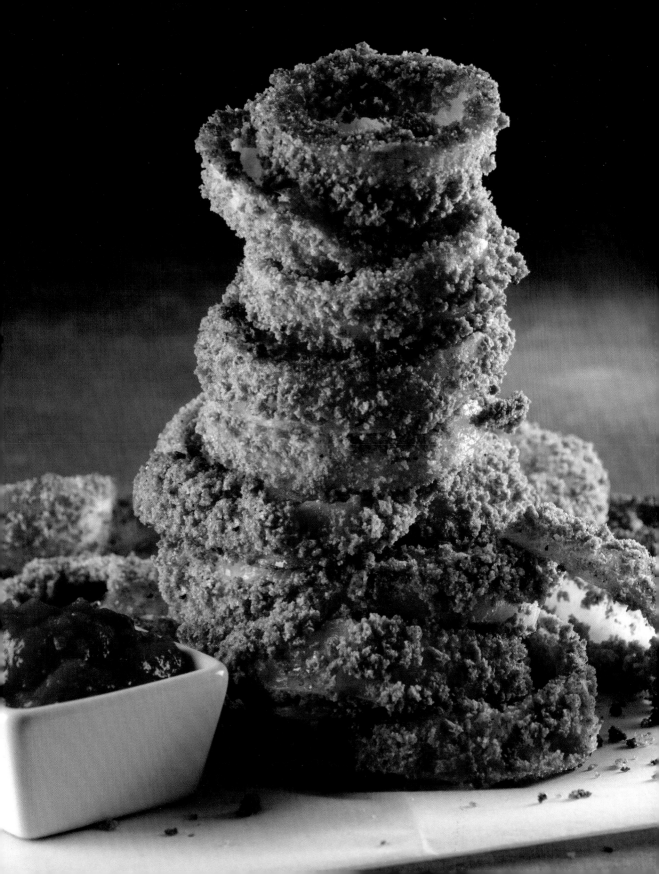

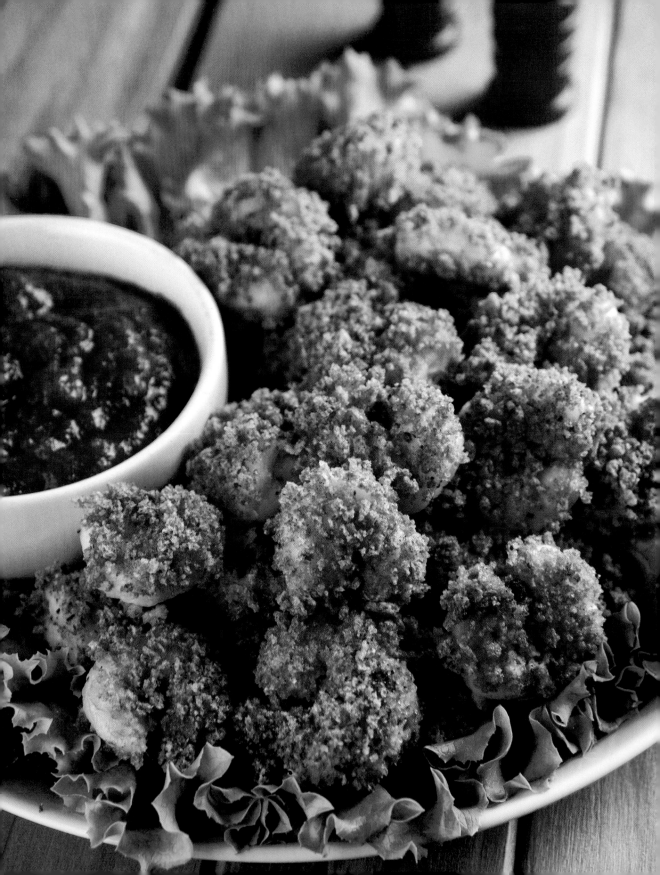

Pop 'Til You Drop Popcorn Shrimp

5i **30m** These things are as delicious as they are low in calories . . . only around 14 calories each!

½ **cup whole-wheat panko breadcrumbs**

1 **teaspoon garlic powder**

½ **teaspoon chili powder**

¼ **teaspoon salt**

⅛ **teaspoon black pepper**

12 **ounces (about 36) raw medium shrimp, peeled, tails removed, deveined**

¼ **cup egg whites (about 2 large eggs' worth)**

Optional dip: Clean & Hungry Ketchup (recipe and store-bought alternatives on page 343)

¼th of recipe (about 9 shrimp): 122 calories, 1g total fat (<0.5g sat fat), 441mg sodium, 7.5g carbs, 1g fiber, 0.5g sugars, 18.5g protein

You'll Need: baking sheet, nonstick spray, 2 wide bowls
Prep: 15 minutes • **Cook:** 10 minutes

1. Preheat oven to 400 degrees. Spray a baking sheet with nonstick spray.
2. In a wide bowl, mix breadcrumbs with seasonings.
3. Place shrimp in another wide bowl. Top with egg whites, and toss to coat.
4. One at a time, shake shrimp to remove excess egg and coat with seasoned crumbs. Lay on the baking sheet, evenly spaced.
5. Bake for 5 minutes.
6. Flip shrimp. Bake until cooked through and crispy, about 5 more minutes.

MAKES 4 SERVINGS

Chew on This . . .

We don't skimp on shrimp. It's the most eaten seafood here in America!

Calamari Me Right Now

184 cal

5i This one tastes EXACTLY like the fried restaurant appetizer, but it's way lower in calories. Find more HG "faux-frys" on page 363!

¾ cup whole-wheat panko breadcrumbs

1 teaspoon grated Parmesan cheese

1 teaspoon onion powder

1 teaspoon garlic powder

1 teaspoon Italian seasoning

½ teaspoon salt

¼ teaspoon black pepper

½ cup egg whites (about 4 large eggs' worth)

1 pound raw calamari rings (not breaded)

2 tablespoons whole-wheat flour

Optional dip: Clean & Hungry Marinara Sauce (recipe and store-bought alternatives on page 336)

Optional garnish: lemon wedges

¼th of recipe (about 1¼ cups): 184 calories, 2g total fat (0.5g sat fat), 403mg sodium, 17.5g carbs, 2g fiber, 1g sugars, 22g protein

You'll Need: 2 baking sheets, nonstick spray, 2 wide bowls, large sealable plastic bag
Prep: 30 minutes • **Cook:** 20 minutes

1. Preheat oven to 375 degrees. Spray 2 baking sheets with nonstick spray.

2. In a wide bowl, combine breadcrumbs, Parm, and seasonings. Mix well.

3. Place egg whites in another wide bowl.

4. Add calamari to a large sealable plastic bag. Sprinkle with flour. Seal bag, and shake to coat.

5. Add calamari to the bowl of egg whites, and gently toss to coat.

6. One at a time, shake calamari to remove excess egg whites, and lightly coat with breadcrumbs.

7. Evenly place on the baking sheets, and top with any remaining breadcrumbs.

8. Bake for 10 minutes.

9. Carefully remove baking sheets, and return them to the oven on the opposite racks.

10. Bake until lightly browned and cooked through, about 10 more minutes.

MAKES 4 SERVINGS

Chew on This...

Calamari is more than a beloved appetizer. Fishermen use it as fish bait. Lucky fish!

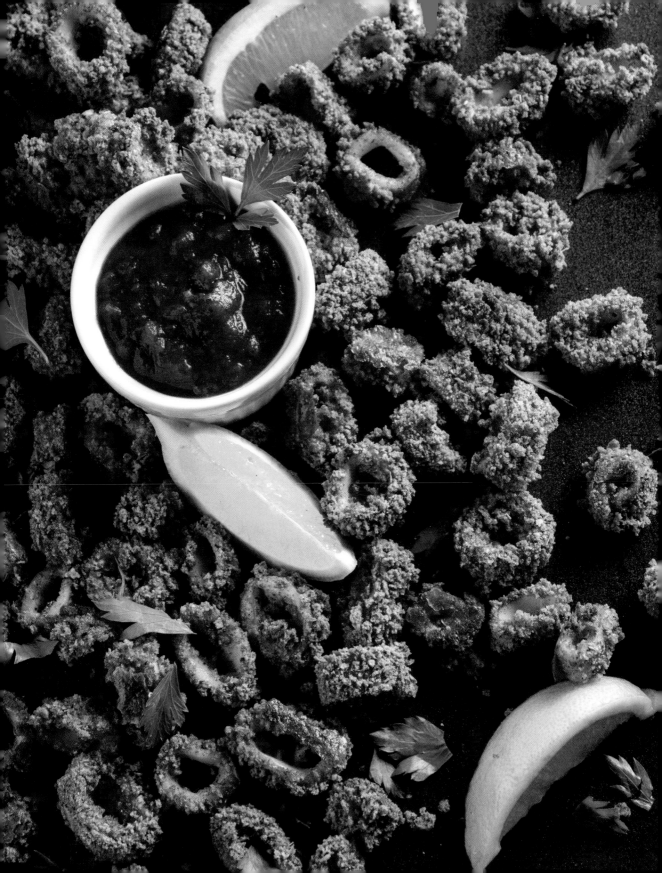

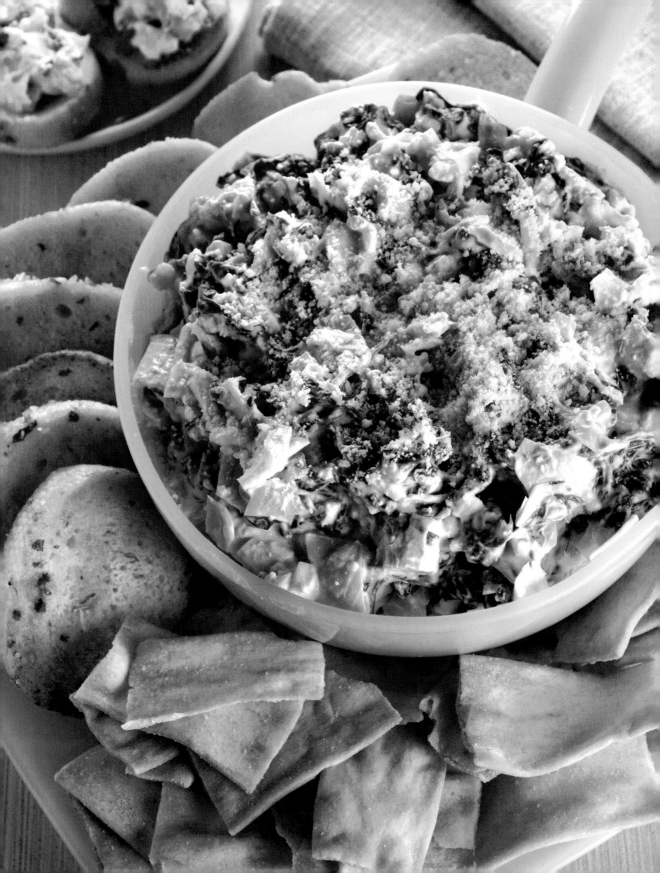

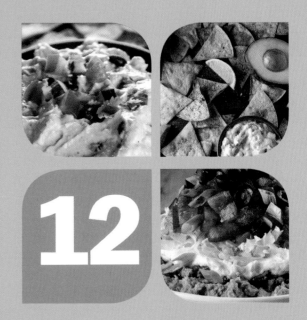

Party Hearty!

Why, oh why do classic party foods have to be SO loaded with fat and calories?! From cheesy nachos to creamy dips, they're pretty much ALL bad news. But no need to serve just celery and carrot sticks at your next shindig. (Your pals might never come back!) Just whip up these surprisingly guilt-free party snacks, and prepare for praise . . .

Reconstructed Nachos

245 cal

30m · V · GF   This is such a fun and delicious take on traditional nachos! Make a few batches for your next party. For more nacho-ish nibbles, check out my Tater Tot-chos (page 183).

Four 6-inch corn tortillas

¼ cup refried beans

⅛ teaspoon ground cumin

⅛ teaspoon chili powder

½ cup shredded reduced-fat Mexican-blend cheese

2 tablespoons seeded and chopped jalapeño pepper

¼ cup Clean & Hungry Salsa (recipe and store-bought alternatives on page 334)

2 tablespoons light sour cream

2 tablespoons chopped scallions

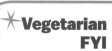

Vegetarian FYI

Not all refried beans are vegetarian friendly. If you avoid animal products, check the can's ingredient list.

½ of recipe (2 loaded tortillas): 245 calories, 9g total fat (4g sat fat), 438mg sodium, 30g carbs, 4.5g fiber, 4g sugars, 12g protein

You'll Need: baking sheet, nonstick spray, small bowl

Prep: 10 minutes • **Cook:** 20 minutes

1. Preheat oven to 400 degrees. Spray a baking sheet with nonstick spray.

2. Lay tortillas on the sheet, and lightly spray with nonstick spray.

3. Bake for 5 minutes.

4. Flip tortillas. Bake until crispy, 3 to 5 minutes.

5. In a small bowl, mix seasonings into beans. Evenly spread onto the tortillas.

6. Sprinkle with cheese, and top with jalapeño pepper.

7. Bake until beans are hot and cheese has melted, 5 to 7 minutes.

8. Top with salsa, sour cream, and scallions.

MAKES 2 SERVINGS

Chew on This . . .

Talk about a happy accident! Some Americans walked into a restaurant in Mexico, and the head chef was nowhere to be found . . . The maître d' threw together some ingredients, and nachos were born.

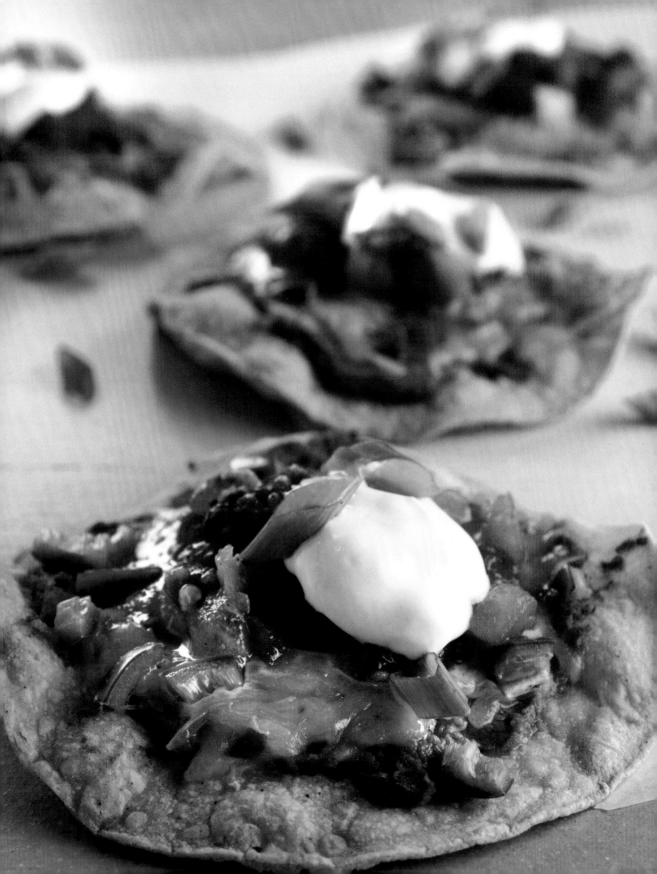

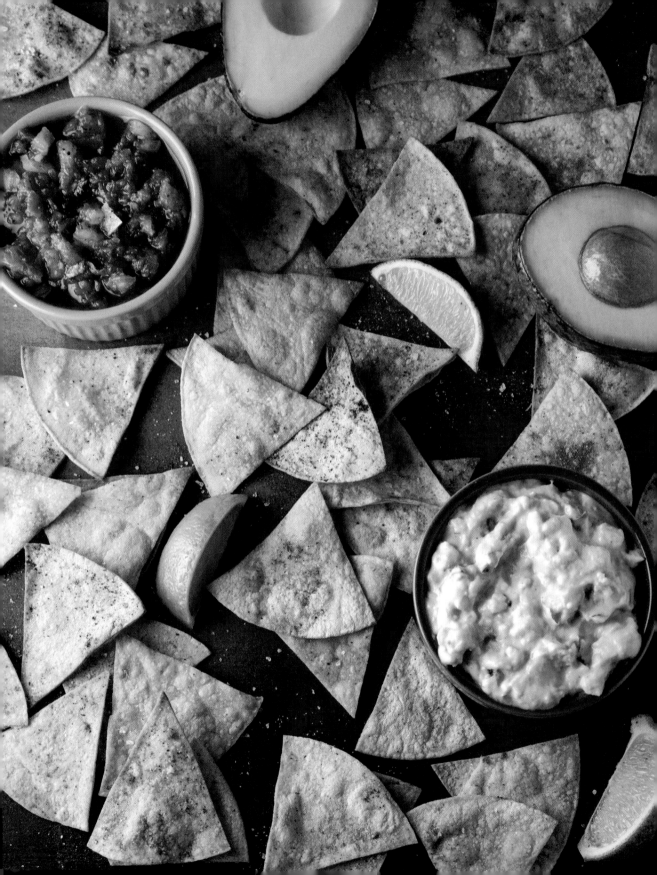

Crispy Crunchy Tortilla Chips

103 cal

5i **15m** **V** **GF** Dip these chips in everything! Clean & Hungry Salsa (page 334), Trop 'Til You Drop Island Salsa (page 207), or one of the many dips on the following pages! Multiply the recipe to serve a crowd . . .

Four 6-inch corn tortillas

¼ teaspoon ground cumin

¼ teaspoon chili powder

¼ teaspoon salt

½ of recipe (12 chips): 103 calories, 1.5g total fat (0g sat fat), 307mg sodium, 20.5g carbs, 2.5g fiber, 1g sugars, 2g protein

You'll Need: baking sheet, nonstick spray

Prep: 5 minutes • **Cook:** 10 minutes

1. Preheat oven to 400 degrees. Spray a baking sheet lightly with nonstick spray.

2. Cut tortillas in half. Cut each half into thirds, for a total of 24 wedges.

3. Lay wedges on the sheet. Spray with nonstick spray, and sprinkle with seasonings.

4. Bake for 5 minutes.

5. Carefully flip wedges. Bake until lightly browned and crispy, about 3 minutes.

MAKES 2 SERVINGS

Chew on This . . .

Potato chips may be the top-selling salty snack, but tortilla chips are increasing in sales at a speedy pace . . .

Ultimate Ate-Layer Dip

  Why stop at seven layers? This dip has EIGHT!

One 16-ounce can refried beans

¼ teaspoon chili powder

¾ teaspoon ground cumin

½ teaspoon onion powder

½ teaspoon garlic powder

8 ounces raw extra-lean ground beef (4% fat or less)

¼ teaspoon salt

1 cup fat-free plain Greek yogurt

½ cup shredded reduced-fat Mexican-blend cheese

2 cups shredded lettuce

1 cup chopped tomatoes

¼ cup chopped scallions

¼ cup sliced black olives

⅛th of recipe (about ¾ cup): 150 calories, 4g total fat (1.5g sat fat), 419mg sodium, 13.5g carbs, 3.5g fiber, 2.5g sugars, 14.5g protein

You'll Need: medium bowl, large skillet, nonstick spray, 8-inch by 8-inch baking pan

Prep: 15 minutes • **Cook:** 5 minutes

1. In a medium bowl, combine beans, chili powder, ½ teaspoon cumin, and ¼ teaspoon each onion powder and garlic powder. Mix well.

2. Bring a large skillet sprayed with nonstick spray to medium-high heat. Add beef, salt, and remaining ¼ teaspoon each cumin, onion powder, and garlic powder. Cook and crumble until fully cooked, about 5 minutes.

3. Spread seasoned beans into an 8-inch by 8-inch baking pan, and evenly layer remaining ingredients: beef, yogurt, cheese, lettuce, tomatoes, scallions, and olives. Serve cold or at room temperature.

MAKES 8 SERVINGS

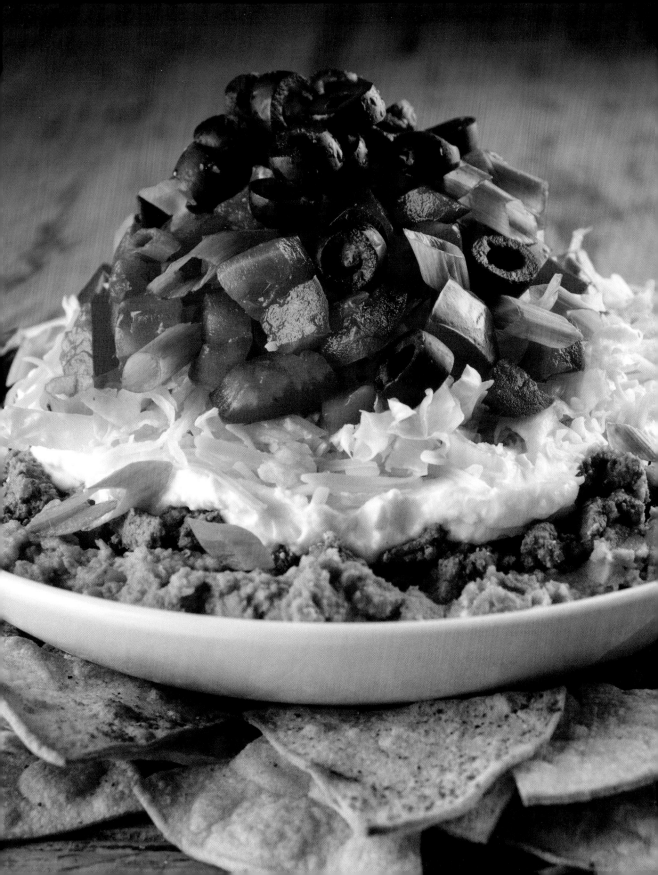

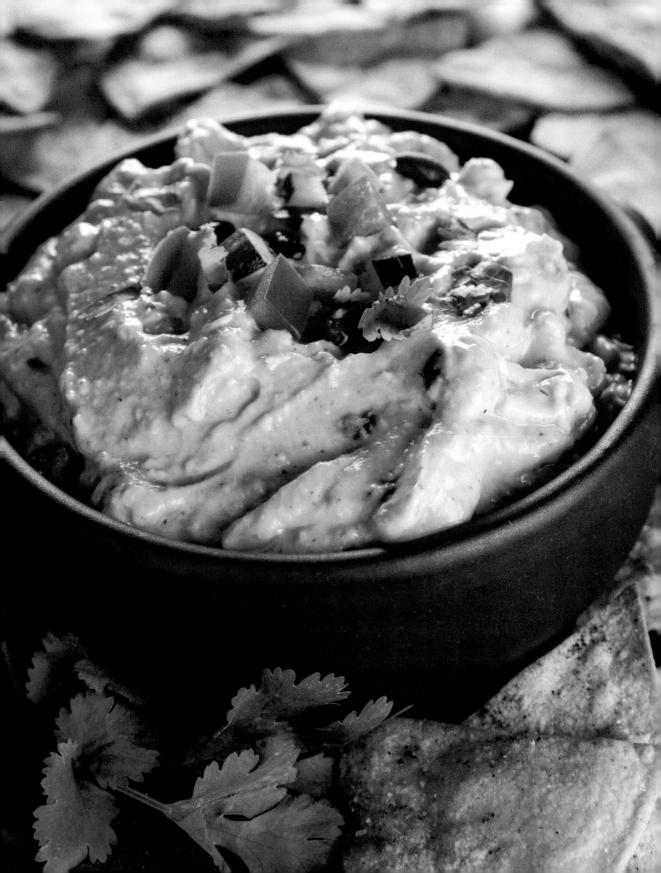

Best in the Southwest Guac Dip

73 cal

🕐15m Ⓥ ⒼⒻ My trick for super-sizing guacamole? Mix in fat-free Greek yogurt and extra veggies! This stuff is insane . . . I love it SO much!

8 ounces mashed avocado (about 1 cup or 2 small avocados' worth)

1 cup fat-free plain Greek yogurt

1 teaspoon lime juice

¾ teaspoon garlic powder

¾ teaspoon chili powder

½ teaspoon salt

¼ cup canned black beans, drained and rinsed

¼ cup chopped red bell pepper

¼ cup finely chopped red onion

2 tablespoons finely chopped fresh cilantro

⅛th of recipe (about ¼ cup): 73 calories, 4g total fat (0.5g sat fat), 180mg sodium, 6g carbs, 2.5g fiber, 2g sugars, 4g protein

You'll Need: medium bowl

Prep: 10 minutes

1. In a medium bowl, combine avocado, yogurt, lime juice, and seasonings. Mix until smooth and uniform.
2. Stir in remaining ingredients.
3. Cover and refrigerate until ready to serve.

MAKES 8 SERVINGS

Chew on This . . .

On Super Bowl Sunday alone, an estimated 139 million pounds of avocado is consumed. Yowsa!

Let's Get Tropical Guacamole

68 cal

   Obsession confession: I once ate an entire batch of this in 24 hours! It's THAT good . . .

8 ounces mashed avocado (about 1 cup or 2 small avocados' worth)

⅔ cup fat-free plain Greek yogurt

1 teaspoon lime juice

½ teaspoon garlic powder

½ teaspoon ground cumin

½ teaspoon salt

½ cup finely chopped mango

¼ cup finely chopped red onion

¼ cup peeled and finely chopped jicama

2 tablespoons finely chopped fresh cilantro

⅛th of recipe (about ¼ cup): 68 calories, 4g total fat (0.5g sat fat), 156mg sodium, 6g carbs, 2.5g fiber, 2.5g sugars, 2.5g protein

You'll Need: medium bowl

Prep: 10 minutes

1. In a medium bowl, combine avocado, yogurt, lime juice, and seasonings. Mix until mostly smooth and uniform.

2. Stir in remaining ingredients.

3. Cover and refrigerate until ready to serve.

MAKES 8 SERVINGS

Chew on This . . .

An avocado tree is more likely to bear fruit with a complementary avocado tree nearby. How romantic!

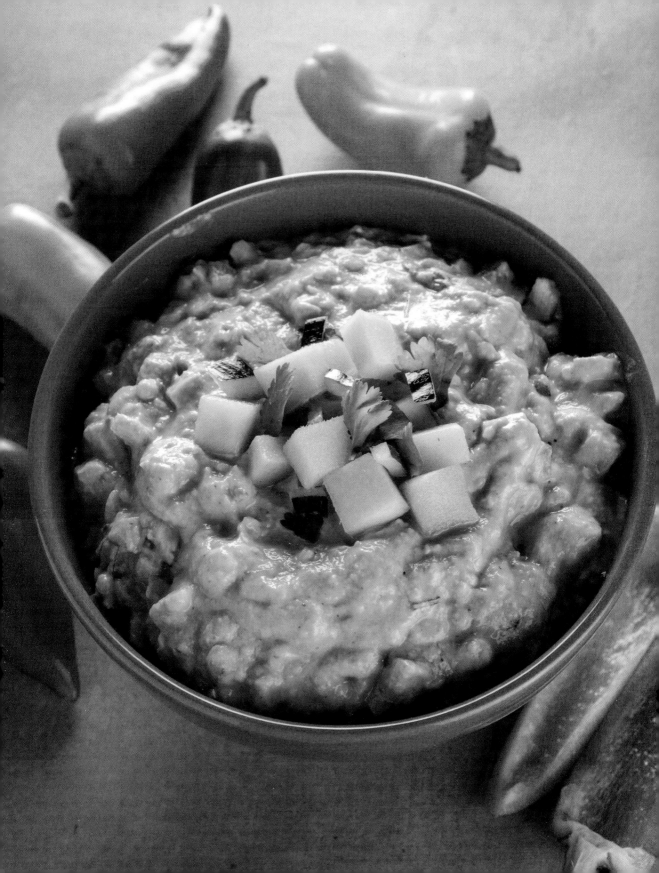

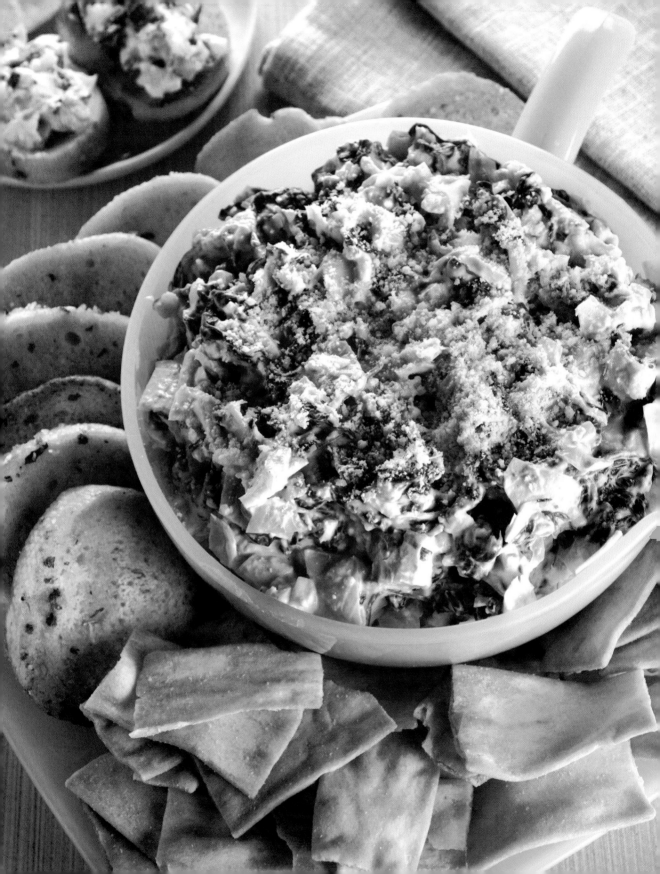

For the Win
Spinach Artichoke Dip

73 cal

This ooey-gooey dip is outrageously delicious! Your party guests will never guess it's guilt-free . . .

½ cup fat-free plain Greek yogurt

½ cup light/reduced-fat cream cheese

¼ teaspoon each salt and black pepper

One 14-ounce can artichoke hearts packed in water, drained and chopped

½ cup shredded part-skim mozzarella cheese

3 tablespoons grated Parmesan cheese

1 cup finely chopped onion

¼ cup finely chopped shallots

10 cups chopped spinach

1 teaspoon chopped garlic

1⁄12th of recipe (about ¼ cup): 73 calories, 3.5g total fat (2g sat fat), 283mg sodium, 5.5g carbs, 1.5g fiber, 2g sugars, 5.5g protein

You'll Need: 8-inch by 8-inch baking pan, nonstick spray, large bowl, extra-large skillet

Prep: 25 minutes • **Cook:** 30 minutes

1. Preheat oven to 350 degrees. Spray an 8-inch by 8-inch baking pan with nonstick spray.

2. In a large bowl, combine yogurt, cream cheese, salt, and pepper. Mix until smooth. Stir in chopped artichoke hearts, mozzarella, and 2 tablespoons Parm.

3. Bring an extra-large skillet sprayed with nonstick spray to medium-high heat. Add onion and shallots. Cook and stir until softened, about 3 minutes.

4. Add spinach and garlic to the skillet. Cook and stir until spinach has wilted and garlic is fragrant, about 2 minutes. Pat dry, if necessary.

5. Add skillet contents to the large bowl. Mix thoroughly.

6. Transfer mixture to the baking pan. Sprinkle with remaining 1 tablespoon Parm. Bake until hot and bubbly, 20 to 25 minutes.

MAKES 12 SERVINGS

Chew on This . . .

Artichokes are a known aphrodisiac. You'll be feeling the love once you try this dip!

OMG! Caramelized Onion Dip

75 cal

V **GF** There are a bazillion ways to enjoy this decadent dip. Get creative! And if you love onions, don't miss the Caramelized Onion Mashies (page 100), Caramelized Onion Cauli-Crust Pizza (page 110), and Caramelized Onion Chickpea Burgers (page 157).

1 cup fat-free plain Greek yogurt

¼ cup light/reduced-fat cream cheese, room temperature

1 tablespoon whipped butter

4 cups chopped sweet onions

½ teaspoon salt

¼ teaspoon cayenne pepper

1½ teaspoons chopped garlic

1 teaspoon Dijon mustard

1 teaspoon balsamic vinegar

⅛th of recipe (about 3 tablespoons): 75 calories, 2g total fat (1.5g sat fat), 212mg sodium, 9.5g carbs, 1.5g fiber, 5g sugars, 4.5g protein

You'll Need: large bowl, extra-large skillet

Prep: 20 minutes • **Cook:** 45 minutes

1. In a large bowl, combine yogurt with cream cheese. Stir until smooth.

2. Melt butter in an extra-large skillet over medium-high heat. Add onions, and sprinkle with salt and cayenne pepper. Stirring frequently, cook for 10 minutes.

3. Reduce heat to medium low. Stirring often, cook until caramelized, 25 to 30 minutes.

4. Add garlic, mustard, and vinegar to the skillet. Cook and stir until garlic is fragrant, about 2 minutes.

5. Add skillet contents to the large bowl, and stir until uniform.

6. Serve warm or chilled.

MAKES 8 SERVINGS

Chew on This...

The average American eats 20 pounds of onions per year. Good thing that's not all at once. (Imagine the smell of that breath!)

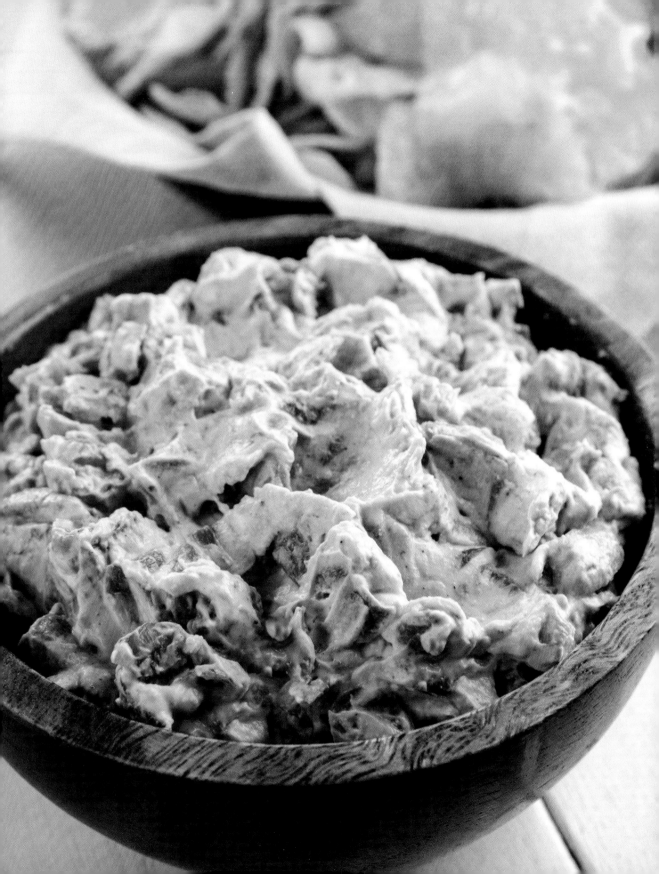

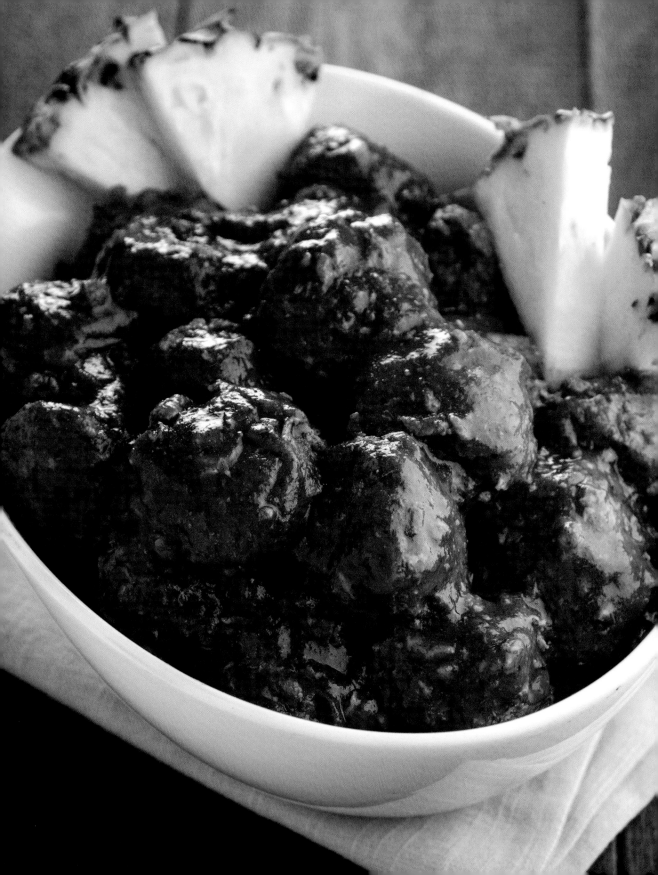

Party-Time Pineapple BBQ Meatballs

263 cal

30m These sweet 'n savory meatballs are spot on. The texture, the sauce . . . Perfect! Also check out my Skillet Swedish Meatball Madness on page 81.

1 cup canned crushed pineapple packed in juice (not drained)

1 cup Clean & Hungry BBQ Sauce (recipe and store-bought alternatives on page 335)

1 pound raw extra-lean ground beef (4% fat or less)

¼ cup whole-wheat panko breadcrumbs

¼ cup egg whites (about 2 large eggs' worth)

2 tablespoons finely chopped fresh cilantro

½ teaspoon garlic powder

½ teaspoon onion powder

¼ teaspoon each salt and black pepper

¼th of recipe (5 meatballs with about ¼ cup sauce):
263 calories, 5g total fat (2g sat fat), 557mg sodium, 25g carbs, 2g fiber, 17g sugars, 27.5g protein

You'll Need: medium bowl, large bowl, extra-large skillet with a lid, nonstick spray
Prep: 15 minutes • **Cook:** 15 minutes

1. Thoroughly drain the juice from the pineapple into a medium bowl. Add ¾ cup BBQ sauce, and mix until uniform.

2. Place drained pineapple in a large bowl. Add remaining ingredients, including remaining ¼ cup BBQ sauce. Mix until uniform.

3. Firmly and evenly form beef mixture into 20 meatballs.

4. Bring an extra-large skillet sprayed with nonstick spray to medium-high heat. Place meatballs in the skillet. Cook and rotate until browned on all sides, about 5 minutes.

5. Reduce heat to medium low. Carefully add BBQ sauce mixture, coating the meatballs. Cover and cook for 10 minutes, or until meatballs are cooked through.

MAKES 4 SERVINGS

Chew on This . . .

Almost every culture has its own version of meatballs. There are Spanish albondigas, Dutch bitterballen, Chinese lion's heads . . . and now Hungry Girl Party-Time Pineapple BBQ Meatballs!

Zucchini-Bottomed Pizza Bites

142 cal

(5i) (30m) (V) (GF) I love pizza so much that I literally cannot stop creating pizza-licious recipes. My Pizza-fied Meatloaf (page 74), White Pizza-fied Grilled Cheese (page 172), and all the recipes in Chapter 4 (You Wanna Pizza Me?) are some great examples!

8 ounces (about 1 medium) zucchini

3 tablespoons canned crushed tomatoes

⅛ teaspoon garlic powder

⅛ teaspoon onion powder

⅛ teaspoon Italian seasoning

Dash each salt and black pepper

3 tablespoons shredded part-skim mozzarella cheese

2 teaspoons grated Parmesan cheese

Optional toppings: red pepper flakes, fresh basil

Entire recipe: 142 calories, 6.5g total fat (3.5g sat fat), 503mg sodium, 11.5g carbs, 3g fiber, 7.5g sugars, 11.5g protein

You'll Need: baking sheet, nonstick spray, small bowl

Prep: 10 minutes • **Cook:** 15 minutes

1. Preheat oven to 400 degrees. Spray a baking sheet with nonstick spray.

2. Slice off and discard the stem ends of the zucchini. Slice into ½-inch rounds, and place on the baking sheet. Bake for 5 minutes.

3. Flip zucchini. Bake until mostly softened and lightly browned, about 5 more minutes.

4. Meanwhile, in a small bowl, combine crushed tomatoes with seasonings. Mix well.

5. Blot excess moisture from zucchini. Top with seasoned tomatoes, and sprinkle with both types of cheese.

6. Bake until tomatoes are hot and mozzarella has melted, about 3 minutes.

MAKES 1 SERVING

Chew on This . . .

Zucchini isn't the strangest thing to happen to pizza. Pizza-flavored potato chips, ice cream, and beer all existed at some point!

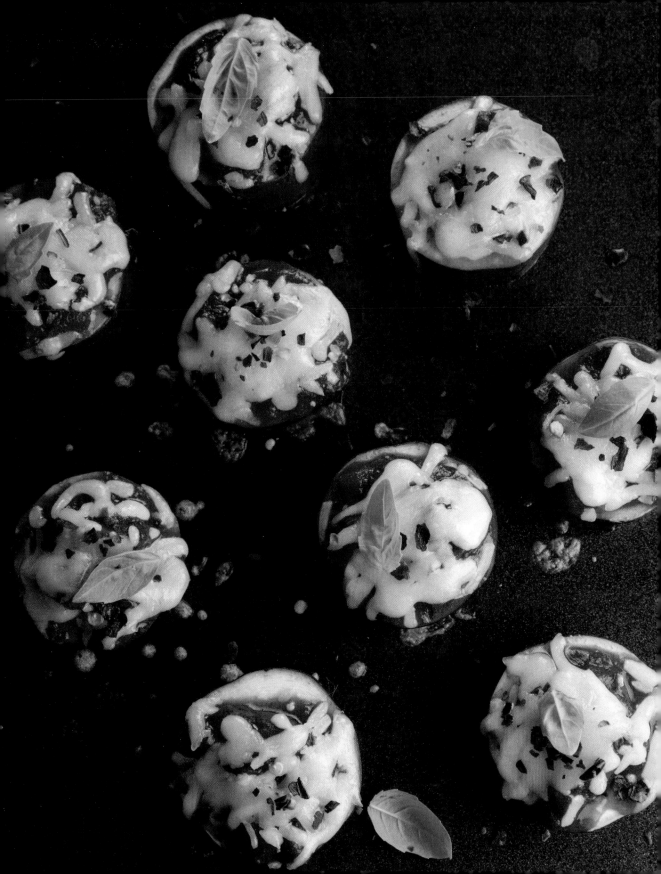

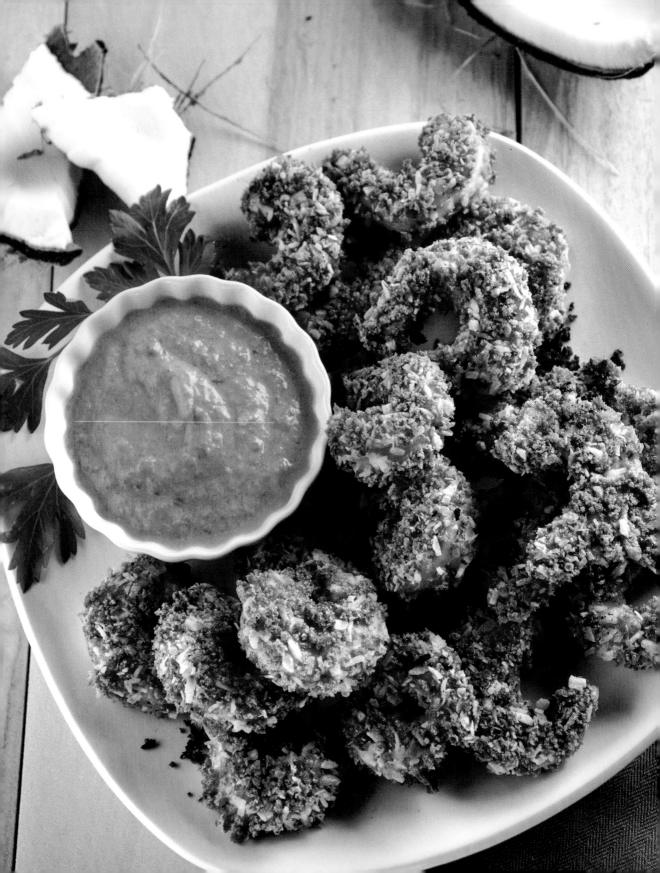

Coco' Loco Coconut Shrimp

177 cal

30m This dish screams decadence, but it's a total calorie bargain. Try it with my Clean & Hungry Creamy Fresh Sriracha (page 340)!

¼ cup egg whites (about 2 large eggs' worth)

¼ teaspoon coconut extract

½ cup whole-wheat panko breadcrumbs

⅓ cup unsweetened shredded coconut

1 packet natural no-calorie sweetener

½ teaspoon chili powder

¼ teaspoon garlic powder

⅛ teaspoon each salt and black pepper

12 ounces (about 24) raw large shrimp, peeled, tails removed, deveined

2 tablespoons whole-wheat flour

¼th of recipe (about 6 shrimp): 177 calories, 5g total fat (3.5g sat fat), 369mg sodium, 12g carbs, 2g fiber, 1g sugars, 19g protein

You'll Need: baking sheet, nonstick spray, 2 wide bowls, large sealable plastic bag

Prep: 15 minutes • **Cook:** 15 minutes

1. Preheat oven to 400 degrees. Spray a baking sheet with nonstick spray.

2. In a wide bowl, mix egg whites with coconut extract.

3. In another wide bowl, combine breadcrumbs, shredded coconut, sweetener, and seasonings. Mix well.

4. Place shrimp in a large sealable plastic bag. Sprinkle with flour. Seal bag, and shake to coat.

5. One at a time, coat shrimp with egg mixture, shake to remove excess, and lightly coat with breadcrumb mixture. Evenly place on the baking sheet.

6. Top shrimp with any remaining breadcrumbs mixture.

7. Bake for 6 minutes.

8. Flip shrimp. Bake until cooked through and crispy, about 6 more minutes.

MAKES 4 SERVINGS

Chew on This...

Betcha thought there was only one . . . There are actually over 1,300 types of coconut!

Easy Cheesy Stuffed Mushrooms

83 cal

V **GF**   Three flavorful cheeses are in each of these savory stuffed mushrooms. So much yum!

16 medium baby bella mushrooms (each about 2 inches wide)

½ cup finely chopped onion

2 teaspoons chopped garlic

⅛ teaspoon cayenne pepper

1½ cups chopped spinach

½ cup light/low-fat ricotta cheese

2 tablespoons shredded part-skim mozzarella cheese

¼ teaspoon onion powder

¼ teaspoon salt

⅛ teaspoon black pepper

⅛ teaspoon ground nutmeg

2 teaspoons grated Parmesan cheese

¼th of recipe (4 stuffed mushrooms): 83 calories, 2.5g total fat (1.5g sat fat), 251mg sodium, 9g carbs, 1.5g fiber, 4.5g sugars, 7.5g protein

You'll Need: baking sheet, nonstick spray, large skillet, medium bowl

Prep: 20 minutes • **Cook:** 25 minutes

1. Preheat oven to 350 degrees. Spray a baking sheet with nonstick spray.

2. Remove stems from mushrooms, and finely chop.

3. Place mushroom caps on the sheet, rounded sides down. Bake until tender, 12 to 14 minutes.

4. Meanwhile, bring a large skillet sprayed with nonstick spray to medium heat. Add chopped mushroom stems, onion, garlic, and cayenne pepper. Cook and stir until veggies have mostly softened and lightly browned, about 3 minutes.

5. Add spinach to the skillet. Cook and stir until wilted, about 2 minutes. Remove from heat, and pat dry, if needed.

6. In a medium bowl, combine all remaining ingredients *except* Parm. Mix thoroughly. Add mixture to the skillet, and stir well.

7. Pat mushroom caps dry. Evenly fill with veggie-cheese mixture. Sprinkle with Parm.

8. Bake until filling is hot and bubbly, 8 to 10 minutes.

MAKES 4 SERVINGS

Chew on This . . .

Eat like an Egyptian . . . Some sources say they once believed mushrooms were the plant of immortality!

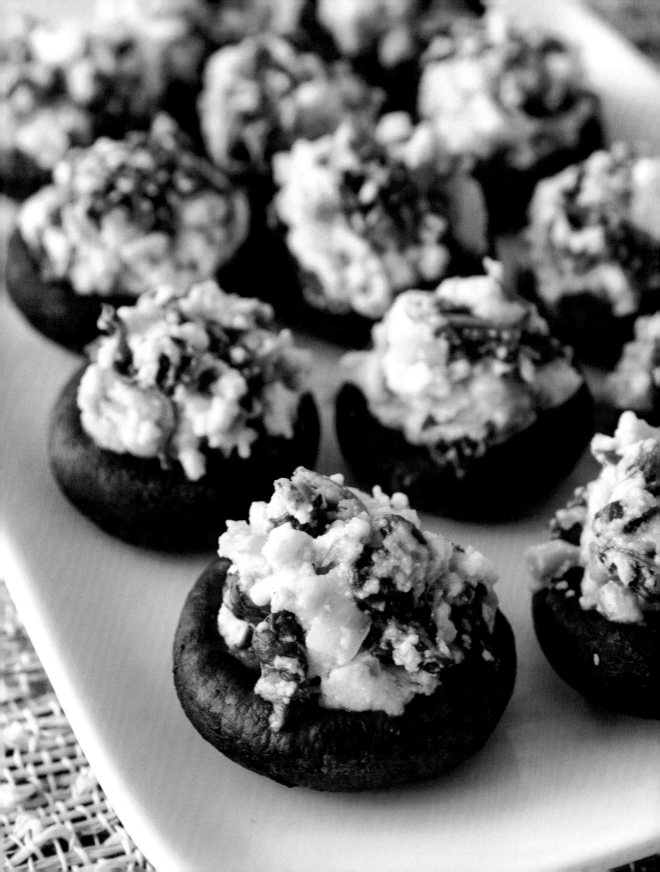

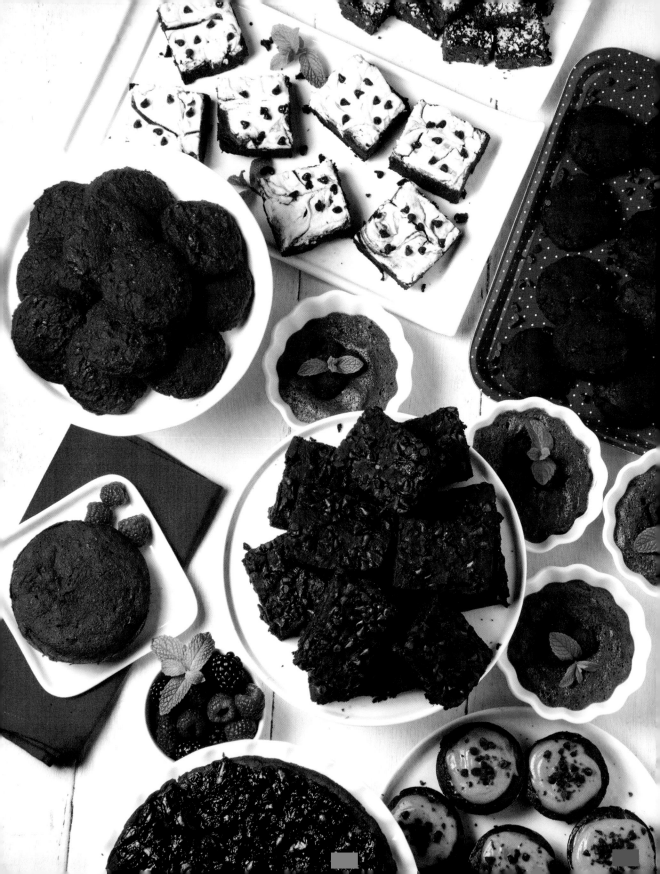

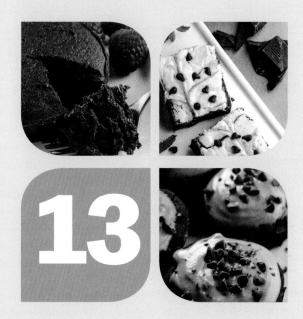

13

Choc' It to Me!

Chocolate consistently ranks as one of the most craved foods in existence. The average American consumes around 9½ pounds of it each year! Of course, it's no surprise that chocolate treats are often sugary, fat heavy, and loaded with calories. Good news: The following pages are filled with healthy chocolate goodies, each under 200 calories per serving!

Bam Bam BrownieZ

97 cal

V I was skeptical about making brownies with zucchini, but it totally works! The dark cocoa really gives them a rich, decadent flavor. Fudgy fantasticness!

1 pound (about 2 medium) zucchini

1½ cups whole-wheat flour

½ cup unsweetened dark cocoa powder

½ cup Truvia spoonable no-calorie sweetener (or another natural brand about twice as sweet as sugar)

1½ teaspoons baking soda

¼ teaspoon salt

½ cup canned pure pumpkin

½ cup egg whites (about 4 large eggs' worth)

½ cup unsweetened vanilla almond milk

1 tablespoon vanilla extract

½ cup mini (or chopped) semi-sweet chocolate chips

¹⁄₁₆th of pan: 97 calories, 3g total fat (1.5g sat fat), 175mg sodium, 22g carbs, 3g fiber, 5g sugars, 3.5g protein

You'll Need: 9-inch by 13-inch baking pan, nonstick spray, box or hand grater, large bowl, medium bowl, whisk

Prep: 20 minutes • **Cook:** 30 minutes • **Cool:** 1 hour

1. Preheat oven to 350 degrees. Spray a 9-inch by 13-inch baking pan with nonstick spray.

2. Peel and shred zucchini.

3. In a large bowl, combine flour, cocoa powder, sweetener, baking soda, and salt. Mix well.

4. In a medium bowl, combine pumpkin, egg whites, almond milk, and vanilla extract. Whisk until uniform.

5. Add contents of the medium bowl to the large bowl, and stir until smooth and uniform. (Batter will be thick.)

6. Fold in shredded zucchini and ¼ cup chocolate chips.

7. Spread mixture into the baking pan, and smooth out the top.

8. Sprinkle with remaining ¼ cup chocolate chips, and lightly press to adhere.

9. Bake until a toothpick (or knife) inserted into the center comes out mostly clean, 25 to 30 minutes.

10. Let cool completely, about 1 hour.

MAKES 16 SERVINGS

Chew on This . . .

Reportedly, the largest brownie ever made weighed an astonishing 4,000 pounds. That's approximately 8,446,000 calories. Eeeks!

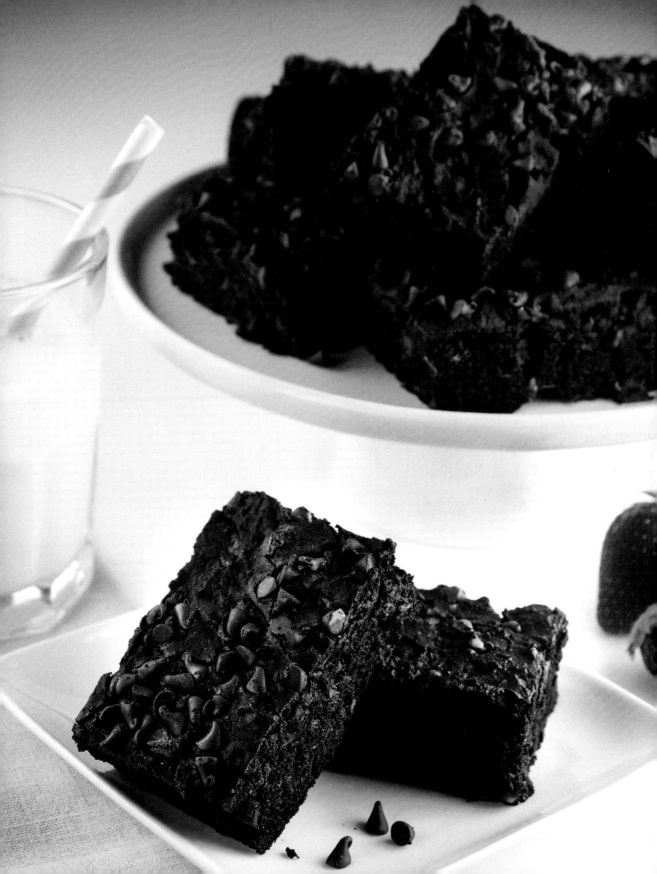

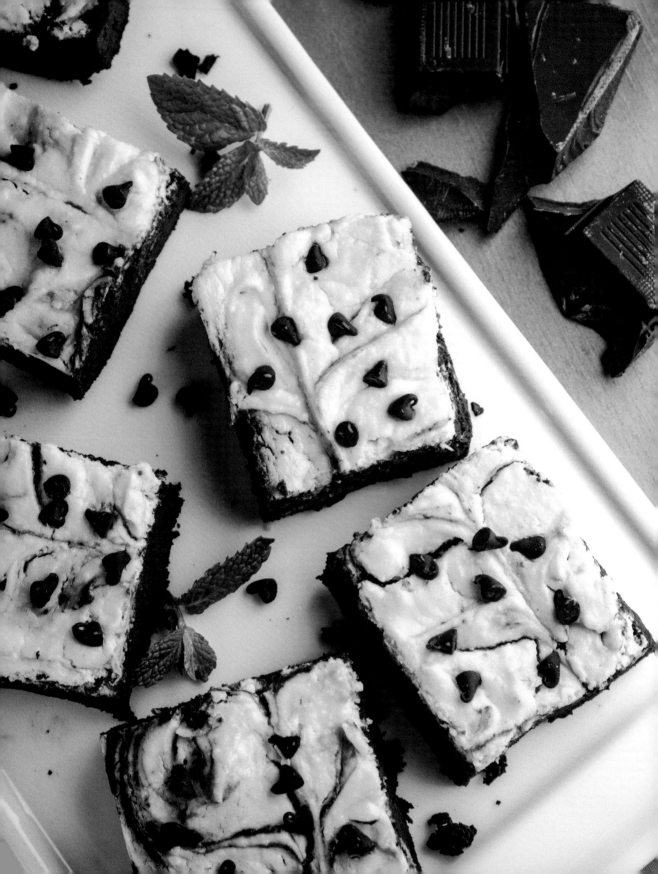

Three Cheers for Cheesecake Brownies

136 cal

v I promise, you cannot taste the black beans in these cheesecake-topped brownies. They're awesome!

BROWNIES

One 15-ounce can black beans, drained and rinsed

½ cup unsweetened cocoa powder

⅓ cup unsweetened applesauce

¼ cup canned pure pumpkin

¼ cup egg whites (about 2 large eggs' worth)

¼ cup whole-wheat flour

¼ cup Truvia spoonable no-calorie sweetener (or another natural brand about twice as sweet as sugar)

1 teaspoon vanilla extract

¾ teaspoon baking powder

¼ teaspoon salt

1 tablespoon mini (or chopped) semi-sweet chocolate chips

TOPPING

½ cup light/reduced-fat cream cheese, room temperature

½ cup light/low-fat ricotta cheese

1 tablespoon Truvia spoonable no-calorie sweetener (or another natural brand about twice as sweet as sugar)

1 teaspoon vanilla extract

1 tablespoon mini (or chopped) semi-sweet chocolate chips

⅑th of pan: 136 calories, 5g total fat (3g sat fat), 303mg sodium, 24g carbs, 4.5g fiber, 4.5g sugars, 7g protein

You'll Need: 8-inch by 8-inch baking pan, nonstick spray, food processor, large bowl, electric mixer

Prep: 20 minutes • **Cook:** 30 minutes • **Cool:** 1 hour

1. Preheat oven to 350 degrees. Spray an 8-inch by 8-inch baking pan with nonstick spray.

2. Place all brownie ingredients *except* chocolate chips in a food processor. Puree until completely smooth and uniform.

3. Fold in chocolate chips.

4. Spread batter into the baking pan, and smooth out the top.

5. In a large bowl, stir cream cheese until smooth. Add all remaining topping ingredients *except* chocolate chips. With an electric mixer set to medium speed, beat until smooth, 1 to 2 minutes.

6. Spoon topping over the brownie batter in dollops. Swirl topping into the batter with a knife. Top with chocolate chips, and lightly press to adhere.

7. Bake until a toothpick (or knife) inserted into the center comes out mostly clean, 25 to 30 minutes.

8. Let cool completely, about 1 hour.

MAKES 9 SERVINGS

Chew on This . . .

It's rumored that cheesecake was served to athletes for energy at early Olympic games. Not sure about you, but I wouldn't be in any shape to run a race after eating a big hunk of cheesecake!

Coconutty Chocolate Fudge

51 cal

V **GF**   This may be the best HG fudge ever! Okay, maybe it's tied with my Nutty for Peanut Butter Fudge Bites on page 322. Both are incredible!

¼ cup pitted dried dates

One 15-ounce can black beans, drained and rinsed

½ cup unsweetened cocoa powder

⅓ cup canned pure pumpkin

¼ cup unsweetened applesauce

¼ cup egg whites (about 2 large eggs' worth)

2 tablespoons coconut flour

2 tablespoons Truvia spoonable no-calorie sweetener (or another natural brand about twice as sweet as sugar)

1 teaspoon baking powder

½ teaspoon coconut extract

¼ teaspoon vanilla extract

¼ teaspoon salt

3 tablespoons mini (or chopped) semi-sweet chocolate chips

2 tablespoons unsweetened shredded coconut

½₀th of pan: 51 calories, 1.5g total fat (1g sat fat), 109mg sodium, 9.5g carbs, 2.5g fiber, 3g sugars, 2g protein

You'll Need: 8-inch by 8-inch baking pan, nonstick spray, 2 small bowls (1 microwave-safe), food processor

Prep: 25 minutes • **Cook:** 40 minutes •
Cool: 1 hour • **Chill:** 2 hours

1. Preheat oven to 350 degrees. Spray an 8-inch by 8-inch baking pan with nonstick spray.

2. Place dates in a small bowl with ½ cup warm water. Soak until softened, 5 to 10 minutes. Drain excess liquid.

3. In a food processor, combine dates with all remaining ingredients *except* chocolate chips and shredded coconut. Puree until completely smooth and uniform.

4. In a small microwave-safe bowl, microwave chocolate chips at 50 percent power for 1½ minutes, or until melted.

5. Add melted chocolate to the food processor, and puree until completely blended.

6. Fold in 1 tablespoon shredded coconut. Spread batter into the baking pan, and smooth out the top.

7. Sprinkle with remaining 1 tablespoon shredded coconut, and lightly press to adhere. Bake until a toothpick (or knife) inserted into the center comes out mostly clean, 30 to 35 minutes.

8. Let cool completely, about 1 hour.

9. Cover and refrigerate until completely chilled, at least 2 hours. (This fudge tastes best when chilled overnight; it's even good slightly frozen!)

MAKES 20 SERVINGS

Chew on This . . .

A tiny island in Michigan considers itself the fudge capital of the world, with upwards of a dozen fudge shops within 3.75 square miles. Who's up for a trip to fudge island?!

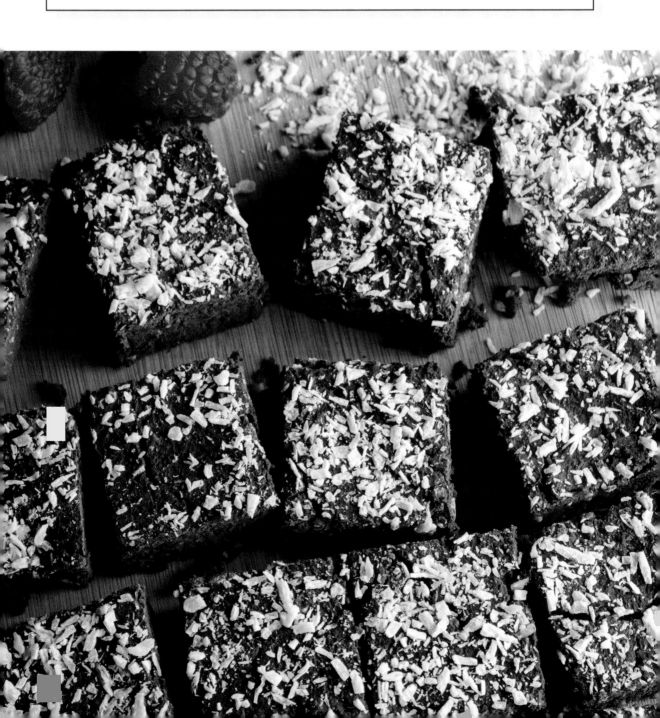

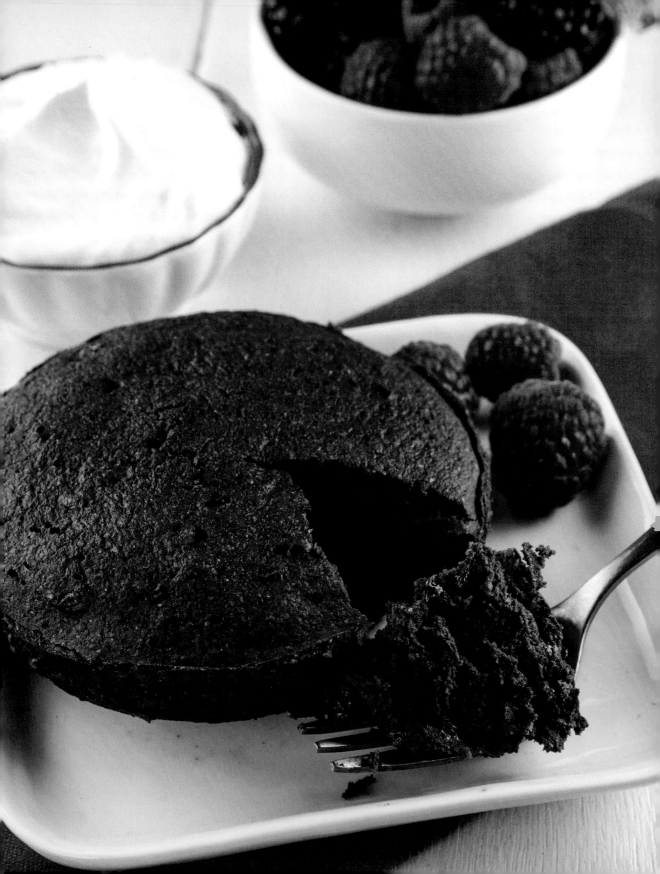

Double Chocolate Mug Cake

190 cal

🕐30m ⓥ Can't trust yourself around a multi-serving cake? Whip up this single-serving cake in minutes! Moist, flavorful, and all-around amazing.

2 tablespoons whole-wheat flour

2 tablespoons unsweetened cocoa powder

3 packets natural no-calorie sweetener

¼ teaspoon baking powder

2 tablespoons unsweetened vanilla almond milk

2 tablespoons egg whites (about 1 large egg's worth)

2 tablespoons fat-free plain Greek yogurt

½ teaspoon vanilla extract

2 teaspoons mini (or chopped) semi-sweet chocolate chips

Entire recipe: 190 calories, 4.5g total fat (2g sat fat), 208mg sodium, 27.5g carbs, 6g fiber, 7g sugars, 11g protein

You'll Need: large microwave-safe mug, nonstick spray

Prep: 5 minutes • **Cook:** 5 minutes • **Cool:** 15 minutes

1. Spray a large microwave-safe mug with nonstick spray. Add flour, cocoa powder, sweetener, and baking powder. Mix well.

2. Add all remaining ingredients *except* chocolate chips. Stir until uniform.

3. Fold in chocolate chips.

4. Microwave for 2½ minutes, or until set.

5. Immediately run a knife along the edges to help separate the cake from the mug.

6. Gently shake mug to release cake, and plate, right side up.

7. Let cool completely, about 15 minutes.

MAKES 1 SERVING

Chew on This . . .

Studies have found that the scent of chocolate triggers relaxation. I'd buy a chocolate candle if I didn't think it would make me hungry every time I burned it!

Fab 'n Flourless Black Forest Cake

V **GF** Chocolate and cherries are quite the dynamic duo! Once again, black beans fly under the radar . . .

CAKE

One 15-ounce can black beans, drained and rinsed

½ cup unsweetened cocoa powder

½ cup egg whites (about 4 large eggs' worth)

⅓ cup unsweetened applesauce

⅓ cup canned pure pumpkin

¼ cup Truvia spoonable no-calorie sweetener (or another natural brand about twice as sweet as sugar)

1½ teaspoons baking powder

1 teaspoon vanilla extract

¼ teaspoon salt

2 tablespoons mini (or chopped) semi-sweet chocolate chips

TOPPING

1 tablespoon arrowroot powder

1½ cups frozen pitted dark sweet cherries (no sugar added), thawed, drained, chopped

1 tablespoon Truvia spoonable no-calorie sweetener (or another natural brand about twice as sweet as sugar)

⅛ teaspoon vanilla extract

Dash salt

⅛th of cake: 117 calories, 2g total fat (1g sat fat), 331mg sodium, 27.5g carbs, 5.5g fiber, 7.5g sugars, 6g protein

You'll Need: 9-inch round cake pan, foil, nonstick spray, food processor, medium nonstick pot, medium bowl

Prep: 20 minutes • **Cook:** 40 minutes •
Cool: 1 hour • **Chill:** 1 hour

1. Preheat oven to 350 degrees. Line a 9-inch round cake pan with foil, and generously spray with nonstick spray.

2. Place all cake ingredients *except* chocolate chips in a food processor. Puree until completely smooth and uniform.

3. Fold chocolate chips into cake batter.

4. Spread batter into the baking pan, and smooth out the top.

5. Bake until a toothpick (or knife) inserted into the center comes out mostly clean, 35 to 40 minutes.

6. Meanwhile, make the topping. Combine arrowroot powder with ⅓ cup water in a medium nonstick pot. Stir to dissolve. Add remaining topping ingredients. Mix well.

7. Set heat to medium. Stirring frequently, cook until thick and gooey, 5 to 7 minutes.

8. Transfer topping to a medium bowl. Once cool, cover and refrigerate.

9. Let cake cool completely, about 1 hour.

10. Evenly top cake with topping.

11. Refrigerate until chilled, at least 1 hour.

MAKES 8 SERVINGS

Chew on This . . .

In Mayan times, cocoa beans were a valuable form of currency! This chocolate cake is pretty priceless . . .

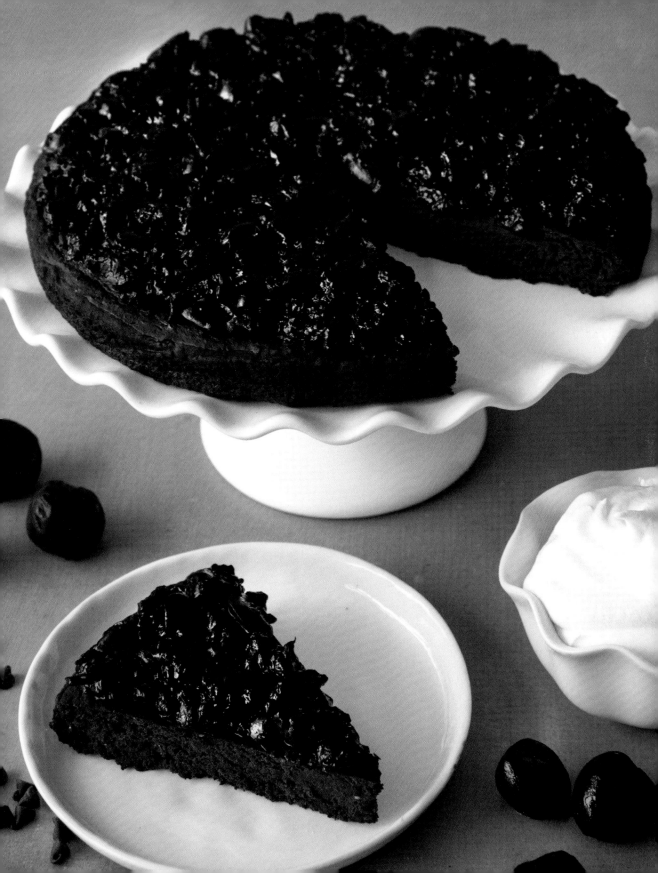

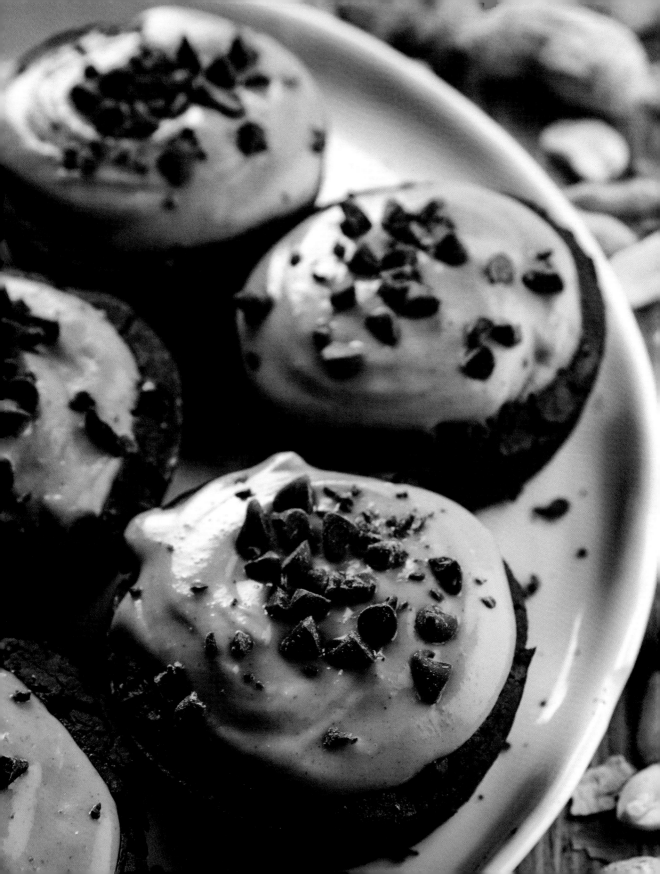

PB for Me Flourless Chocolate Cupcakes

132 cal

V **GF** Portion-controlled chocolate cake with a gooey peanut butter topping? Hello, deliciousness! Find more PB recipes on page 363!

CUPCAKES

One 15-ounce can black beans, drained and rinsed

½ cup unsweetened cocoa powder

½ cup egg whites (about 4 large eggs' worth)

⅓ cup unsweetened applesauce

⅓ cup canned pure pumpkin

¼ cup Truvia spoonable no-calorie sweetener (or another natural brand that's about twice as sweet as sugar)

1½ teaspoons baking powder

1 teaspoon vanilla extract

¼ teaspoon salt

2 tablespoons mini (or chopped) semi-sweet chocolate chips

TOPPING

2½ tablespoons powdered peanut butter or defatted peanut flour

3 tablespoons unsweetened vanilla almond milk

1 tablespoon creamy peanut butter (no sugar added)

2½ teaspoons honey

1 tablespoon mini (or chopped) semi-sweet chocolate chips, crushed

⅛th of recipe (1 cupcake): 132 calories, 3.5g total fat (1.5g sat fat), 325mg sodium, 25g carbs, 5.5g fiber, 7g sugars, 7g protein

You'll Need: 12-cup muffin pan, nonstick spray, food processor, small microwave-safe bowl

Prep: 15 minutes • **Cook:** 40 minutes • **Cool:** 1 hour

1. Preheat oven to 350 degrees. Generously spray 8 cups of a 12-cup muffin pan with nonstick spray.

2. Place all cupcake ingredients *except* chocolate chips in a food processor. Puree until completely smooth and uniform.

3. Fold in chocolate chips.

4. Evenly distribute batter into the 8 cups of the muffin pan, and smooth out the tops.

5. Bake until a toothpick (or knife) inserted into the center of a cupcake comes out mostly clean, 35 to 40 minutes.

6. Let cool completely, about 1 hour.

7. To make the topping, in a small microwave-safe bowl, combine powdered peanut butter/peanut flour with almond milk. Stir until uniform. Add creamy peanut butter and honey. Microwave for 15 seconds, or until melted. Stir until smooth and uniform.

8. Spread topping onto cupcakes, and sprinkle with crushed chocolate chips.

MAKES 8 SERVINGS

Chew on This...

When it comes to peanut butter, women tend to go for creamy, while men prefer chunky. Who knew?

Mmmm, Chocolate Mousse

  Creamy, dreamy, chocolatey deliciousness! Dark cocoa does it again . . .

½ cup egg whites (about 4 large eggs' worth), room temperature

½ teaspoon cream of tartar

2 packets natural no-calorie sweetener

3 tablespoons mini (or chopped) semi-sweet chocolate chips

1 teaspoon vanilla extract

¼ cup fat-free plain Greek yogurt

2 tablespoons unsweetened dark cocoa powder

Optional topping: raspberries

¼th of recipe (about ½ cup): 89 calories, 3.5g total fat (2.5g sat fat), 81mg sodium, 9.5g carbs, 1g fiber, 6.5g sugars, 5.5g protein

You'll Need: large bowl, electric mixer, medium microwave-safe bowl, 4 small bowls

Prep: 15 minutes • **Cook:** 5 minutes • **Chill:** 4 hours

1. Place room-temp egg whites in a large bowl. With an electric mixer set to high speed, beat until fluffy and slightly stiff, about 4 minutes.

2. Continue to beat while adding cream of tartar and 1 sweetener packet. Beat until stiff peaks form, 2 to 3 minutes.

3. In a medium microwave-safe bowl, combine chocolate chips, vanilla extract, and 1 tablespoon water. Microwave at 50 percent power for 30 seconds, or until melted. Stir well. Add Greek yogurt, cocoa powder, and remaining sweetener packet. Mix until uniform.

4. Gently fold contents of the medium bowl into the large bowl. Evenly distribute mixture among four small bowls.

5. Refrigerate until chilled and set, about 4 hours.

MAKES 4 SERVINGS

Chew on This . . .

The first written record of chocolate mousse in the US appears to come from an 1892 food exposition held at Madison Square Garden in New York City. Go, NYC!

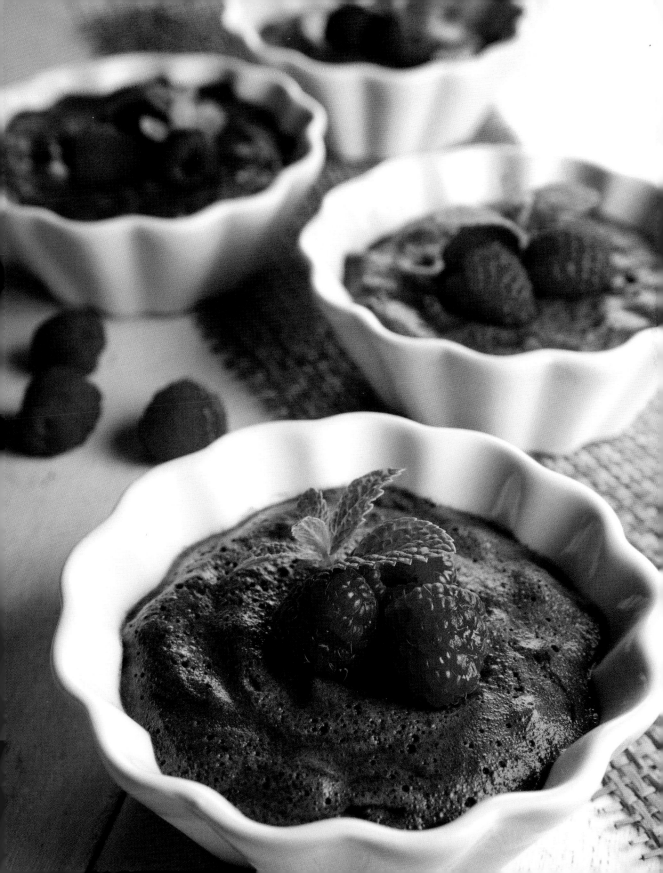

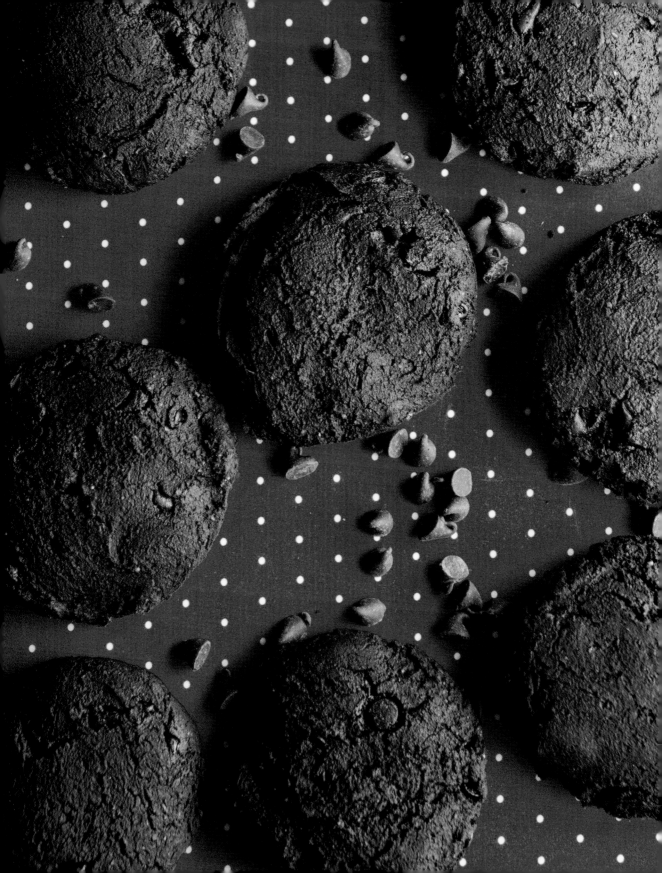

Lookie Lookie Chocolate Fudge Cookies

56 cal

30m **V** These chewy cookies get much of their richness from avocado, but all you'll taste is rich chocolate flavor. Promise!

3 ounces avocado (about ⅓ cup or 1 small avocado's worth)

⅓ cup egg whites (about 3 large eggs' worth)

3 tablespoons Truvia spoonable no-calorie sweetener (or another natural brand about twice as sweet as sugar)

2 tablespoons canned pure pumpkin

1 teaspoon vanilla extract

½ cup unsweetened cocoa powder

⅓ cup whole-wheat flour

½ teaspoon baking soda

3 tablespoons mini (or chopped) semi-sweet chocolate chips

¹⁄₁₂th of recipe (1 cookie): 56 calories, 2.5g total fat (1g sat fat), 65mg sodium, 10.5g carbs, 2g fiber, 2g sugars, 2g protein

You'll Need: baking sheet, wax or parchment paper, small blender or food processor, medium-large bowl, whisk

Prep: 15 minutes • **Cook:** 15 minutes

1. Preheat oven to 350 degrees. Line a baking sheet with wax or parchment paper.

2. In a small blender or food processor, puree avocado until smooth.

3. In a medium-large bowl, combine pureed avocado, egg whites, sweetener, pumpkin, and vanilla extract. Whisk until uniform.

4. Gradually stir in cocoa powder, flour, and baking soda. Stir until just mixed and uniform.

5. Fold in chocolate chips.

6. Evenly distribute mixture into 12 mounds on the baking sheet, about 1½ tablespoons each. Use the back of a spoon to spread and flatten into 2-inch circles.

7. Bake until a toothpick inserted into the center of a cookie comes out clean, 10 to 12 minutes.

MAKES 12 SERVINGS

Freeze It: Baked Goods Edition

To Freeze: Once cool, tightly wrap each serving in foil or plastic wrap. Place individually wrapped treats in a sealable container or bag, seal, and store in the freezer.

To Thaw: Unwrap a treat, and place on a microwave-safe plate. Microwave at 50 percent power for 45 seconds, or until it reaches your desired temperature. Alternatively, refrigerate overnight to thaw.

Double Chocolate Cakies

48 cal

V Obsession confession: These started out as donut holes but didn't hold their shape. But since they were SO delicious, I embraced their flatness and renamed them cakies!

¾ cup whole-wheat flour

⅓ cup unsweetened cocoa powder

3 tablespoons Truvia spoonable no-calorie sweetener (or another natural brand that's about twice as sweet as sugar)

½ teaspoon baking powder

⅛ teaspoon baking soda

⅛ teaspoon salt

½ cup unsweetened vanilla almond milk

½ cup fat-free plain Greek yogurt

⅓ cup canned pure pumpkin

¼ cup egg whites (about 2 large eggs' worth)

¾ teaspoon vanilla extract

3 tablespoons mini (or chopped) semi-sweet chocolate chips

⅟₁₆th of recipe (1 cakie): 48 calories, 1g total fat (0.5g sat fat), 57mg sodium, 10g carbs, 1.5g fiber, 2g sugars, 2.5g protein

You'll Need: baking sheet, nonstick spray, large bowl, medium bowl, whisk

Prep: 15 minutes • **Cook:** 10 minutes • **Cool:** 15 minutes

1. Preheat oven to 350 degrees. Spray a baking sheet with nonstick spray.

2. In a large bowl, combine flour, cocoa powder, sweetener, baking powder, baking soda, and salt. Mix well.

3. In a medium bowl, combine almond milk, yogurt, pumpkin, egg whites, and vanilla extract. Whisk until uniform.

4. Add contents of the medium bowl to the large bowl, and stir until smooth and uniform. (Batter will be thick.)

5. Fold in chocolate chips. Spoon batter onto the sheet in 16 evenly sized mounds. Use the back of a spoon to spread and flatten into 2-inch circles.

6. Bake until a toothpick inserted into the center of a "cakie" comes out mostly clean, about 10 minutes.

7. Let cool completely, about 15 minutes.

MAKES 16 SERVINGS

Chew on This...

A restaurant in New York offers a super-schmancy sundae made with one of the world's most expensive types of chocolate. It requires a reservation two days in advance, includes edible gold, and costs $1,000! Thanks, but no thanks . . .

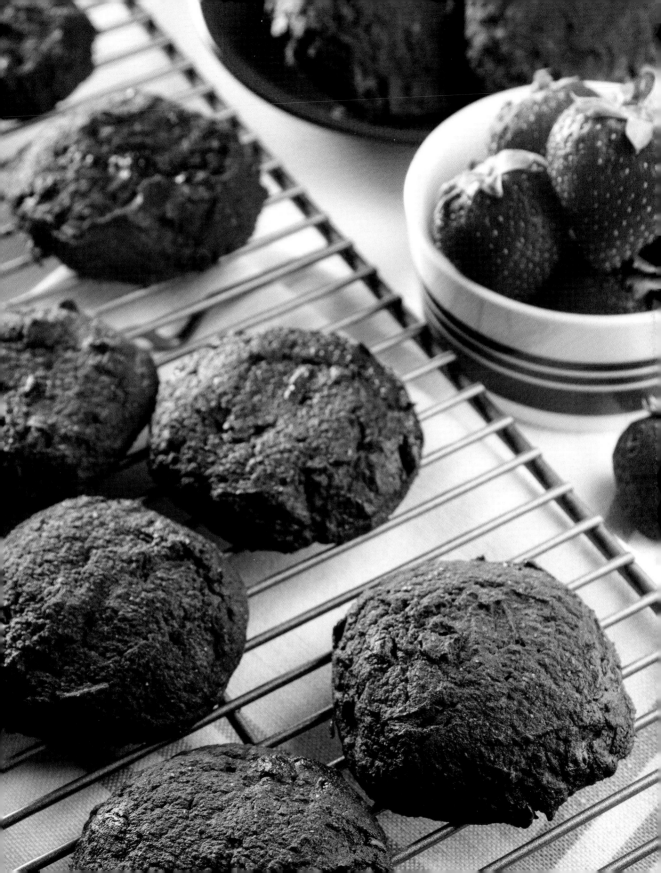

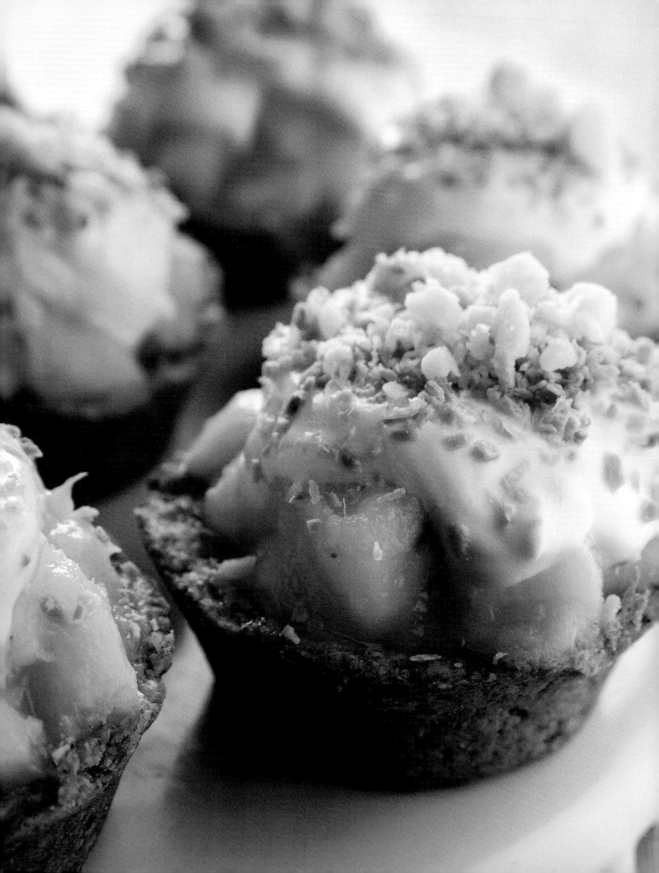

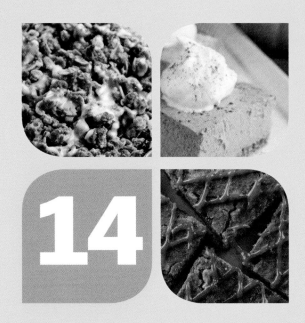

Totally Desserted!

Chocolate isn't the only type of dessert we're obsessed with! From fruit-pie cravings to peanut-butter passions, America's got a huge sweet tooth. Well, just forget about all the over-caloried temptations out there. These lightened-up desserts will blow your sweets-lovin' mind . . .

Sweet Cinnamon Cakies

41 cal

V These cake-like cookies are so delicious, they're practically addictive . . . and only 41 calories each!

1 cup whole-wheat flour

3 tablespoons Truvia spoonable no-calorie sweetener (or another natural brand about twice as sweet as sugar)

1 teaspoon pumpkin pie spice

½ teaspoon baking powder

⅛ teaspoon baking soda

⅛ teaspoon salt

½ cup unsweetened vanilla almond milk

½ cup fat-free plain Greek yogurt

⅓ cup canned pure pumpkin

¼ cup egg whites (about 2 large eggs' worth)

½ teaspoon vanilla extract

¼ teaspoon maple extract

1 tablespoon whipped butter

1 teaspoon cinnamon

¹⁄₁₆th of recipe (1 cakie): 41 calories, 0.5g total fat (<0.5g sat fat), 62mg sodium, 9g carbs, 1g fiber, 0.5g sugars, 2g protein

You'll Need: baking sheet, nonstick spray, large bowl, medium bowl, whisk, 2 small bowls (one microwave-safe)

Prep: 20 minutes • **Cook:** 10 minutes • **Cool:** 15 minutes

1. Preheat oven to 350 degrees. Spray a baking sheet with nonstick spray.

2. In a large bowl, combine flour with 2½ tablespoons sweetener. Add pumpkin pie spice, baking powder, baking soda, and salt. Mix well.

3. In a medium bowl, combine almond milk, yogurt, pumpkin, egg whites, and both extracts. Whisk until uniform.

4. Add contents of the medium bowl to the large bowl, and stir until smooth and uniform. (Batter will be thick.)

5. Spoon batter onto the sheet in 16 evenly sized mounds. Use the back of a spoon to spread and flatten into 2-inch circles.

6. Bake until a toothpick inserted into the center of a "cakie" comes out mostly clean, about 10 minutes.

7. Let cool completely, about 15 minutes.

8. In a small microwave-safe bowl, microwave butter for 30 seconds, or until melted.

9. In a small bowl, mix cinnamon with remaining ½ tablespoon sweetener.

10. Brush cakies with melted butter, and sprinkle with cinnamon mixture.

MAKES 16 SERVINGS

Chew on This . . .

People love their bite-sized sweets! Google searches for mini desserts grew 82 percent from December 2015 to January 2016.

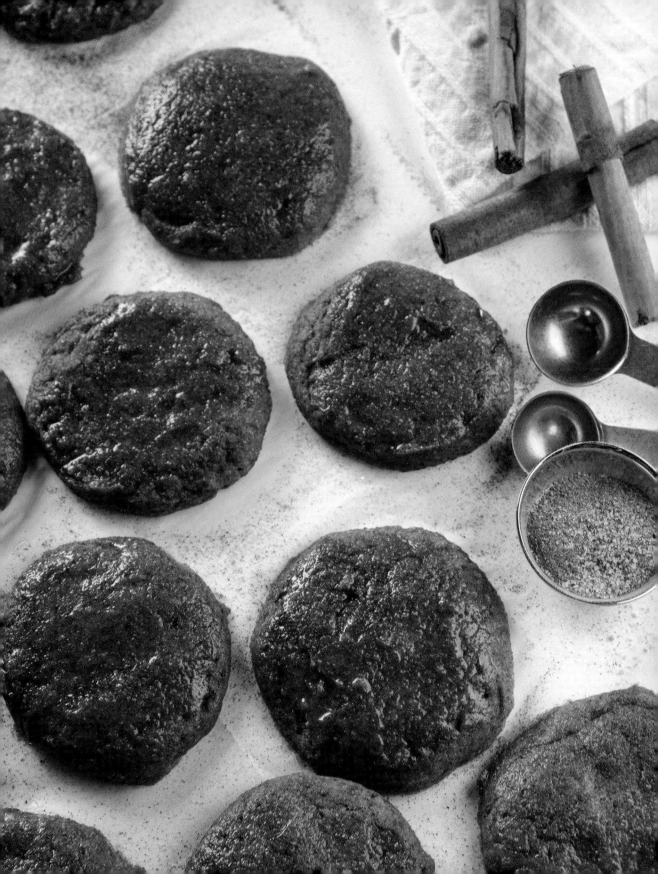

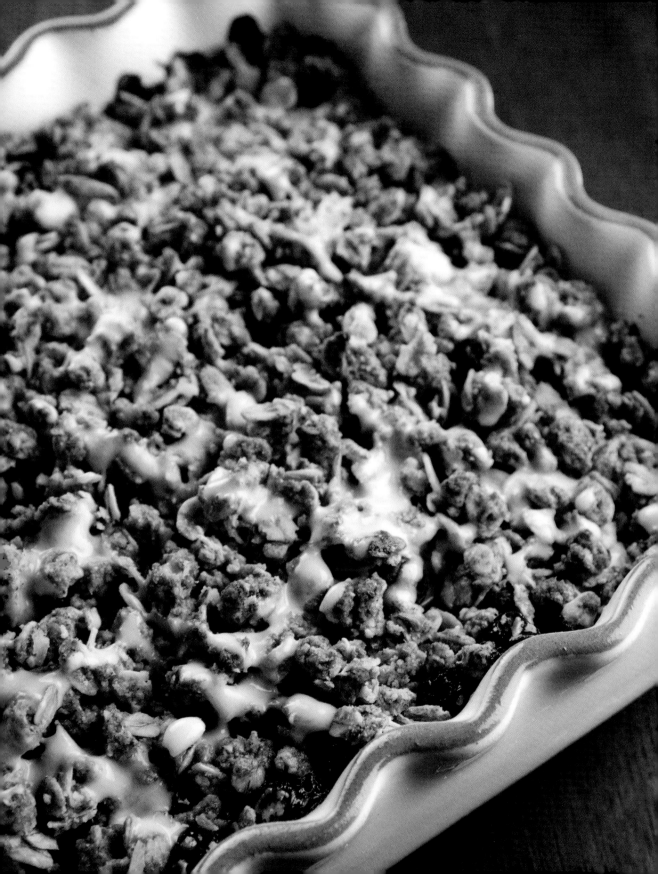

Bigtime Blueberry Crumble

193 cal

V The pie-like filling, the cream-cheese drizzle, the crumbly topping . . . This recipe is out of this world!

FILLING

6 cups blueberries (fresh or thawed from frozen and drained)

¼ cup arrowroot powder

2 tablespoons Truvia spoonable calorie-free sweetener (or another natural brand that's about twice as sweet as sugar)

2 teaspoons lemon juice

1 teaspoon vanilla extract

¼ teaspoon cinnamon

⅛ teaspoon salt

TOPPING

½ cup old-fashioned oats

¼ cup whole-wheat flour

2 tablespoons whipped butter

2 tablespoons unsweetened applesauce

2 teaspoons Truvia spoonable calorie-free sweetener (or another natural brand that's about twice as sweet as sugar)

¼ teaspoon cinnamon

¼ teaspoon baking powder

⅛ teaspoon salt

ICING

2 tablespoons light/reduced-fat cream cheese

1 tablespoon honey

¼ teaspoon vanilla extract

⅙th of pan (about ¾ cup): 193 calories, 4g total fat (2g sat fat), 158mg sodium, 44g carbs, 5g fiber, 18.5g sugars, 3g protein

You'll Need: 8-inch by 8-inch baking pan, nonstick spray, large bowl, medium bowl, small microwave-safe bowl

Prep: 15 minutes • **Cook:** 40 minutes • **Cool:** 1 hour • **Chill:** 2 hours

1. Preheat oven to 375 degrees. Spray an 8-inch by 8-inch baking pan with nonstick spray.

2. Place blueberries in a large bowl. Sprinkle/top with remaining filling ingredients, and stir to coat.

3. Transfer filling to the baking pan.

4. Combine topping ingredients in a medium bowl. Mash and stir until uniform and crumbly.

5. Break topping into pieces, and sprinkle over filling.

6. Bake until topping is golden brown and filling is bubbly, 35 to 40 minutes.

7. Let cool for 1 hour.

8. Refrigerate until thickened and chilled, at least 2 hours.

9. In a small microwave-safe bowl, combine icing ingredients. Mix well. Microwave at 50 percent power for 15 seconds, or until melted.

10. Drizzle icing over topping.

MAKES 6 SERVINGS

Tropical Pineapple Cutie Pies

198 cal

V **GF** These treats can totally double as breakfast. After all, they're made with oats, fruit, and yogurt! Creamy, fruity deliciousness . . .

CRUST

1 cup old-fashioned oats

¼ cup whipped butter

¼ cup unsweetened applesauce

3 tablespoons powdered peanut butter or defatted peanut flour

2 packets natural no-calorie sweetener

1 teaspoon cinnamon

¼ teaspoon salt

FILLING

¾ cup chopped mango

1 tablespoon arrowroot powder

1 packet natural no-calorie sweetener

½ teaspoon coconut extract

2 cups chopped pineapple

TOPPING

1 tablespoon unsweetened shredded coconut

1 cup fat-free plain Greek yogurt

2 packets natural no-calorie sweetener

1 teaspoon vanilla extract

⅓ ounce (about 2 tablespoons) chopped macadamia nuts

⅙th of recipe (1 mini pie): 198 calories, 7.5g total fat (3.5g sat fat), 156mg sodium, 25.5g carbs, 3.5g fiber, 11.5g sugars, 8g protein

You'll Need: 12-cup muffin pan, nonstick spray, small blender or food processor, small microwave-safe bowl, large bowl, medium nonstick pot, skillet, medium bowl

Prep: 30 minutes • **Cook:** 15 minutes • **Cool:** 20 minutes • **Chill:** 2 hours

1. Preheat oven to 350 degrees. Spray 6 cups of a 12-cup muffin pan with nonstick spray.

2. In a small blender/food processor, pulse oats to the consistency of coarse flour.

3. In a small microwave-safe bowl, microwave butter for 30 seconds, or until melted.

4. In a large bowl, combine ground oats, melted butter, and remaining crust ingredients. Mix until uniform with the consistency of wet sand.

5. Evenly distribute crust among the 6 cups of the muffin pan, using your hands or a flat utensil to firmly press and form the crusts. Press it into the edges and up along the sides.

6. Bake until firm, about 10 minutes. Let cool completely, about 20 minutes.

7. Clean blender/processor. Add all filling ingredients *except* pineapple. Add 1 tablespoon water. Puree until smooth.

8. Transfer filling mixture to a medium nonstick pot. Set heat to medium. Cook and stir until thickened, about 2 minutes. Remove pot from heat, and stir in pineapple. Evenly distribute among pie crusts. Cover and refrigerate until chilled, at least 2 hours.

9. Bring a skillet to medium heat. Cook and stir coconut until lightly browned, about 2 minutes.

10. In a medium bowl, mix yogurt, sweetener, and vanilla extract. Dollop yogurt over pies. Sprinkle with macadamia nuts and coconut.

MAKES 6 SERVINGS

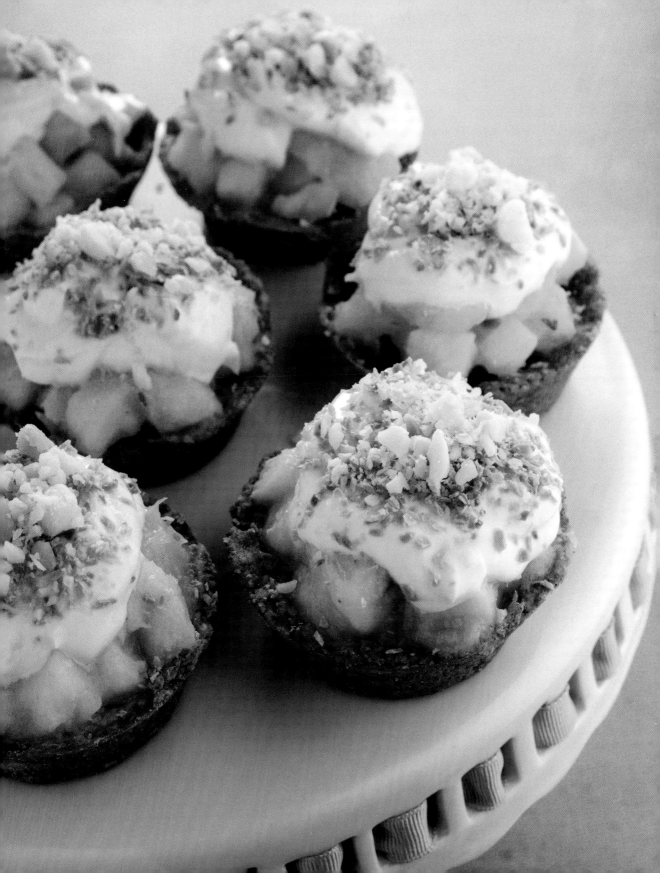

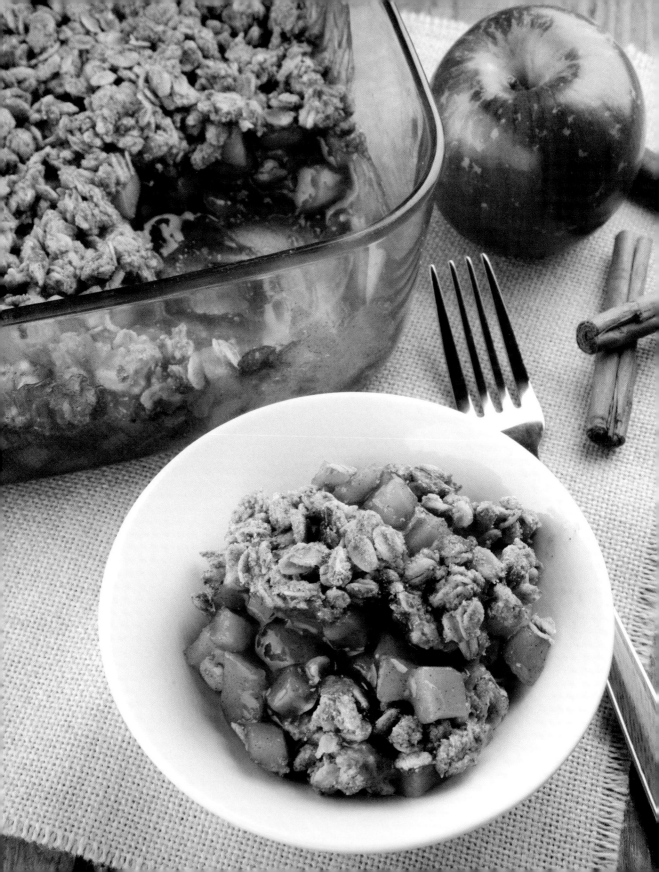

Tumbly Crumbly
Spiced Apple Bake

175 cal

 Apple pie lovers: Meet your new favorite dessert. I'm obsessed!

FILLING

6 cups peeled and chopped Fuji or Gala apples

¼ cup arrowroot powder

2 tablespoons Truvia spoonable no-calorie sweetener (or another natural brand that's about twice as sweet as sugar)

1 tablespoon lemon juice

2 teaspoons vanilla extract

1½ teaspoons cinnamon

¾ teaspoon pumpkin pie spice

⅛ teaspoon salt

TOPPING

½ cup old-fashioned oats

¼ cup whole-wheat flour

2 tablespoons whipped butter

2 tablespoons unsweetened applesauce

2 teaspoons Truvia spoonable calorie-free sweetener (or another natural brand that's about twice as sweet as sugar)

¼ teaspoon cinnamon

¼ teaspoon baking powder

⅛ teaspoon salt

1 ounce (about ¼ cup) chopped walnuts

⅙th of pan: 175 calories, 6g total fat (1.5g sat fat), 135mg sodium, 34.5g carbs, 3.5g fiber, 12g sugars, 2.5g protein

You'll Need: 8-inch by 8-inch baking pan, nonstick spray, large bowl, medium bowl

Prep: 20 minutes • **Cook:** 1 hour • **Cool:** 1 hour

1. Preheat oven to 350 degrees. Spray an 8-inch by 8-inch baking pan with nonstick spray.

2. Place apples in a large bowl. Sprinkle/top with remaining filling ingredients, and stir to coat. Transfer to the baking pan.

3. In a medium bowl, combine all topping ingredients *except* walnuts. Mash and stir until uniform and crumbly. Stir in walnuts.

4. Break topping into pieces, and sprinkle over filling.

5. Bake until topping is golden brown and filling is bubbly, about 1 hour.

6. Let cool completely, about 1 hour.

MAKES 6 SERVINGS

The Great Pumpkin Cheesecake Bars

161 cal

V **GF** Can't decide between perfectly spiced pumpkin pie and creamy, dreamy cheesecake? No need to choose! These bars satisfy both cravings . . .

CRUST

1 cup old-fashioned oats

¼ cup whipped butter

¼ cup unsweetened applesauce

3 tablespoons powdered peanut butter or defatted peanut flour

2 teaspoons Truvia spoonable calorie-free sweetener (or another natural brand that's about twice as sweet as sugar)

1 teaspoon cinnamon

¼ teaspoon salt

FILLING

One 8-ounce tub light/reduced-fat cream cheese, room temperature

1 cup fat-free plain Greek yogurt

¾ cup canned pure pumpkin

3 tablespoons Truvia spoonable calorie-free sweetener (or another natural brand that's about twice as sweet as sugar)

2 tablespoons egg whites (about 1 large egg's worth)

2 teaspoons vanilla extract

1½ teaspoons arrowroot powder

1½ teaspoons cinnamon

½ teaspoon pumpkin pie spice

⅛ teaspoon salt

Optional topping: natural light whipped topping

⅑th of pan: 161 calories, 9g total fat (5g sat fat), 261mg sodium, 18g carbs, 2.5g fiber, 4g sugars, 7.5g protein

You'll Need: 8-inch by 8-inch baking pan, nonstick spray, small blender or food processor, small microwave-safe bowl, 2 large bowls, electric mixer

Prep: 15 minutes • **Cook:** 55 minutes • **Cool:** 1 hour and 20 minutes • **Chill:** 2 hours

1. Preheat oven to 350 degrees. Spray an 8-inch by 8-inch baking pan with nonstick spray.

2. In a small blender or food processor, pulse oats to the consistency of coarse flour.

3. In a small microwave-safe bowl, microwave butter for 20 seconds, or until melted.

4. In a large bowl, combine ground oats, melted butter, and remaining crust ingredients. Mix until uniform with the consistency of wet sand.

5. Evenly distribute along the bottom of the baking pan, using your hands or a flat utensil to firmly press and form the crust. Press it into the edges of the pan.

6. Bake until firm, about 10 minutes.

7. Let cool completely, about 20 minutes.

8. Meanwhile, reduce oven temperature to 300 degrees, and prepare filling. In a large bowl, combine cream cheese with yogurt. With an electric mixer set to medium speed, beat until smooth and uniform, about 2 minutes.

9. Set mixer to low speed. Continue to beat while gradually adding remaining filling ingredients. Beat until just mixed, about 1 minute.

10. Top crust with filling, and smooth out the top. Bake until firm, about 40 minutes.

11. Let cool completely, about 1 hour.

12. Refrigerate until chilled, at least 2 hours.

MAKES 9 SERVINGS

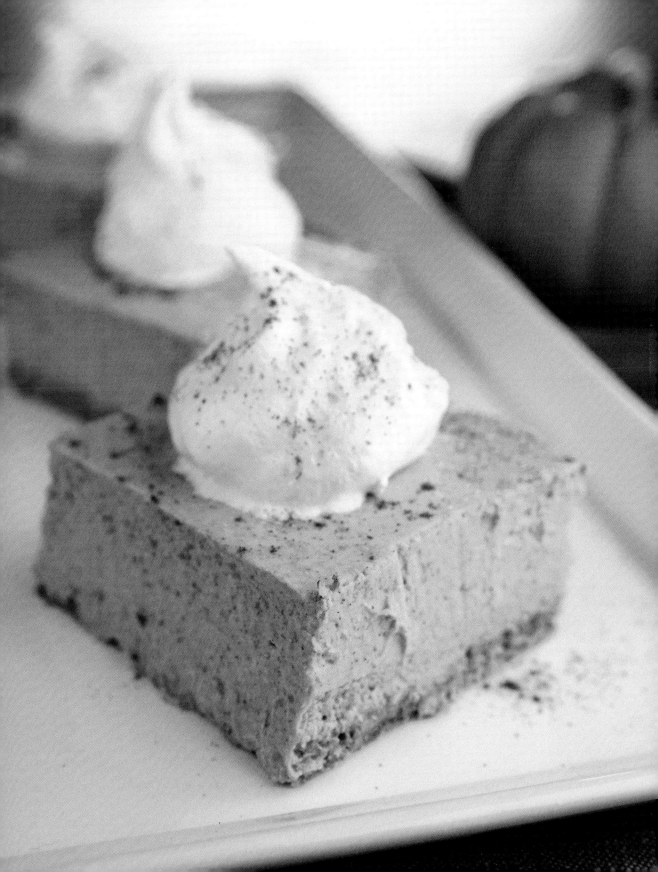

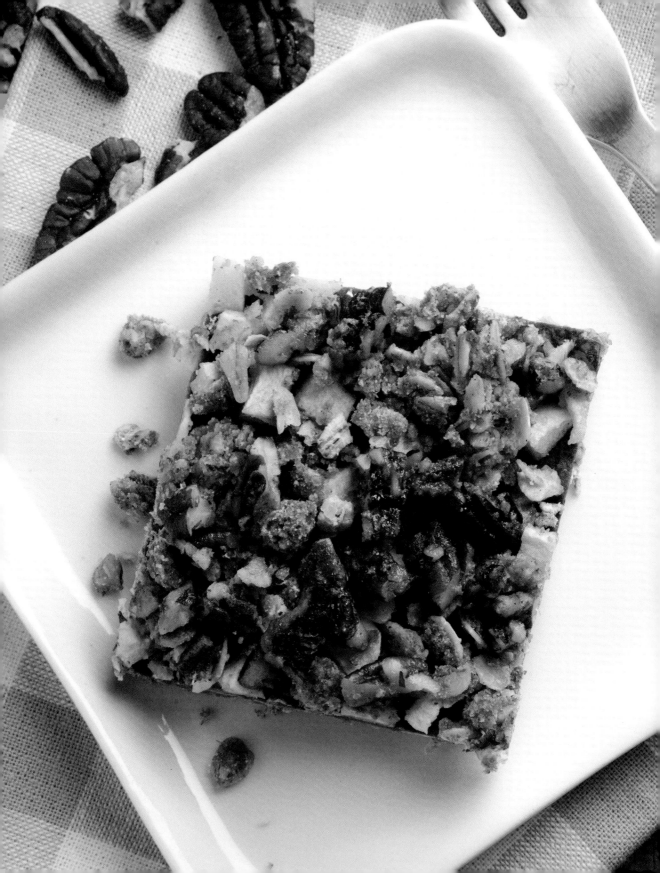

Pump Up the Pecan Apple Streusel Bars

152 cal

V Obsession confession: These started as simple pumpkin streusel bars, but they were missing some sweetness and crunch. So I added apples and pecans, and the rest is history!

DOUGH

1½ cups old-fashioned oats

¾ cup whole-wheat flour

⅓ cup whipped butter

¼ cup unsweetened applesauce

2 tablespoons Truvia spoonable no-calorie sweetener (or another natural brand about twice as sweet as sugar)

1 teaspoon pumpkin pie spice

½ teaspoon baking powder

¼ teaspoon salt

FILLING

1½ tablespoons arrowroot powder

1 cup canned pure pumpkin

2 tablespoons Truvia spoonable no-calorie sweetener (or another natural brand about twice as sweet as sugar)

1½ teaspoons cinnamon

1 cup peeled and finely chopped Granny Smith apple

TOPPING

2 tablespoons whipped butter

1½ teaspoons Truvia spoonable no-calorie sweetener (or another natural brand about twice as sweet as sugar)

2 ounces (about ½ cup) finely chopped pecans

¹⁄₁₂th of pan: 152 calories, 8g total fat (2.5g sat fat), 101mg sodium, 22g carbs, 3.5g fiber, 2.5g sugars, 3g protein

You'll Need: 9-inch by 13-inch baking pan, nonstick spray, large bowl, medium bowl, small bowl

Prep: 20 minutes • **Cook:** 30 minutes • **Cool:** 10 minutes

1. Preheat oven to 375 degrees. Spray a 9-inch by 13-inch baking pan with nonstick spray.

2. Combine dough ingredients in a large bowl. Mash and stir until uniform and crumbly.

3. Spread three-quarters of the dough (about 2½ cups) into the baking pan, pressing firmly into an even layer.

4. In a medium bowl, combine arrowroot powder with 2 tablespoons water. Stir to dissolve. Add all remaining filling ingredients *except* apple. Mix well.

5. Pour filling mixture into the pan, and smooth out the top. Evenly top with apple.

6. Break remaining dough into pieces, and sprinkle over the filling.

7. To make the topping, place butter in a small bowl. Stir in sweetener. Add pecans, and stir to coat.

8. Sprinkle topping over filling.

9. Bake until topping is golden brown and filling is bubbly, 25 to 30 minutes.

10. Let cool for 10 minutes before slicing.

MAKES 12 SERVINGS

Jazzy Razzy Streusel Bars

122 cal

V These fruit-filled bars are perfect for potluck parties. They're delicious and impressive but so easy to make!

DOUGH

1½ cups old-fashioned oats

¾ cup whole-wheat flour

⅓ cup whipped butter

¼ cup unsweetened applesauce

2 tablespoons Truvia spoonable no-calorie sweetener (or another natural brand about twice as sweet as sugar)

1 teaspoon cinnamon

½ teaspoon baking powder

¼ teaspoon salt

FILLING

2 tablespoons Truvia spoonable no-calorie sweetener (or another natural brand about twice as sweet as sugar)

1½ tablespoons arrowroot powder

4½ cups raspberries (fresh or thawed from frozen with no sugar added)

⅛ teaspoon salt

¹⁄₁₂th of pan: 122 calories, 4g total fat (1.5g sat fat), 116mg sodium, 23.5g carbs, 5g fiber, 3g sugars, 3g protein

You'll Need: 9-inch by 13-inch baking pan, nonstick spray, 2 large bowls

Prep: 20 minutes • **Cook:** 30 minutes • **Cool:** 1 hour

1. Preheat oven to 375 degrees. Spray a 9-inch by 13-inch baking pan with nonstick spray.

2. Combine dough ingredients in a large bowl. Mash and stir until uniform and crumbly.

3. Spread three-quarters of the dough (about 2½ cups) into the baking pan, pressing firmly into an even layer.

4. To make the filling, in a second large bowl, mix sweetener with arrowroot powder. Add raspberries and salt, and stir to coat.

5. Evenly pour filling over the dough in the pan. Break remaining dough into pieces, and sprinkle over the filling.

6. Bake until topping is golden brown and filling is bubbly, 25 to 30 minutes.

7. Let cool completely, about 1 hour.

MAKES 12 SERVINGS

Chew on This . . .

Fans of raspberries might feel that the west coast is the best coast—nearly all of America's berries come from Washington, California, and Oregon.

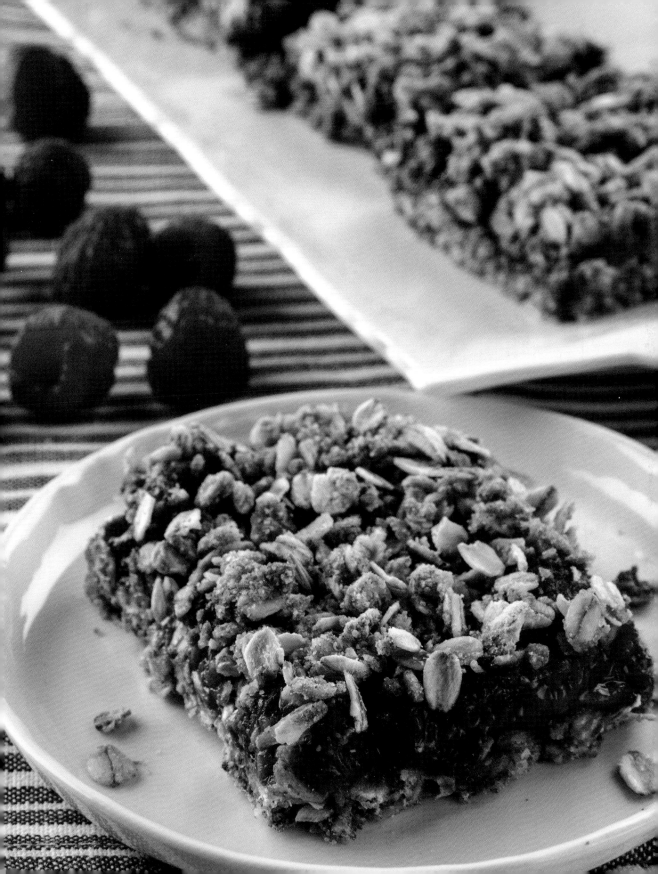

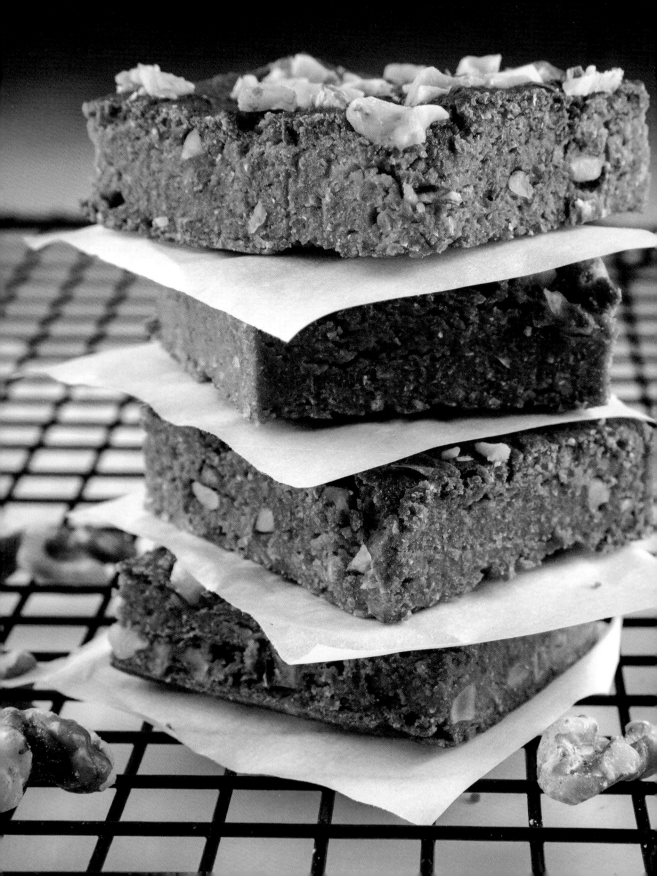

My Oh My Maple Nut Blondies

117 cal

V Chickpeas are the secret ingredient in these incredible blondies. Serve 'em to friends, and see if anyone can guess what they're made with! (My experience: NO ONE can.)

One 15-ounce can chickpeas (garbanzo beans), drained and rinsed

¼ cup plus 2 tablespoons whole-wheat flour

⅓ cup unsweetened applesauce

¼ cup egg whites (about 2 large eggs' worth)

3 tablespoons Truvia spoonable no-calorie sweetener (or another natural brand about twice as sweet as sugar)

2 tablespoons creamy peanut butter (no sugar added)

2 tablespoons canned pure pumpkin

1½ tablespoons maple extract

1 teaspoon vanilla extract

¾ teaspoon baking powder

¼ teaspoon salt

1 ounce (about ¼ cup) finely chopped walnuts

⅑th of pan: 117 calories, 4.5g total fat (0.5g sat fat), 193mg sodium, 17.5g carbs, 3.5g fiber, 2g sugars, 5g protein

You'll Need: 8-inch by 8-inch baking pan, nonstick spray, food processor

Prep: 15 minutes • **Cook:** 30 minutes • **Cool:** 1 hour

1. Preheat oven to 350 degrees. Spray an 8-inch by 8-inch baking pan with nonstick spray.

2. Place all ingredients *except* walnuts in a food processor. Puree until completely smooth and uniform.

3. Fold in ½ ounce (about 2 tablespoons) walnuts.

4. Spread mixture into the baking pan, and smooth out the top.

5. Evenly top with remaining ½ ounce (about 2 tablespoons) walnuts, and lightly press to adhere.

6. Bake until a toothpick (or knife) inserted into the center comes out mostly clean, 25 to 30 minutes.

7. Let cool completely, about 1 hour.

MAKES 9 SERVINGS

Chew on This . . .

These blondies are so good it should be illegal. Speaking of illegitimate things, a handful of crooks once stole 18 million dollars' worth of maple syrup from a Canadian warehouse!

Nutty for Peanut Butter Fudge Bites

55 cal

V **GF** How can these be so good and yet so low in calories!? Even I have a hard time understanding it! Fudge lovers: Also check out page 290's Coconutty Chocolate Fudge.

¼ cup pitted dried dates

One 15-ounce can chickpeas (garbanzo beans), drained and rinsed

½ cup powdered peanut butter or defatted peanut flour

⅓ cup canned pure pumpkin

¼ cup unsweetened applesauce

¼ cup egg whites (about 2 large eggs' worth)

2 tablespoons coconut flour

2 tablespoons Truvia spoonable no-calorie sweetener (or another natural brand about twice as sweet as sugar)

1 teaspoon baking powder

½ teaspoon vanilla extract

¼ teaspoon salt

2 tablespoons creamy peanut butter (no sugar added)

½ ounce (about 2 tablespoons) chopped peanuts

½₀th of pan: 55 calories, 2g total fat (<0.5g sat fat), 101mg sodium, 8g carbs, 2g fiber, 2g sugars, 3.5g protein

You'll Need: 8-inch by 8-inch baking pan, nonstick spray, small bowl, food processor

Prep: 25 minutes • **Cook:** 35 minutes • **Cool:** 1 hour • **Chill:** 2 hours

1. Preheat oven to 350 degrees. Spray an 8-inch by 8-inch baking pan with nonstick spray.

2. Place dates in a small bowl with ½ cup warm water. Soak until softened, 5 to 10 minutes. Drain excess liquid.

3. In a food processor, combine dates with all remaining ingredients *except* peanut butter and peanuts. Puree until completely smooth and uniform.

4. Spread batter into the baking pan, and smooth out the top.

5. Spoon peanut butter over the batter, and swirl it in with a knife.

6. Sprinkle with peanuts, and lightly press to adhere.

7. Bake until a toothpick (or knife) inserted into the center comes out mostly clean, 30 to 35 minutes.

8. Let cool completely, about 1 hour.

9. Cover and refrigerate until completely chilled, at least 2 hours. (These fudge bites taste best when chilled overnight; they're even good slightly frozen!)

MAKES 20 SERVINGS

Chew on This . . .

The largest slab of fudge was created in Canada and weighed 5,760 pounds. That's more than two Mazda Miatas!

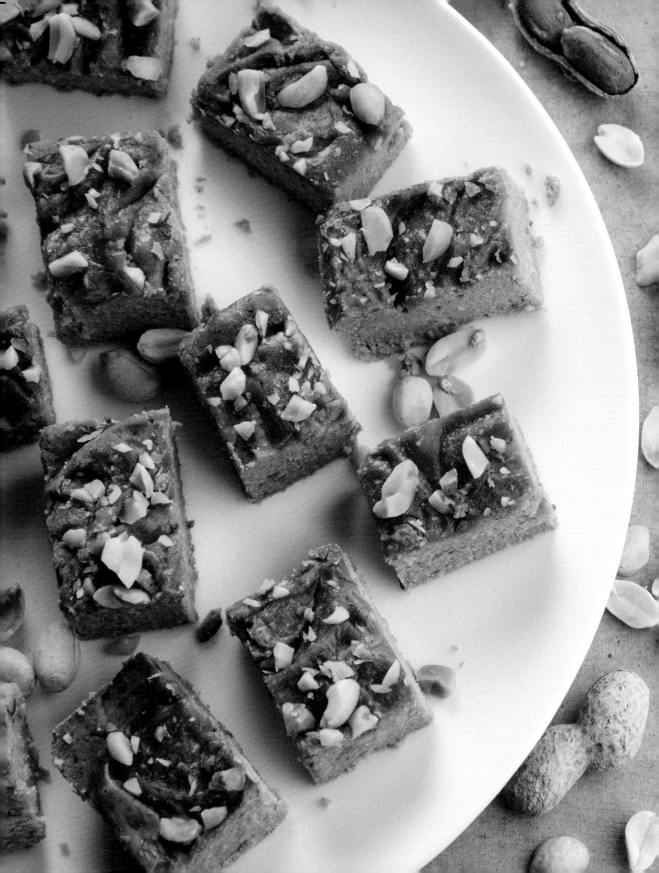

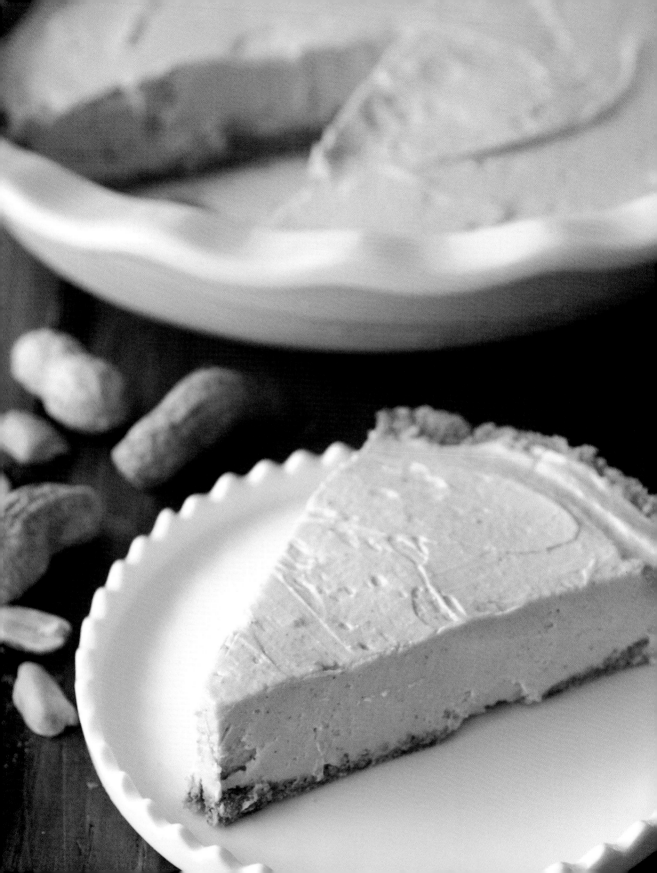

I Dream of Peanut Butter Pie

192 cal

V **GF** Obsession confession: This started out as a frozen pie, but I really wanted to master a refrigerated PB pie. SUCCESS! This pie is fantastic refrigerated or frozen.

CRUST

1 cup old-fashioned oats

¼ cup whipped butter

¼ cup unsweetened applesauce

3 tablespoons powdered peanut butter or defatted peanut flour

2 teaspoons Truvia spoonable calorie-free sweetener (or another natural brand about twice as sweet as sugar)

1 teaspoon cinnamon

¼ teaspoon salt

FILLING

½ cup powdered peanut butter or defatted peanut flour

1½ cups fat-free plain Greek yogurt

½ cup light/reduced-fat cream cheese, room temperature

2 tablespoons creamy peanut butter (no sugar added)

2 tablespoons Truvia spoonable calorie-free sweetener (or another natural brand about twice as sweet as sugar)

1½ teaspoons vanilla extract

⅛ teaspoon salt

⅛th of pie: 192 calories, 10g total fat (4g sat fat), 248mg sodium, 18.5g carbs, 3g fiber, 4g sugars, 12g protein

You'll Need: 9-inch pie pan, nonstick spray, small blender or food processor, small microwave-safe bowl, 2 large bowls

Prep: 15 minutes • **Cook:** 15 minutes • **Cool:** 20 minutes • **Chill:** 4 hours

1. Preheat oven to 350 degrees. Spray a 9-inch pie pan with nonstick spray.

2. Place oats in a small blender or food processor, and pulse until reduced to the consistency of coarse flour.

3. In a small microwave-safe bowl, microwave butter for 30 seconds, or until melted.

4. In a large bowl, combine ground oats, melted butter, and remaining crust ingredients. Mix until uniform with the consistency of wet sand.

5. Evenly distribute mixture along the bottom of the pie pan, using your hands or a flat utensil to firmly press and form the crust. Press it into the edges and up along the sides of the pan.

6. Bake until firm, about 10 minutes. Let cool completely, about 20 minutes.

7. Meanwhile, make the filling. In a second large bowl, combine powdered peanut butter/peanut flour with ⅓ cup water. Stir until uniform.

8. Add all remaining filling ingredients to the bowl. Mix until smooth and uniform.

9. Top crust with filling, and smooth out the top. Refrigerate until firm, at least 4 hours.

MAKES 8 SERVINGS

Chew on This . . .

Each American eats about 3 pounds of peanut butter a year. I've heard that if you put all of that PB together, you could coat the floor of the Grand Canyon!

Lunchbox PB&J Blondies

117 cal

V Kids love these! The freeze-dried strawberries really take things up a notch. Classic flavors, reimagined . . .

BLONDIES

One 15-ounce can chickpeas (garbanzo beans), drained and rinsed

⅓ cup unsweetened applesauce

⅓ cup powdered peanut butter or defatted peanut flour

¼ cup whole-wheat flour

¼ cup egg whites (about 2 large eggs' worth)

3 tablespoons Truvia spoonable no-calorie sweetener (or another natural brand that's about twice as sweet as sugar)

2 tablespoons creamy peanut butter (no sugar added)

2 tablespoons canned pure pumpkin

1½ tablespoons vanilla extract

¾ teaspoon baking powder

¼ teaspoon salt

¾ cup freeze-dried strawberries, chopped

TOPPING

¾ cup frozen strawberries (no sugar added), thawed (not drained)

2¼ teaspoons arrowroot powder

2¼ teaspoons Truvia spoonable no-calorie sweetener (or another natural brand that's about twice as sweet as sugar)

⅑th of pan: 117 calories, 3g total fat (<0.5g sat fat), 202mg sodium, 21.5g carbs, 4g fiber, 4g sugars, 6g protein

You'll Need: 8-inch by 8-inch baking pan, nonstick spray, food processor, medium microwave-safe bowl, plastic bag

Prep: 15 minutes • **Cook:** 30 minutes • **Cool:** 1 hour

1. Preheat oven to 350 degrees. Spray an 8-inch by 8-inch baking pan with nonstick spray.

2. In a food processor, combine all blondie ingredients *except* freeze-dried strawberries. Puree until completely smooth and uniform.

3. Fold in freeze-dried strawberries. Spread batter into the baking pan, and smooth out the top.

4. Bake until a toothpick (or knife) inserted into the center comes out mostly clean, 25 to 30 minutes.

5. Let cool completely, about 1 hour.

6. Meanwhile, make the topping. Clean food processor, and add topping ingredients. Puree until mostly smooth.

7. Transfer topping mixture to a medium microwave-safe bowl. Microwave for 1 minute, or until hot and thickened.

8. Spoon topping into a bottom corner of a plastic bag. Snip off the tip of that corner to create a small hole for piping.

9. Pipe topping over blondies in thin strips.

MAKES 9 SERVINGS

Chew on This . . .

Sources say the average American will eat 1,500 PB&J sandwiches before graduating high school. Around 80 sammies a year? That's crazy!

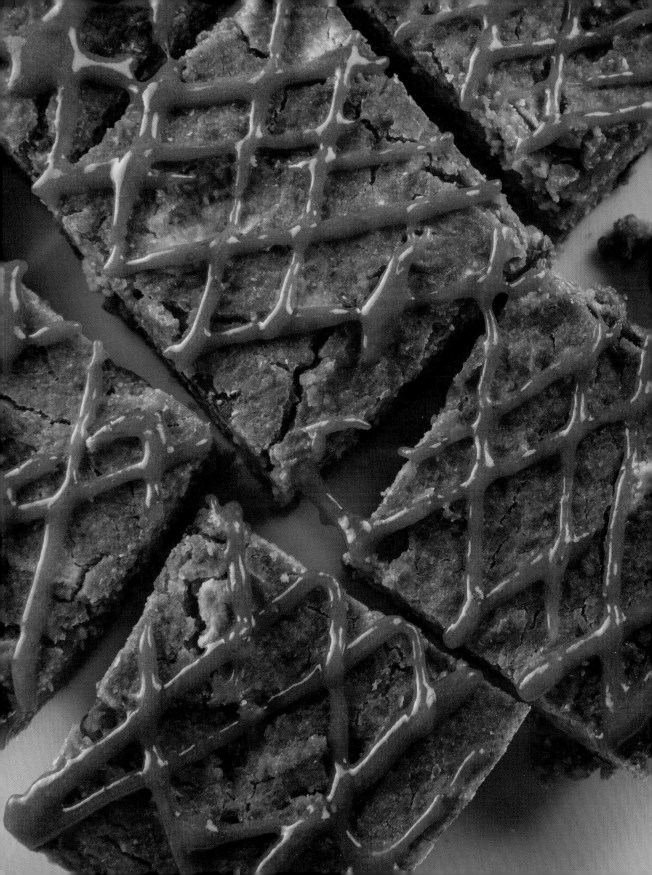

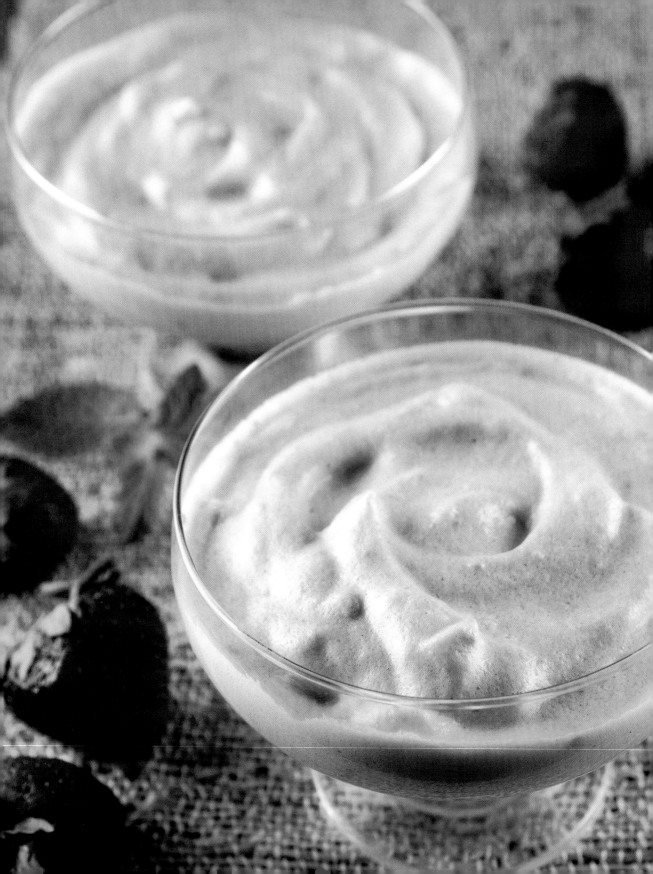

Fluffy PB Mousse

77 cal

5i **V** **GF**   One more PB dessert for the road! You'll FLIP when you taste this super-creamy and good-for-you dessert. More peanut-butter recipes await on page 363!

½ cup egg whites (about 4 large eggs' worth), room temperature

½ teaspoon cream of tartar

2 packets natural no-calorie sweetener

¼ cup fat-free plain Greek yogurt

¼ cup powdered peanut butter or defatted peanut flour

1 tablespoon creamy peanut butter (no sugar added)

¼th of recipe (about ½ cup): 77 calories, 3g total fat (0.5g sat fat), 81mg sodium, 4.5g carbs, 1g fiber, 1.5g sugars, 8.5g protein

You'll Need: large bowl, electric mixer, medium bowl, 4 small bowls

Prep: 15 minutes • **Chill:** 4 hours

1. Place room-temp egg whites in a large bowl. With an electric mixer set to high speed, beat until fluffy and slightly stiff, about 4 minutes.

2. Continue to beat while adding cream of tartar and 1 sweetener packet. Beat until stiff peaks form, 2 to 3 minutes.

3. In a medium bowl, combine Greek yogurt, powdered peanut butter/peanut flour, creamy peanut butter, remaining sweetener packet, and 1 tablespoon water. Mix until uniform.

4. Gently fold contents of the medium bowl into the large bowl.

5. Evenly distribute mixture among four small bowls.

6. Refrigerate until chilled and set, about 4 hours.

MAKES 4 SERVINGS

Chew on This . . .

HG shocker: Peanuts are not actually nuts. They're legumes, which means they're closer in relation to black beans than hazelnuts!

Orange You Glad I Said Banana Pops

44 cal

5i **V** **GF** Obsession confession: It took SO many tries to get these fro-yo pops just right. The trick was switching from mandarin orange segments to OJ! Now they're popsicle perfection . . .

1 cup orange juice

½ cup sliced banana

½ cup fat-free plain Greek yogurt

1 packet natural no-calorie sweetener

1 teaspoon vanilla extract

1 teaspoon orange zest

⅙th of recipe (1 pop): 44 calories, 0g total fat (0g sat fat), 8mg sodium, 8.5g carbs, 0.5g fiber, 6g sugars, 2.5g protein

You'll Need: food processor or blender, 6-piece popsicle mold set

Prep: 5 minutes • **Freeze:** 3 hours

1. Combine all ingredients in a food processor or blender. Blend until completely smooth and uniform, stopping and stirring if needed.

2. Evenly distribute into a 6-piece popsicle mold set, leaving about ½ inch of space at the top. (Pops will expand as they freeze.)

3. Insert popsicle handles. Freeze until solid, at least 3 hours.

MAKES 6 SERVINGS

HG Alternative

If your popsicle mold doesn't contain handles, just cover it with foil after filling it. Then slide popsicle sticks through the foil and into the pops.

Chew on This . . .

Here's a little-known fact: Bananas are technically berries!

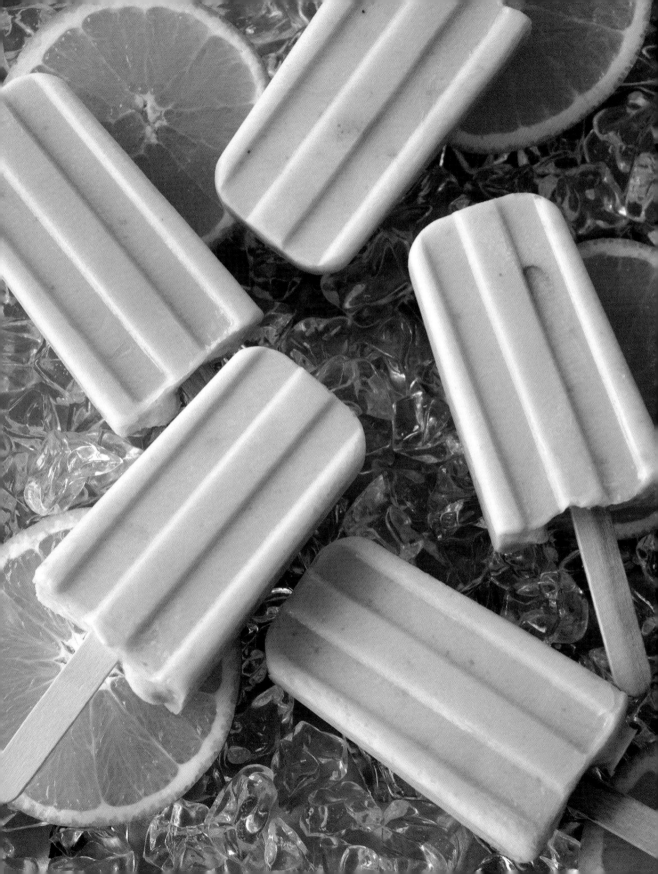

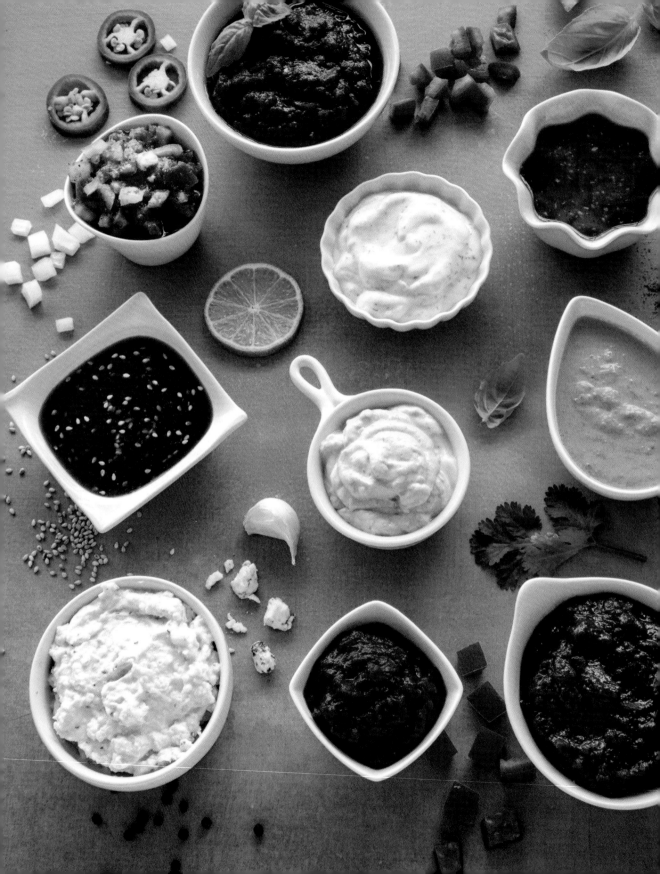

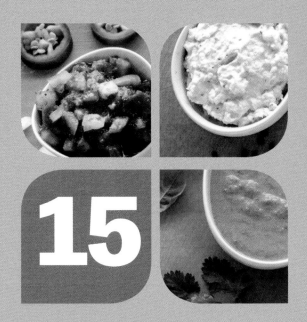

15

Clean & Hungry Staples

When it comes to savory foods that Americans are obsessed with, condiments are the icing on the cake! Store-bought versions are often loaded with calories, sugar, and undesirable ingredients. From sauces to salad dressings, this book wouldn't be complete without these recipe-enhancing staples! BTW, they'll last for up to two weeks in the fridge.

Clean & Hungry Salsa

 30m **V** **GF** This salsa makes pretty much everything taste better—salads, omelettes, chicken . . . your favorite spoon. Whatever you do, don't miss the Trop 'Til You Drop Island Salsa on page 207!

2 cups chopped tomatoes

½ cup finely chopped onion

½ cup finely chopped green bell pepper

2 tablespoons chopped fresh cilantro

2 tablespoons seeded and finely chopped jalapeño pepper

1½ tablespoons lime juice

½ teaspoon each salt and black pepper

½ teaspoon chopped garlic

¼ teaspoon ground cumin

⅛th of recipe (about 2 tablespoons): 7 calories, 0g total fat (0g sat fat), 66mg sodium, 1.5g carbs, 0.5g fiber, 1g sugars, <0.5g protein

You'll Need: medium-large sealable container, blender or food processor

Prep: 20 minutes

1. In a medium-large sealable container, combine all ingredients. Mix until uniform.

2. Transfer half of the mixture to a blender or food processor. Pulse until just pureed.

3. Return pureed mixture to the container. Mix well.

4. Seal, and refrigerate until ready to use.

MAKES 18 SERVINGS

HG Alternatives

Are you a fan of smooth salsa? Puree the entire mixture instead of just half. Prefer a chunky one? Skip the blending process altogether!

Store-Bought Alternatives

Check the refrigerated section for fresh salsa, and watch out for excess sodium!

Clean & Hungry BBQ Sauce

28 cal

15m **V** **GF** This sauce is so flavorful, you won't believe how low in calories and sugar it is. Big win for BBQ lovers!

¾ cup canned crushed tomatoes

¼ cup tomato paste

2 tablespoons apple cider vinegar

1 tablespoon molasses

1 tablespoon honey

1 tablespoon Dijon mustard

1 teaspoon reduced-sodium/lite soy sauce

1 teaspoon garlic powder

1 teaspoon onion powder

¼ teaspoon salt

¼ teaspoon paprika

⅒th of recipe (about 2 tablespoons): 28 calories, 0g total fat (0g sat fat), 151mg sodium, 6g carbs, 0.5g fiber, 4.5g sugars, 0.5g protein

You'll Need: medium-large bowl, whisk, medium-large sealable container

Prep: 10 minutes

1. In a medium-large bowl, combine all ingredients. Whisk until uniform.

2. Transfer sauce to a medium-large sealable container. Seal, and refrigerate until ready to use.

MAKES 10 SERVINGS

Gluten FYI

Some soy sauce contains gluten. If you avoid gluten, read labels carefully. Or grab a product marked gluten-free.

Store-Bought Alternatives

Go for a natural BBQ sauce made with clean (not refined) sweetener, like cane sugar or agave nectar. OrganicVille makes some great ones!

Clean & Hungry
Marinara Sauce

52 cal

5i **15m** **V** **GF** No exaggeration: This sauce is life-changing. It's as good as (if not better than!) the more expensive options on store shelves.

3 cups canned crushed tomatoes

¼ cup tomato paste

1 tablespoon white wine vinegar

2 teaspoons Italian seasoning

½ teaspoon garlic powder

½ teaspoon onion powder

¼ teaspoon salt

⅛ teaspoon black pepper

⅙th of recipe (about ½ cup): 52 calories, 0g total fat (0g sat fat), 354mg sodium, 10.5g carbs, 3g fiber, 5.5g sugars, 2.5g protein

You'll Need: large sealable container

Prep: 5 minutes

1. Combine all ingredients in a large sealable container. Mix until uniform.

2. Seal, and refrigerate until ready to use.

MAKES 6 SERVINGS

Store-Bought Alternatives

Look for a sauce with stats similar to this recipe, made with natural ingredients and no sugar, like the kinds by The Silver Palate and Monte Bene.

Clean & Hungry
Sesame Ginger Dressing

 V **GF** This sweet Asian dressing is incredible, and it doubles as a sauce/marinade . . . Try it!

½ cup plain rice vinegar

¼ cup orange juice

3 tablespoons reduced-sodium/lite soy sauce

1½ tablespoons sesame oil

2 teaspoons crushed ginger

2 teaspoons crushed garlic

1 packet natural no-calorie sweetener

⅛th of recipe (about 2 tablespoons): 32 calories, 2.5g total fat (0.5g sat fat), 204mg sodium, 2g carbs, 0g fiber, 1g sugars, 0.5g protein

You'll Need: medium bowl, whisk, medium sealable container

Prep: 5 minutes

1. In a medium bowl, combine all ingredients. Whisk until uniform.
2. Transfer to a medium sealable container. Seal, and refrigerate until ready to use.

MAKES 8 SERVINGS

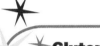

Gluten FYI

Some soy sauce contains gluten. If you avoid gluten, read labels carefully. Or grab a product marked gluten-free.

Chew on This . . .

Rumor has it, 75 percent of all sesame seeds produced in Mexico are purchased by McDonald's for their burger buns!

Clean & Hungry Chunky Blue Cheese Dressing

46 cal

5i **15m** **V** **GF** Three cheers for blue cheese! I highly recommend pairing this dressing with my Bangin' Boneless Buffalo Wings (page 253).

½ cup fat-free plain Greek yogurt

2 tablespoons grated Parmesan cheese

¼ teaspoon each salt and black pepper

½ cup crumbled blue cheese

⅛th of recipe (about 2 tablespoons): 46 calories, 2.5g total fat (1.5g sat fat), 216mg sodium, 1g carbs, 0g fiber, 0.5g sugars, 4g protein

You'll Need: medium sealable container

Prep: 5 minutes

1. In a medium sealable container, combine all ingredients *except* blue cheese. Mix well.

2. Mash and stir blue cheese into the mixture. Seal, and refrigerate until ready to use.

MAKES 8 SERVINGS

Chew on This...

Are you OBSESSED with cheese? There's a word for you: turophile, a.k.a. one who fancies cheese!

Clean & Hungry
Ranch Dressing

50 cal

5i **15m** **V** **GF** This brand-new staple is an instant classic. Great for salads, veggie dipping . . . It's even good with DIY onion rings, like the ones on page 254!

⅓ cup light mayonnaise

¼ cup fat-free plain Greek yogurt

¼ cup fat-free milk

1 teaspoon lemon juice

½ teaspoon garlic powder

½ teaspoon onion powder

½ teaspoon dried dill

¼ teaspoon salt

⅛ teaspoon black pepper

⅙th of recipe (about 2 tablespoons): 50 calories, 3.5g total fat (<0.5g sat fat), 206mg sodium, 2.5g carbs, 0g fiber, 1.5g sugars, 1.5g protein

You'll Need: medium sealable container
Prep: 5 minutes

1. In a medium sealable container, combine all ingredients. Mix until uniform.

2. Seal, and refrigerate until ready to use.

MAKES 6 SERVINGS

Chew on This . . .

The number-one salad dressing in America? It's ranch, by a landslide.

Clean & Hungry
Creamy Fresh Sriracha

V **GF** The appeal of sweet-hot sriracha is a complete phenomenon. Now you can DIY, make it creamy, and avoid unwanted sugar!

1 cup seeded and chopped red jalapeño peppers

1 cup chopped red bell pepper

⅓ cup apple cider vinegar

1 tablespoon chopped garlic

1 packet natural no-calorie sweetener

½ teaspoon salt

¼ cup fat-free plain Greek yogurt

¼ cup light mayonnaise

¹⁄₁₄th of recipe (about 2 tablespoons): 23 calories, 1g total fat (<0.5g sat fat), 117mg sodium, 2g carbs, 0.5g fiber, 1g sugars, 0.5g protein

You'll Need: blender or food processor, small pot, medium sealable container

Prep: 10 minutes • **Cook:** 10 minutes • **Cool:** 30 minutes

1. In a blender or food processor, combine all ingredients *except* yogurt and mayo. Puree until smooth.

2. Transfer to a small pot. Set heat to high, and bring to a boil.

3. Reduce to a simmer. Cook for 5 minutes.

4. Transfer to a medium sealable container. Add yogurt and mayo, and stir until uniform.

5. Let cool completely. Seal, and refrigerate until ready to use.

MAKES 14 SERVINGS

Chew on This . . .

Why is there a rooster on Huy Fong bottled sriracha? It's the founder's Chinese zodiac sign!

Clean & Hungry Special Sauce

24 cal

5i **15m** **V** **GF** This stuff tastes just like a yummy fast-food spread, but it's way better for you. Bonus: It doubles as Russian dressing!

¼ cup light mayonnaise

¼ cup fat-free plain Greek yogurt

2 tablespoons Clean & Hungry Ketchup (recipe and store-bought alternative on page 343)

2 teaspoons yellow mustard

1 teaspoon lemon juice

¼ teaspoon salt

⅛ teaspoon black pepper

¹⁄₁₀th of recipe (about 1 tablespoon): 24 calories, 1.5g total fat (<0.5g sat fat), 132mg sodium, 1.5g carbs, 0g fiber, 1g sugars, 0.5g protein

You'll Need: medium sealable container

Prep: 5 minutes

1. In a medium sealable container, combine all ingredients. Mix until uniform.

2. Seal, and refrigerate until ready to use.

MAKES 10 SERVINGS

Chew on This . . .

McDonald's once lost the recipe for its famous special sauce. You know someone got in trouble for that!

Clean & Hungry Teriyaki Sauce

7 cal

🕐 15m Ⓥ GF If you crave clean Chinese food, you need this recipe in your life! It's got the perfect balance of sweet and salty . . . without having loads of sugar or salt!

¼ cup reduced-sodium/lite soy sauce

3 tablespoons apple cider vinegar

2 packets natural no-calorie sweetener

1½ teaspoons chopped garlic

1½ teaspoons crushed ginger

½ teaspoon xanthan gum

1 teaspoon sesame seeds

¹⁄₁₂th of recipe (about 2 tablespoons): 7 calories, <0.5g total fat (0g sat fat), 184mg sodium, 1g carbs, <0.5g fiber, 0.5g sugars, 0.5g protein

You'll Need: blender or food processor, medium-large sealable container

Prep: 5 minutes

1. In a blender or food processor, combine all ingredients *except* sesame seeds.

2. Add 1 cup water. Blend until uniform and slightly thickened, about 20 seconds.

3. Transfer to a medium-large sealable container, and stir in sesame seeds. (It will be a little frothy at first.)

4. Seal, and refrigerate until ready to use.

MAKES 12 SERVINGS

✶ Gluten FYI

Some brands of soy sauce contain gluten. If you avoid gluten, read labels carefully. Or grab a product marked gluten-free.

Ingredient FYI

Xanthan gum is a natural, plant-based thickener. It gives this sauce a perfect texture. Natural-food stores carry it, as do some mainstream markets. When in doubt, order it online. (I promise; it's worth it!)

Store-Bought Alternatives

Go for teriyaki sauce made with natural ingredients and not too much sugar. Most are higher in calories and sodium than this recipe, so keep that in mind. OrganicVille makes really tasty teriyaki sweetened with agave nectar.

Clean & Hungry Ketchup

14 cal

5i **15m** **V** **GF** Ketchup is one of the most beloved condiments here in the USA! This low-calorie recipe will blow your ketchup-lovin' mind.

½ cup tomato paste

¼ cup canned crushed tomatoes

¼ cup apple cider vinegar

1 tablespoon plus 1 teaspoon honey

½ teaspoon garlic powder

½ teaspoon onion powder

½ teaspoon salt

1/16th of recipe (about 1 tablespoon): 14 calories, 0g total fat (0g sat fat), 88mg sodium, 3.5g carbs, 0.5g fiber, 2.5g sugars, 0.5g protein

You'll Need: medium bowl, whisk, medium sealable container

Prep: 5 minutes

1. Combine all ingredients in a medium bowl.
2. Add 2 tablespoons water, and whisk until smooth and uniform.
3. Transfer to a medium sealable container. Seal, and refrigerate until ready to use.

MAKES 16 SERVINGS

Store-Bought Alternatives

Look for agave-sweetened ketchup. I love the kind by OrganicVille!

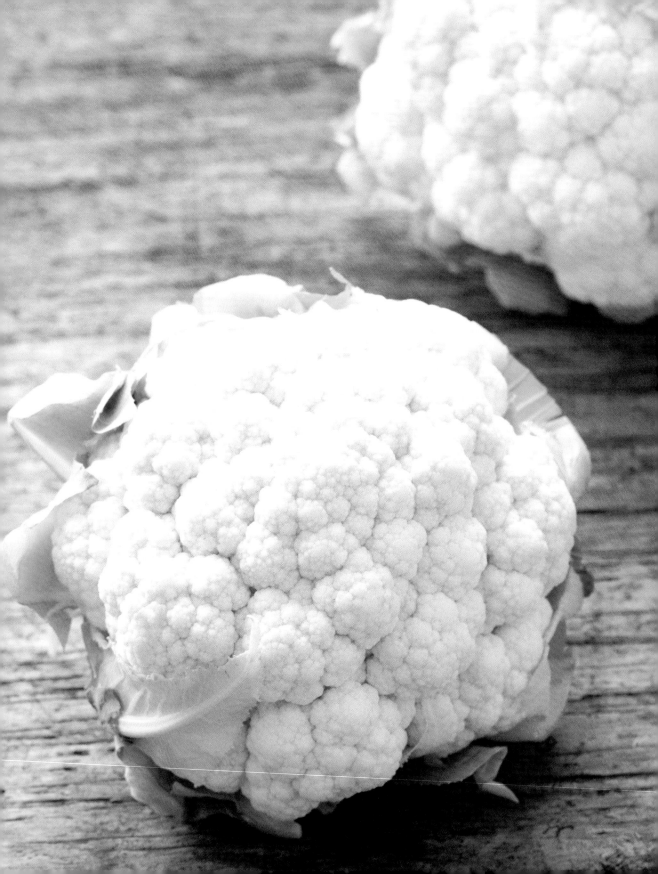

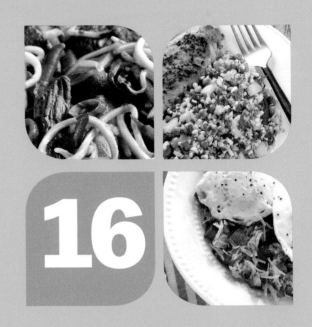

16

How-Tos for Clean & Hungry Obsessions

Cauliflower rice, zucchini noodles, spaghetti squash . . . These foods are Hungry Girl staples! As carb-slashed swaps for heavy starches, they make it possible to enjoy your favorite dishes for way fewer calories. But you've got to know how to find and prepare them. All the info you need is right here . . .

Obsession Essentials: Cauliflower Rice!

Cauliflower rice just may be the best thing since sliced bread. In fact, I think it's BETTER than sliced bread. It tastes GREAT and has a tiny fraction of the carby calories of ordinary rice! Check the freezer aisle and produce section for ready-to-use cauliflower rice, sometimes called cauliflower crumbles. Can't find it? No problem!

From florets to faux grains . . .

A standard blender is all you need. Just pulse roughly chopped cauliflower until reduced to rice-sized pieces. You may occasionally need to stop and stir in order to finish the job. If you're blending more than 2 cups of cauliflower, work in batches.

Want to whip up a big batch to keep on hand?

Great idea! Store uncooked cauliflower rice in an airtight container, and it'll stay fresh for about four days in the fridge. You can also freeze it! To thaw, just let it sit out for several hours, or use the thaw cycle on your microwave. Once thawed, blot away excess moisture.

Just so you know . . .

A head of cauliflower yields around 5 cups roughly chopped cauliflower, which equals about 4 cups raw cauliflower rice.

Flip to page 362 for a full list of recipes with cauliflower rice!

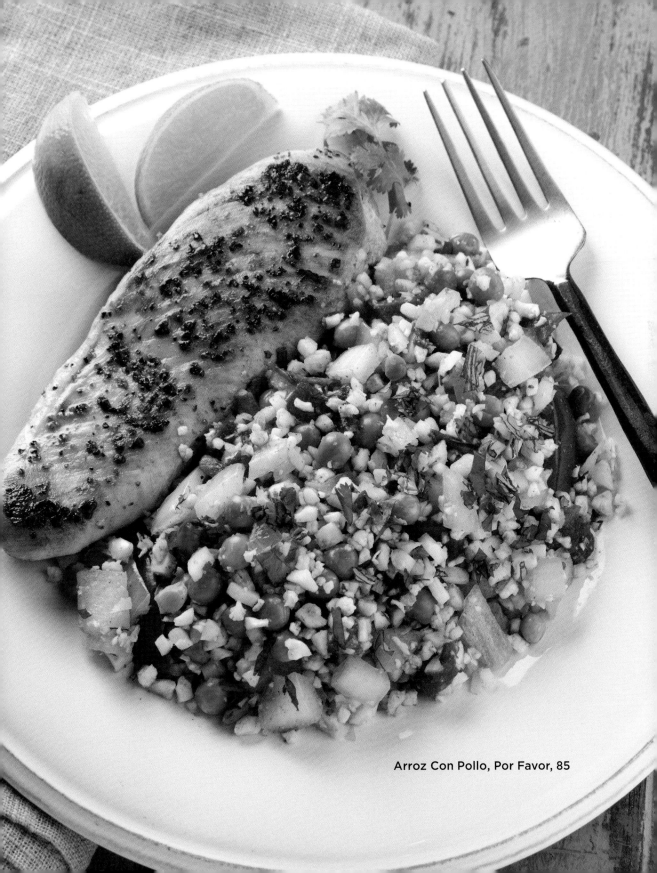

Arroz Con Pollo, Por Favor, 85

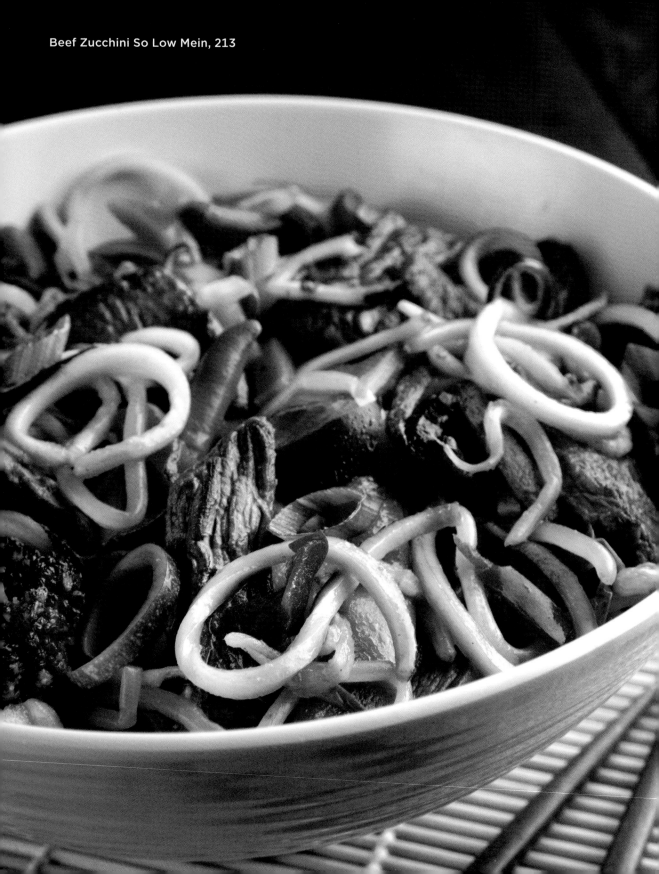

Obsession Essentials: Zucchini Noodles!

Spiralized veggies are among this decade's hottest healthy-eating trends. With so few calories and the perfect texture, they are ON POINT as a pasta swap! Spiralized zucchini is such a phenomenon, you can often find ready-to-cook zucchini noodles in the produce section of the grocery store. Of course, you can easily make your own "z'paghetti." Just get your hands on a spiral veggie slicer (sold online and at places like Bed Bath & Beyond), and follow these simple steps . . .

1. Cut off and discard zucchini ends.

2. Stick one end of the zucchini into the spiralizer.

3. Twist the zucchini, and watch as oodles of noodles emerge!

4. Roughly chop for shorter noodles.

No spiralizer? No problem! Use a standard veggie peeler to peel the zucchini into thin strips, rotating it after each strip to ensure evenly sized noodles. Roughly chop, if needed.

Just so you know . . .

An 8-ounce (medium) zucchini yields about 1 cup of raw zucchini noodles.

Check out all the zucchini-noodle creations on page 362!

Obsession Essentials: Spaghetti Squash!

Spaghetti squash is Mother Nature's noodle! But how exactly do you turn that clunky yellow gourd into noodle strands? I've got a cooking method for every kitchen personality type . . .

"I Want It NOW!", a.k.a. In the Microwave

You'll Need: extra-large microwave-safe bowl, strainer

Prep: 15 minutes • **Cook:** 20 minutes

Microwave squash for 6 minutes, or until soft enough to cut.

Once cool enough to handle, halve lengthwise; scoop out and discard seeds. Place one half in an extra-large microwave-safe bowl, cut side down.

Add ¼ cup water. Cover and cook for 7 minutes, or until soft. Repeat with remaining squash half.

"I Want It Easy!", a.k.a. In a Slow Cooker

You'll Need: slow cooker, strainer

Prep: 10 minutes • **Cook:** 2½ hours

Place whole squash in a slow cooker with ½ cup water. Cover and cook on high for 2½ hours, or until squash is soft. You're free this whole time to do whatever you like—read a book, do some yoga, watch a movie, take a nap, whatever.

Slice squash in half lengthwise; scoop out and discard seeds.

"I Want It Old-School!", a.k.a. In the Oven

You'll Need: large baking pan, strainer

Prep: 15 minutes • **Cook:** 50 minutes

Preheat oven to 400 degrees.

Microwave squash for 6 minutes, or until soft enough to cut.

Once cool enough to handle, halve lengthwise; scoop out and discard seeds.

Fill a large baking pan with ½ inch water, and place squash halves in the pan, cut sides down. Bake until tender, about 40 minutes.

Once cooked . . .

Use a fork to scrape out the strands. Place in a strainer to drain excess moisture. Thoroughly blot dry, removing as much moisture as possible.

If not eating immediately, let cool completely; then cover and refrigerate.

Just so you know . . .

A 4-pound squash yields about 5 cups cooked squash . . . sometimes more!

Flip to page 363 for all the spaghetti-squash recipes!

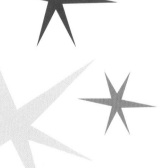

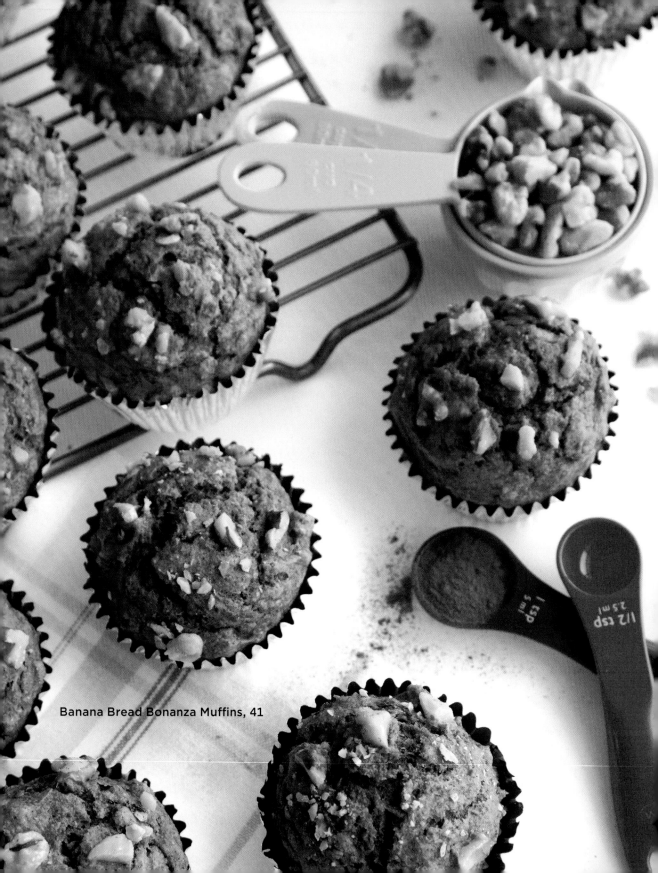

Banana Bread Bonanza Muffins, 41

17

Shop It Up!
Grocery Guide &
Ingredient FAQs

New to the world of clean eating? First things first: Always buy natural. Every ingredient in this cookbook is available in natural varieties. If you aren't sure if the item is natural, check the ingredient list for anything questionable. Or just stick to shopping at natural-food markets. Now, here are some helpful tips & tricks when it comes to staple HG ingredients!

Unsweetened Vanilla Almond Milk

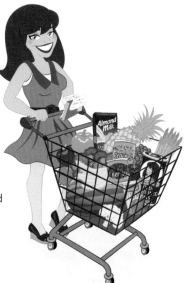

With around 35 calories per cup, this creamy, dreamy milk swap has less than half the calories of dairy milk, and it's virtually sugar-free. (Fat-free dairy milk is still a good choice, and it's used in certain recipes where the flavor of vanilla almond isn't quite right.) Look for almond milk in refrigerated cartons as well as shelf-stable containers.

Favorite brands: Blue Diamond Almond Breeze (refrigerated or shelf stable) and Silk (refrigerated or shelf stable).

Almond Milk FAQ!

"I don't like almonds. Can I use something instead of almond milk?"

Almond milk doesn't taste overly nutty; try it and see! But if you'd still prefer to avoid it, there are alternatives. Unsweetened cashew milk and unsweetened coconut milk both have calorie counts similar to the almond milk, making them perfect swaps. (Just don't confuse unsweetened coconut milk with canned lite coconut milk, which is much higher in calories!) Light vanilla soymilk works too, but it's a little higher in calories and contains sugar. And fat-free dairy milk is always an option! It does have around twice as many calories as almond milk, though, so keep that in mind when swapping.

What's carrageenan? Carrageenan appears on some labels. It's an FDA-approved natural additive derived from plants. Since it's been linked to stomach inflammation and related concerns, some people prefer to avoid it. Silk (refrigerated or shelf stable) and Whole Foods Market 365 (refrigerated or shelf stable) almond milk are both carrageenan-free.

Cheese

Be a blockhead! Let me clarify: If you prefer cheese that's completely free of preservatives, you may want to stick with block-style cheese. Cheese that comes pre-crumbled, pre-shredded, pre-sliced, or pre-grated sometimes contains anti-caking agents and mold inhibitors, such as cellulose, silica, and calcium sorbate. You can always crumble, shred, slice, or grate the cheese yourself.

Favorite brands: Sargento and Cabot

Eggs, Poultry & Meat

Heads up! If you're someone who spends extra money on eggs and poultry marked "no added hormones," know this: Federal regulations prohibit the use of hormones in *any* poultry. So if it's an egg or poultry product in a USA grocery store, chances are it's free of added hormones (or it's breaking the law).

Egg FAQ!

"Why do many of these recipes call for egg whites only? Can I use whole eggs instead?"

Cooking with egg whites is a fantastic way to cut calories without sacrificing taste. While fat is essential, frankly, I'd rather get it from things like cheese, avocado, nuts, and chocolate! Of course, there are exceptions . . . like my Spaghetti Squash Your Hunger B-fast Bowl (page 22) and Fried Rice for Breakfast Bowl (page 25)!

If you want to use whole eggs in recipes that call for just the whites, simply measure out the appropriate amount. (The recipes call for egg whites by the cup, not the number.) And for each ¼ cup of egg whites you swap out for whole eggs, add about 55 calories and 6 grams of fat to the total nutritionals. Then do the math to figure out how it affects each serving.

Ground Meat FAQ!

"Why do these recipes call for extra-lean ground beef but lean ground turkey?"

Extra-lean meat has considerably fewer calories and fat grams. In the case of extra-lean beef, the meat is flavorful, and the texture is perfect. Extra-lean ground turkey, however, doesn't fare quite as well. It's typically dry and lacks flavor. Splurge on lean ground turkey—it's worth it.

Look for extra-lean ground beef with about 145 calories and 5g fat per 4-ounce serving. It's often labeled as 4% fat or less, or as being at least 96% fat-free.

Choose lean ground turkey with around 160 calories and 7.5g fat per 4-ounce serving. Find labeling that lists 7% fat or less, or at least 93% fat-free.

Seafood

Newsflash! A lot of the raw fish at the seafood counter was previously frozen. And you can often save some money when you buy seafood from the freezer aisle. For the best taste and texture, thaw it in the fridge the night before you cook it.

Curious about the difference between wild and farmed seafood? Wild fish are caught in their natural habitats, and tend to be healthier, as they have less of a chance of contact with pesticides and contaminated materials. Farm-raised fish live in commercial aquatic farms.

Canned Goods

You may have heard about "BPA," a.k.a. Bisphenol A. It's a carbon-based synthetic compound found in the lining of some cans. It's safe as long as the levels are low (which they tend to be in food products), but many companies are eliminating it from their cans as a precaution. If you're concerned, look for products labeled BPA-free.

Nonstick Cooking Spray

This spray helps keep calorie counts down in a major way. If you avoid aerosol containers, no worries. Pompeian and other companies make aerosol-free sprays. Or you can just DIY! Buy a food-safe mist sprayer bottle, and fill it with your favorite oil.

Powdered Peanut Butter and Defatted Peanut Flour

These ingredients are made from defatted peanuts, meaning the excess oil has been squeezed out of the peanuts. They bring rich PB flavor to recipes without adding too many calories. A 2-tablespoon serving has only about 50 calories and 2g fat. The same amount of regular peanut butter has about 200 calories and 16g fat!

Favorite brands: Just Great Stuff Powdered Organic Peanut Butter (made by Betty Lou's), Jif Peanut Powder, and Old Virginia Byrd Mill Light Roast Peanut Flour.

Plain Protein Powder

Whey, casein, and soy are the three most common types of protein powder. Egg-white protein powder is also popular. Whey and egg white are my favorites, because they dissolve well and taste great. But people who avoid dairy will want to skip the whey and casein powders, since they're derived from milk.

Favorite brands: Tera's Whey, Jay Robb, and Quest (All-Purpose Baking Blend).

Semi-Sweet Chocolate Chips

Semi-sweet = less sugar. It also means a higher percentage of pure chocolate than milk chocolate. If you prefer less-refined cane sugar, check out the semi-sweet chips by Enjoy Life and Sunspire. Or skip the sugar—Lily's makes stevia-sweetened dark chocolate chips!

Natural No-Calorie Sweetener Packets

Stevia blends for the win! They taste better than straight stevia, and they're super easy to find. Made with an extract of the stevia plant, they typically include another natural calorie-free ingredient for texture and taste. For example, Truvia is made with erythritol (a naturally occurring sugar alcohol), and SweetLeaf includes inulin (a naturally occurring dietary fiber). If you like your stevia pure, there are plenty of liquid varieties and jars of stevia powder available.

Spoonable Natural No-Calorie Sweetener

When you need more than a few packets, spoonable sweetener is the answer. Truvia is the hands-down Hungry Girl favorite! Stevia in the Raw is also great, but since it's half as sweet as Truvia, you'll need to double the amount called for in the recipe.

Sweetener FAQs!

"Isn't no-calorie sweetener artificial?"

While artificial zero-calorie sweeteners are available, there are PLENTY of natural options as well. Stevia comes from a plant and is 100 percent natural, as are most stevia blends you find in packets and other products. (The ingredients the stevia is blended with? Also natural.)

"Can I use sugar instead?"

Sure you can. If you prefer pure sugar to any substitutes, you'll need to double the amount called for in these recipes. Keep in mind, the calorie and sugar counts will increase significantly. FYI: You might want to stick with unrefined cane sugar. It goes through less chemical processing, and it's often considered more natural than white sugar.

Arrowroot Powder

Also known as arrowroot starch, this is an alternative to cornstarch. It's preferred in the clean-eating world since cornstarch is often made with genetically modified corn. If you're not concerned with GMOs, feel free to use cornstarch instead.

Baking Powder

If you avoid all GMOs, look for baking powder marked GMO-free, like Rumford brand. Baking powder sometimes contains cornstarch, so it may not be GMO-free.

Cauliflower Rice/Crumbles

These fresh and frozen products are handy alternatives to making your own cauli' rice! Green Giant makes refrigerated Cauliflower Crumbles and frozen Riced Cauliflower, and Trader Joe's has cauliflower rice in the freezer and the produce section. For a DIY guide, flip to page 346.

Spiralized Zucchini

Scan the produce aisle for ready-to-use zucchini noodles. They're not exactly a supermarket staple, but they're out there! When in doubt, grab your trusty spiralizer and DIY. How-to guide on page 349.

Visit hungry-girl.com/shopclean to stock up on Hungry Girl favorites via Amazon!

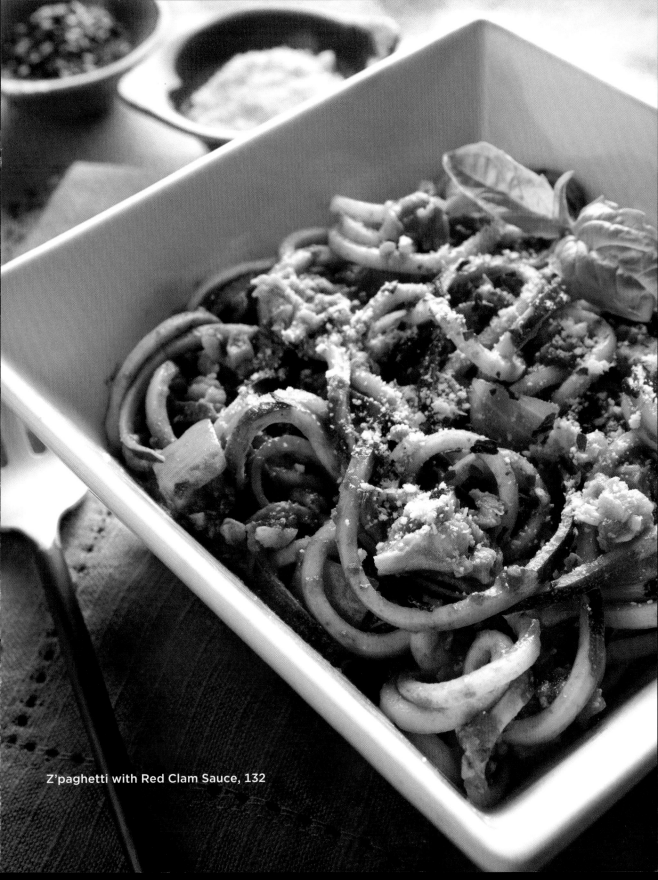

Z'paghetti with Red Clam Sauce, 132

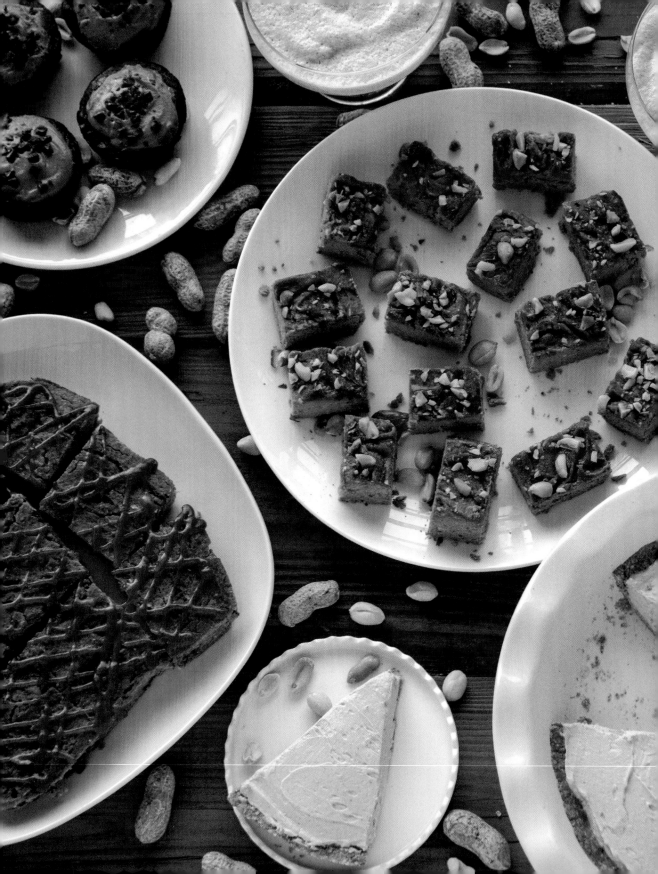

HG Obsessions! Recipes at a Glance

There are even more food obsessions in this book than the chapter names reveal. Love your slow cooker, faux-frying, peanut butter, chicken, holiday foods, and more? Here's a helpful one-stop guide to help you find your favorites. Dig in!

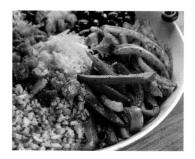

I'm Obsessed with . . .
Cauliflower!

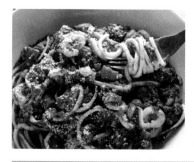

I'm Obsessed with . . .
Zucchini &
Squash Noodles!

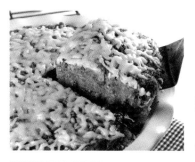

I'm Obsessed with . . .
Spaghetti Squash!

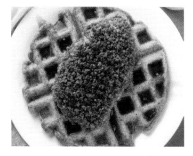

I'm Obsessed with . . .
Faux-Frying!

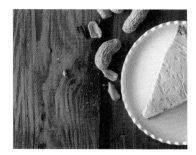

I'm Obsessed with . . .
Peanut Butter!

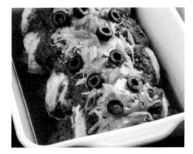

I'm Obsessed with...
Chicken!

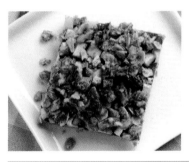

I'm Obsessed with...
Holiday Foods!

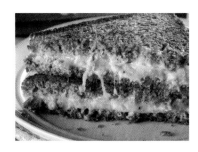

I'm Obsessed with . . .
Cheese!

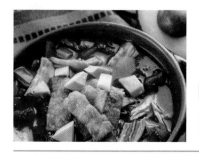

I'm Obsessed with . . .
My Slow Cooker!

There you have it! I hope you LOVE eating these dishes as much as I loved creating them. For more healthy recipes—plus food finds, tips 'n tricks, and more—sign up for the free daily emails at hungry-girl.com.
'Til next time . . .
Chew the right thing!
Lisa :)

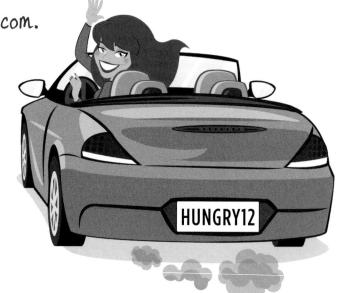

Index